Abortion in India

Abortion in India

Ground Realities

Editors

Leela Visaria
Vimala Ramachandran

Routledge
Taylor & Francis Group
LONDON NEW YORK NEW DELHI

First published 2007
by Routledge
512 Mercantile House, 15 Kasturba Gandhi Marg
New Delhi 110 001

Simultaneously published in the UK
by Routledge
2 Park Square, Milton Park
Abingdon, OX14 4RN

Routledge is an imprint of the Taylor & Francis Group, an informa business

Phototypeset in 10/12 Janson Text by
Star Compugraphics Private Limited
5-CSC, First Floor, Near City Apartments
Vasundhara Enclave, Delhi 110 096

Printed and bound in India by
S. P. Printers
E-120, Sector 7
Noida - 201 301 (U.P.)

British Library Cataloguing and Publication Data
A catalogue record of this book is available from the British Library

ISBN 0-415-42412-7

For

Rushikesh M. Maru

who recognized that abortion was under-researched
and planted the idea of a national study

Contents

List of Illustrations

Tables

Figures

Boxes

Glossary

AAP–I	Abortion Assessment Project–India
ACF	Abortion Care Facility
ANC	Ante Natal Care
ANM	Auxiliary Nurse Midwife
BAMS	Bachelor of Ayurvedic Medicine and Surgery
BPL	Below Poverty Line
CEHAT	Centre for Enquiry into Health and Allied Themes
CFPC	Comprehensive Family Planning Centre
CHC	Community Health Centre
CHV	Community Health Volunteer
CPA	Consumer Protection Act
Cu-T	Copper-T
D&C	Dilation and Curettage
DDG (SG)	Deputy Director General for Safeguards
DE/DC	Dilation and Evacuation/Dilation and Curettage
DHMS	Diploma in Homeopathy Medicine and Surgery
DWCRA	Development of Women and Children in Rural Areas
EVA	Electric Vacuum Aspiration
FGD	Focus Group Discussion
FOGSI	Federation of Obstetrician and Gynaecologist Society of India
GIDR	Gujarat Institute of Development Research
GOI	Government of India
GP	General Practitioner
ICMR	Indian Council of Medical Research
ICPD	International Conference on Population Development
IEC	Information, Education and Communication
IIHMR	Indian Institute of Health Management Research
IIPS	International Institute of Population Sciences
ISM	Indian Systems of Medicine
IUD	Intra-Uterine Device

MASUM	Mahila Sarvangeen Utkarsha Mandal
MBBS	Bachelor of Medicine and Surgery
MIDS	Madras Institute of Development Studies
MOHFW	Ministry of Health and Family Welfare
MR	Menstrual Regulation
MTP	Medical Termination of Pregnancy
MVA	Manual Vacuum Aspiration
NFHS	National Family Health Study
NGO	Non-Governmental Organisation
OB/GN	Obstetrician/Gynaecologist
OBC	Other Backward Class
OPD	Out Patient Department
ORC	Opinion Research Corporation
PF	Provident Fund
PHC	Primary Health Centre
PNDT	Pre-natal Diagnostic Techniques
RCH	Reproductive and Child Health
RH	Reproductive Health
RMP	Rural Medical Practitioners
RUWSEC	Rural Women's Social Education Centre
SC	Scheduled Caste
TAC	Technical Advisory Committee
UFWC	Urban Family Welfare Centre
UNFPA	United Nations Population Fund
VHN	Village Health Nurse
WHO	World Health Organization

Preface

Vimala Ramachandran and Ravi Duggal

Abortion remains a sensitive matter in most countries, receiving considerable international attention not only as a public health concern but also as an ethical/moral/religious issue. Public discussion on abortion in India has either centred on declining sex ratios and sex-selective abortion or on the proliferation of clinics across urban areas. Unfortunately, there is much less public debate on abortion-related morbidity and mortality despite several national programmes and campaigns for safe motherhood. 'Abortion is also a singularly difficult topic to research; even legal "abortion seeking" remains a private, sensitive act with negative moral and emotional connotations that sets it apart from other reproductive health treatment seeking. It is not surprising then that much of available literature in India focuses on the secondary analysis of official data or on the study of easily accessible urban hospital populations.'[1] Therefore, attempting a nationwide research study on the quantitative and qualitative aspects of abortion, from both the provider's as well as women's perspective, was not easy.

Given the volatile nature of this issue, especially in a world where ethnic, religious and community identities have gained greater legitimacy in politics, researchers and activists have shied away from initiating a public debate on abortion. Some argue that this may push the clock back and women will face a setback in reproductive rights. This concern acquired a sense of urgency in light of the US government–led threat to withdraw support for research on abortion and support to international (including multilateral agencies like UNFPA), organisations that work on abortion and related issues.

The post-ICPD Cairo (September 1994) conference period created a new window of opportunity in India. The Government of India's decision in the post-Cairo phase (1996) to introduce a more comprehensive Reproductive and Child Health (RCH) programme in place of vertical safe motherhood, child survival and family planning programmes gave women's health advocates an opportunity to re-establish the importance of a holistic approach.

The 2001 Census jolted the government and civil society alike—an alarming decline in the juvenile sex ratio from 971 in 1981 to 945 in 1991 and 927 in 2001 made national as well as international headlines. The release of the provisional figures was followed by a series of national and regional meetings to understand this alarming trend and evolve policy instruments to reverse it. This led to a renewed interest in enforcing the Prenatal Diagnostic Techniques (Regulation and Prevention of Misuse) Act (the PNDT Act) enacted in 1994 by the Government of India for the regulation of the use of prenatal diagnostic techniques that prevents their misuse for the purpose of prenatal sex determination leading to female foeticide.

Given the above trend in India, there was a feeling that this was an opportune time to initiate a nationwide debate on abortion. While the climate was favourable to initiate debate among key stakeholders, a lack of reliable information, wide regional variations, rural-urban differences and a thin research base has made it difficult for policy-makers, administrators and women's health advocates to develop strategic interventions. There is little dialogue between different stakeholders and it is not uncommon to see registered service providers, unregistered/untrained practitioners, women's health advocates, the population control lobby, public health advocates and others working at cross-purposes.

To fill the gap in our understanding of the ground reality with respect to induced abortion in India and to create an evidence-based body of knowledge, the Abortion Assessment Project–India (AAP–I) was designed as a multicentric research study. This study was designed in collaboration with India's Ministry of Health and Family Welfare and funded jointly by the Ford Foundation, the Rockefeller Foundation and the MacArthur Foundation. The project was housed in CEHAT, Mumbai and HealthWatch, Jaipur. The main objectives of the project were:

- to review government policy towards abortion care, the availability of funds, its flow and policy/programme environment in the country, including family planning and abortion care;

- to assess and analyse abortion services, including organization, management facilities, technology, registration, training, certification and utilization in the public and private sector;
- study user perspectives with special focus on women's perceptions of quality, availability, accessibility (including barriers to utilization of safe abortion facilities), confidentiality, consent, post-abortion contraception and attitude of service providers;
- study social, economic and cultural factors that influence decision making: impact of changing social values, male responsibility, family dynamics and decision-making;
- document costing and finance issues related to the above; and
- estimate the rate of abortion, resultant morbidity and mortality and reasons for induced abortion.

At the outset, it was acknowledged that abortion was a sensitive issue and also that a vast number of service providers were not registered. Given the prevalent political and administrative climate in the country, certification/registration was contentious; unregistered providers may not be willing to talk unless the researchers ensured complete confidentiality. This necessitated that the study adhere to strict ethical criteria and ensure confidentiality, crucial not only to gain the confidence of service providers, but also to create a non-threatening environment for inquiry. Therefore, the study did not rely on researchers alone, but tried to work with social groups that had established a rapport with women. We were aware of the need to design data/information-gathering tools to facilitate data collection in a gentle and non-judgemental manner.

A technical advisory committee consisting of researchers, providers and nominees of GOI and ICMR was constituted to guide and monitor the project.[2] All proposals, research protocols and ethical guidelines were reviewed and approved by TAC. The following stakeholders were represented in TAC: policymakers and administrators involved in the decision-making process related to medical standards for abortion care (MOHFW, GOI and ICMR); the medical community represented by FOGSI; family planning service providers (Parivar Seva Sanstha); community-based organisations and women's health advocates; social science and medical researchers; and demographers and family-planning advocates (members of the population lobby).

An Ethics Committee[3] was constituted to review all proposals and protocols from an ethics standpoint. This provided assistance and training on ethical aspects to IECs of partner institutions and researchers whenever needed; monitored ethical concerns through review of reports submitted by researchers and through field visits as and when required; provided inputs on ethics in project workshops and meetings; and addressed ethical dilemmas faced by researchers and act as a sounding board.

When the project began, all the collaborating institutions came together and agreed on a code of ethics to be followed during the course of the study and in the dissemination of study findings. The following important protocols were agreed upon: informed consent would be procured; the identities of the respondents—abortion seekers as well as abortion providers—would be protected; data would be presented only in tabulated form; and, if narratives were used, the identities of the respondents would be camouflaged. An important decision taken was that the data collected through this study would be available for use of researchers, women's health advocates, the government and any other stakeholder. To this end, tabulated data and the reports would be made available on the CEHAT website. A separate budget provision was made to ensure the implementation of the code of ethics developed by CEHAT and discussed and finalised by the TAC.

Given the prevailing situation of abortion services and the changing perception and values of the community, the national assessment study not only covered a wide geographic area but also tried to capture the various dimensions of the problem. There were five dimensions to this study:

- an overview paper on policy related issues;
- a series of working papers based on existing data/research;
- a multi-centric facility survey in six states, namely Rajasthan, Haryana, Kerala, Madhya Pradesh, Mizoram and Orissa;
- qualitative studies on specific issues to complement the multi-centric studies; and
- community based studies (among other issues) to estimate the abortion rate in Maharashtra and Tamil Nadu.

We hoped that such a five-pronged approach would capture the complex situation as it obtains on the ground, provide policymakers, administrators and medical professionals with valuable insights into abortion care, and help identify areas for public policy intervention and advocacy. The project that commenced in August 2000[4] was completed in December 2004.

This edited volume brings together the qualitative studies. We hope to come forward with another volume with the findings of the six facilities surveys and the main findings of the community-based studies.

Cehat, Mumbai
January 2006

Notes

1. Bela Ganatra, 'Abortion Research in India: What We Know and What We Need to Know', in Radhika Ramasubban and Shireen J. Jejeebhoy (eds), *Women's Reproductive Health in India*, Jaipur and New Delhi: Rawat Publications, 2000.
2. TAC Members: Kamini Rao (FOGSI), Leela Visaria (HealthWatch), Manisha Gupte (MASUM), Padmini Swaminathan (MIDS), R. N. Gupta (ICMR), Ravi Duggal (CEHAT), Saramma Thomas Mathai (Consultant in Maternal and Child Health), Sudarshan Iyengar (GIDR), Sudha Tiwari (Parivar Seva Sanstha), Thelma Narayan (Community Health Cell), Vimala Ramachandran (HealthWatch) and Narika Namshum (MOHFW, GOI).
3. Ethics Consultative Group: Dr Sudarshan Iyengar (representing the TAC), Dr S. V. Joga Rao (National Law School of India University, Bangalore), Dr Sanjay Gupte (Chairperson, Ethics and Medico-Legal Committee, FOGSI, Pune), Dr Vasantha Muthuswami (expert on Bio-Medical Ethics DDG (SG), Indian Council of Medical Research, New Delhi), Dr Ritu Priya (researcher and academician, Jawaharlal Nehru University, New Delhi), Padma Prakash (Deputy Editor, *Economic and Political Weekly*, Mumbai), Dr V. R. Muraleedharan (researcher and academician, Department of Humanities, Indian Institute of Technology, Chennai) and Dr Amar Jesani (independent researcher and ethicist, Mumbai).
4. The study was designed in 1998–99 by a team led by Vimala Ramachandran, then a visiting faculty at IIHMR, Jaipur. The late Dr Rushekesh Maru, then Director, Indian Institute of Health Management Research, Jaipur (IIHMR) negotiated a planning grant with Michael Koenig of Ford Foundation to prepare a proposal for an abortion assessment project after consulting important stakeholders in India.

I

Abortion Use and Practice: Evidence, Challenges and Emerging Issues

Leela Visaria, Vimala Ramachandran,
Bela Ganatra and Shveta Kalyanwala

India is a pioneer in legalising induced abortion (through the Medical Termination of Pregnancy [MTP] Act of 1971) under which a woman can legally have an abortion if the pregnancy carries the risk of grave physical injury or endangers her mental health, if it is the result of contraceptive failure in a married woman, if it is the consequence of rape, or if it is likely to result in the birth of a child with physical or mental abnormalities. In such circumstances, abortion is permitted up to 20 weeks of pregnancy without any need for spousal consent (MOHFW 1971, 1975). While, according to the Ministry of Health and Family Welfare (MOHFW), about 5.4 lakh MTPs were performed in the country in 1996–97,[1] an estimated '6.7 million abortions per year are performed in other than registered and government-recognised institutions, often by untrained persons in unhygienic conditions' (Khan et al. 1998).

Despite an intensive national campaign for safe motherhood and the attention given to unsafe abortion in the 1960s and early 1970s, which led to the legalisation of abortion, morbidity and mortality due to unsafe abortion have remained 'a serious problem for Indian women 28 years after abortion was legalised in India' (Johnston 1999). However, in the last decade, researchers on the basis of field studies have drawn the attention of policymakers and administrators to a range of abortion-related issues such as lack of access and safety, poor quality of care during abortion and the lack of post-abortion follow-up (Bandewar 2000; Khan et al. 1994; *Manushi* 2002; Varkey et al. 2000). The comprehensive Reproductive and Child Health (RCH) programme initiated in India post-Cairo has also included abortion in its package and aims to work towards making it safe (HealthWatch Trust 1999). However, in the absence of evaluation, it is not easy to assess the extent to which the components of the RCH package have been implemented.

While these few studies have brought to light the fact that access to safe abortion has been very limited, much deeper and varied studies are needed to understand issues such as regional and rural-urban differences, the reasons for abortion, the decision-making process, the pathways to abortion and the role of providers. There is also a need to initiate a debate on safe abortion among key stakeholders and to bring various constituencies of policymakers, administrators and women's health advocates on a common platform to develop strategic interventions to improve access to safe abortion.

The Abortion Assessment Project–India (AAP–I) ventured to fill the gap by creating an evidence-based body of knowledge on all facets of induced abortion. This multi-centric research project, which began in August 2000, was managed jointly by CEHAT (Mumbai) and HealthWatch (New Delhi). The result is this collection of essays, *Ground Realities*, which is the first of a three-volume series entitled *Abortion in India*, relating to eight qualitative research studies that were coordinated by HealthWatch as part of the larger project. In addition, this volume includes a synthesis of the findings of a multi-centric study on informal providers of abortion that was coordinated by HealthWatch and Ipas in collaboration with seven NGO (non-government organisation) partners from different parts of the country.

In addition to the in-depth studies, the AAP–I project also collected and analysed information on a range of abortion-related issues.The project commissioned a review of the government policy towards abortion care, the availability of funds, and the policy/programme environment in the country, including family planning and abortion care. Along with several partners, multi-centric studies were conducted to assess and analyse abortion services, including issues such as organisation, management, facilities, technology, registration, training, certification and the utilisation of both the public and private sector. Further, community-based surveys were conducted in Tamil Nadu and Maharashtra in order to estimate, at the state level, the rate of abortion, the resultant morbidity and mortality and the reasons for induced abortion. These various components were designed to provide a comprehensive understanding of the abortion issue in India.[2]

Using various qualitative research methods, sometimes supplemented with quantitative data, the studies included in this volume explore a range of such diverse issues as the reasons for seeking abortion, decision-making pathways, intergenerational differences in abortion-seeking, the selection and perspectives of abortion providers and the quality of care received during and after abortion.[3] It is important to note here that in view of the sensitivity of the subject being explored, all our partners (see Appendix, Table 1.1 for geographic area, the focus of each of the studies and the names of principal investigators) constituted an institutional ethics committee to review the research tools and ensure adherence to the ethical guidelines of the project.

This introductory chapter attempts to highlight some of the salient issues that emerge from the eight qualitative studies on induced abortion along with the multi-centric study of informal providers of abortion. On the basis of the findings, we identify and discuss the challenges before us in the provision of safe abortion to all who seek it, the gaps that exist in our understanding of the issue and the advocacy strategies that are needed.

The major findings of the studies are highlighted in this chapter under the following heads: (a) Reasons for Seeking Abortion, (b) Decision-Making Pathways, (c) Differences across Generations, (d) Selection of Providers, (e) Quality of Care (during and after abortion), (f) Providers' Perceptions (about the legality of abortion and on why women seek abortion) and (g) Challenges and Emerging Issues. In this last section, an additional issue that has been brought on board with field-based findings is that of female-selective abortion.[4]

Reasons for Seeking Abortion

The reasons for seeking abortion appear to range from such proximate causes as the desire to limit family size or to space pregnancies, the preference for sons and medical compulsions, to more distant determinants like poverty, violence and local belief systems.

Limiting Family Size and Spacing Pregnancies

The most common reason for seeking abortion among married women was limiting family size. This reason was cited by the majority of women in the study areas of Maharashtra (Radkar), Gujarat (Barua),

Andhra Pradesh (Prakasamma) and Tamil Nadu (Balasubramanian, Ravindran and Mishra) who were asked to indicate situations in which they would seek or had actually sought abortion.

A very short interval between conceptions was also cited as a reason for abortion. During postpartum amenorrhoea and while breastfeeding the child, some women become pregnant without realising it. In such cases, abortion served as a viable way to avoid having another child so quickly after the previous one. In Tamil Nadu (Anandhi), for instance, younger women viewed frequent childbirth as shameful and resorted to abortion as a spacing method to increase the inter-birth interval.

Although less common, another (contraceptive-related) reason for abortion cited by some women in Tamil Nadu (Anandhi), Andhra Pradesh (Prakasamma), Gujarat (Barua) and Maharashtra (Radkar) was conception immediately after marriage. This reason was cited despite the pressure young brides are usually under to prove their fertility as quickly aspossible.

Inadequate Use of Contraception

Non-use of contraception rather than contraceptive failure seemed to be the chief reason why unwanted pregnancy tended to occur. Actual contraceptive failure appeared to be rare and was cited by only one study respondent in Andhra Pradesh, who reported tubectomy failure as the reason for conception and subsequent abortion.

Incomplete Knowledge of Contraception

Incomplete information about contraception is a major factor affecting its use. Although knowledge of sterilisation as a method of limiting family size was common, knowledge of reversible methods such as condoms, oral pills and the intra-uterine device (IUD) for spacing births was either inadequate or inaccurate. For example, 29 of the 66 women who were interviewed in one of the two Tamil Nadu studies (Balasubramanian et al.) did know about reversible methods. Also, since such knowledge is usually based on information received through health outreach activities and not on the lived experiences of people, it does not translate into actual practice and women tended either to be irregular in their use of such methods of reversible contraception or discontinued their use after some time.

Fear of some methods, their irregular supply, objection by families to their use and the fear of side effects were also some reasons why women tended to resist the use of reversible contraceptives. For example, a belief that oral pills 'dry up the blood in [the] body', thereby preventing women from doing hard physical labour, was reported in Tamil Nadu (Anandhi), while women in the Andhra Pradesh study area quoted an irregular supply of oral pills as the main reason for not using them.

While many women admit that condoms are the safest method of contraception, husbands are not particularly enthusiastic about using them. As reported in a Tamil Nadu study (Balasubramanian et al.), men tended to be inconsistent and irregular in the use of condoms, which, many complained, interfered with their sexual pleasure.[5] As for the IUD, some women rejected its use because they claimed it caused pain and discomfort. This perception, shared by women in various settings, may be an outcome of poor quality of care, especially if IUDs were inserted without proper pelvic examination or when basic hygienic conditions were compromised, leading to infection.

Female Sterilisation as First and Final Method of Contraception

Rather than put up with the real or imagined inconveniences of contraceptive use, women in some study areas preferred to have themselves sterilised after giving birth to the desired number of children. However, since desired family size is measured in terms of surviving children, couples typically wait for a few years to ensure that enough children have survived. Not surprisingly, women who get pregnant during this period tend to seek abortion—a better option, according to them, than relying on the IUD or oral pills. Women interviewed in one of the Maharashtra studies (Morankar et al). also indicated a preference for abortion, saying that it allowed them to resume routine work almost immediately as there was no need for too much post-abortion rest.

Perception of Low Risk for Becoming Pregnant

Some women, who have infrequent sexual contact, either because their children are grown up or married or because their husbands are often away for long periods, do not expect occasional sexual contact to lead to pregnancy. If they do become pregnant, most tend to opt for abortion.

Perception that Abortion is Safe

All the qualitative studies were conducted in states where the availability of safe abortion services was reasonably good, especially for married women. Perhaps due to this, many of the women interviewed believed that abortion did not have any long-term adverse health consequences and was therefore a 'safer' option compared to IUDs and other spacing methods of contraception.

Abortion for Desired Sex Composition of Children

Though most studies did not tackle the topic of sex-selective abortion directly, it is clear that in some study areas couples and their extended families chose abortion to not only limit family size but also to achieve the desired sex composition of children. The widespread internalisation of a preference for sons was clearly indicated in the studies conducted in Gujarat (Visaria; Barua), Maharashtra (Radkar) and to a certain extent in Tamil Nadu (Anandhi), which demonstrate that couples resorted to female-selective abortions after undergoing a sex-determination test. A preference for sons is explained in terms of the need to ensure 'support in old age', to 'continue the family line' (as expressed in a Maharashtra study: 'producing an heir is the prime duty of women') and for the 'performance of death rites'.

In almost all the study areas, the availability of ultrasound facilities, coupled with the knowledge that sex-selective abortion is illegal, meant that women went to different facilities to ascertain the sex of the foetus and for abortions. Women and service providers seemed to be more knowledgeable about the new Prenatal Diagnostic Techniques (PNDT) (Prevention) Act than details of the MTP Act—a point that was clearly reflected in the spirited turn that group discussions took whenever sex selection was discussed. Women cited helplessness as their excuse for flouting the law, claiming that their status in the family and sometimes the very survival of their marriage depended on their ability to produce sons. Although the discussion in most studies was in terms of perceptions, one Maharashtra study (Radkar) indicated that 8 out of 70 (or 11 per cent) reported abortions could be deemed sex-selective. Further, Radkar observed: 'Women who go for sex determination follow it up with the abortion of the female foetus. Everyone seemed to know at least some women who had done this'. According to one of the Gujarat studies (Barua), 10 out of 62 or 16 per cent of abortions were performed after a sex-determination test and the confirmation of a female foetus.

Even in areas where abortion was generally frowned upon, as was reported from Maharashtra (Morankar et al.), family and community approval was readily granted in the case of women who had or conceived only female children. Thus, no social stigma was attached to a woman who underwent sex-selective abortion because she was already the mother of several daughters. Women from Gujarat and Haryana (Visaria) also reported that while they were not comfortable with abortion per se, son preference was so strongly entrenched in the psyche of men and women that they had no objection when it was done for the sake of 'family honour' which was linked with having a son.

Sometimes, as reported in Tamil Nadu (Balasubramanian et al.), a female child was aborted to avoid expected violence against the mother for delivering a girl. Further, if a woman were to conceive while her male child was still young, she would not hesitate to abort the second child if its birth were to threaten the provision of special care and attention that she felt her existing male child required.[6]

On 'Medical Advice'

While some of the studies highlighted that occasionally abortions were performed for medical reasons, such as when a woman's life was threatened or when there was fear of the foetus being abnormal, in a Gujarat study (Barua) a divergence was noted in the reasons cited by women and by abortion service providers. While providers indicated that the 'medical reasons' for which they conducted abortions rarely included an ill-formed foetus, some women respondents claimed that they had undergone abortions on foetus-related 'medical advice'. It is a moot point whether the terminology used by the women was a euphemism for sex-selective abortion.

Economic Situations, Work and Poverty

Poverty, as a reason for seeking abortion, crops up both in the two Tamil Nadu studies and the study based in Karnataka (Nagraj and Nagraj). The study on pharmaceutical industry workers in

Tamil Nadu (Anandhi) shows that almost all units employing young women insist on a contract which clearly debars them from getting married during the contract period if unmarried at the time of employment, and from becoming pregnant if already married.

The rise in the incidence of abortion among unmarried young women is thus significant on two counts: one, it coincides with their increasing employment in the industrial sector; and two, it seems to be a conscious reproductive choice emerging from their role as providers in the family. Unfortunately, far from empowering them, it serves only as a means to negotiate the disempowering conditions of their work and production relations. Likewise, for some married women the pressures of childcare coupled with the responsibility of supporting their families are primary reasons for resorting to abortion.

The Karnataka study, which focuses on women engaged in either *beedi* rolling or agricultural work and belonging to the lower socio-economic srata of the population, shows that many more younger and literate women than older or illiterate ones undergo induced abortion. It is likely that the younger and more literate women are better exposed to mass media and urban influences, which in turn influence their reproductive behaviour.

In one Tamil Nadu study area (Balasubramanian et al.), on the other hand, poverty compels some younger women to resort to abortion. A concomitant reason given is that, by and large, they do not have access to any social support during and after pregnancy. As one woman said: 'I aborted two pregnancies, my third and fifth one. My family's economic situation was very bad at that time, and I was also not keeping well.' Another woman's husband decided that they should terminate the pregnancy '...because I would not be able to stand all day in the shop during my pregnancy and that would affect the sales and our income'.

Physical and Psychological Violence

Women in several study areas spoke of being pressured into having an abortion by their husbands or conjugal family members. Pregnancy was likely to accentuate both physical and verbal violence if the husband did not want the child (for example, in the case a later order birth or that of a girl child), or if he suspected that the child was not his. In such instances, violence became a way of demonstrating his power over her. In a Tamil Nadu study (Balasubramanian et al.), some women claimed that abortion was the only way they could negotiate the cycle of domestic violence that another pregnancy might bring on. In a Gujarat study (Barua) also, women reported using abortion as a way to settle family disputes or to use abortion as a means to retaliate or protest against violence.

Sometimes, violence in the form of non-consensual sex played a role in women becoming pregnant. Threats of violence, accusations of infidelity and promiscuity as well as actual physical abuse were often used to ensure marital sexual relations, often against the women's wishes. In such cases, contraceptive use was unlikely. Some women reported that sometimes husbands compelled them to give in to their sexual demands by saying that they would pay for an abortion if necessary.

Myths about Conception

An interesting finding in Tamil Nadu was that women sometimes cited conception during certain inauspicious months as a reason for abortion. In both the Tamil Nadu study areas the prevalence of a myth that a child born from a third pregnancy would not survive (three being an unlucky number) meant that women who became pregnant for the third time were forced to terminate their pregnancy. If, perchance, the pregnancy happened to coincide with some accident or injury to the breadwinner or the head of the family, such a pregnancy was regarded as an ill omen. For instance, a woman was asked: 'Is your unborn baby's life worth more than that of your husband?'

While such myths probably exist in other regions as well, no other study except the Tamil Nadu one made such reference. In this context, it might be interesting to explore whether there are any intergenerational differences and changing sexual practices among younger, better educated women who have a relatively more scientific understanding of conception.

Abortion among Single, Divorced or Separated Women

Though no study focused directly on why or when unmarried, divorced or separated women resorted to abortion, or whether having a child outside of wedlock was an option for them, according to women in the study areas of Maharashtra, Tamil Nadu and Andhra Pradesh, pregnancy outside marriage had to be aborted in order to preserve family honour. In fact, some women covered by the Maharashtra study (Morankar et al.) said that since such a pregnancy was the result of women's immoral behaviour, possibly even a 'sin', it had to be terminated. However, there was also some sympathy for such women and some community members conceded that pregnancy could also result from rape or violence or be caused by someone known to and trusted by the women. But on the whole, abortions outside the framework of marriage were characterised by secrecy, shame and stigma.

The multi-centric study of informal providers of abortion conducted in seven locations clearly indicated that, in most areas, such providers were used by unmarried girls or widowed women because they could be trusted to maintain confidentiality, even though they charged substantially more while providing services to this category of clients.

Decision-making Pathways

While all studies identified the various socio-cultural factors that influence the decision to abort, a few also collected information on the processes involved before arriving at such a decision. For instance, a Maharashtra study (Radkar) delineated the stages of decision-making women went through once they discovered they were pregnant and wanted to abort the foetus. They first tried out home remedies that are part of every community's folklore, such as eating fruits and foods that are considered 'hot' (papaya, jackfruit) or imbibing various concoctions, including headache tablets. If menstruation still did not resume, women were likely to attempt invasive methods like inserting a sharp instrument in their vagina in the hope that bleeding might start. However, the study did not throw light on the extent to which such invasive methods were practised. When discussing their decision-making pathways, women often tended to mix up facts with hearsay. Interestingly, some of the women who were part of an urban Gujarat study (Barua) claimed that they directly approached the chemist for drugs that would induce abortion.

While making a decision to abort is relatively easy in the case of married women, the same cannot be said for women who conceive out of wedlock. Typically, widowed, separated, divorced or never-married women first inform their parents or partners about the pregnancy and it is they who take the decision about whether and how to go about seeking abortion. In the case of an unmarried young girl, parents try their best to get her married to the boy who is responsible for her pregnancy. A Maharashtra study (Morankar et al.) explores in some detail how this is negotiated between the two families. When marriage is not possible, the next option is to take the girl to an informal provider (in the belief that such providers are more reliable in terms of maintaining secrecy and confidentiality). If both options fail or if the parents cannot afford the cost, the girl is sent off for a few days to a distant place and abortion is sought in a formal facility.

The situation of widowed or divorced women is somewhat different. If pregnancy occurs while the woman is residing with her in-laws, it is not possible to hide her condition from them. The blame is placed squarely on the woman, even if the man responsible for the pregnancy is of their acquaintance or is a family member. Abortion is then sought to 'preserve the honour of the village'. Responding to a hypothetical vignette, some respondents in Maharashtra (Morankar et al.) even indicated that such women should commit suicide or leave the village.

Making decisions about abortion is both a dynamic and a complex process. It is therefore important to understand with whom women discuss their pregnancy, whom they consult, whose permission they seek, or who compels them to undergo abortion. Apart from factors such as caste, education, landholding and/or economic status that influence the decision-making process, the reasons for seeking abortion also play a role in determining who takes the decision. While several studies in this volume address this issue, nearly half the cases in one Maharashtra study (Radkar) said that it was the women themselves who, either on their own or jointly with their husbands, made the decision to abort; in the rest it was the husband who took the decision. The extended family was also seen to be closely involved. As one woman pointed out: 'If they (family members, especially mother-in-law and sister-in-law) don't approve of the abortion, how will I get the required rest? Who will look after my children when I am away in the hospital?'

In Gujarat and Haryana women stated that if they conceived a female child, the pressure to abort from the extended conjugal family was enormous, particularly if they already had one or two daughters. In such cases, the decision to abort was almost entirely that of the husband and/or the mother-in-law; the woman herself usually had no say in the matter. However, the influence of in-laws on the decision-making process varied, depending on the social stratum to which the woman belonged. While women from higher social groups were required to both inform and consult their in-laws, women from scheduled castes and other backward communities said that they had to obtain only their husband's consent. The natal family rarely had any say in matters relating to abortion, sex determination or sex-selective termination of pregnancy, though a Tamil Nadu study (Balasubramanian et al.) reveals that even when the decision to abort was taken by the husband and parents-in-law, women were likely to be asked to approach their natal family for money or to pawn their personal assets such as jewellery to take care of the expenses, especially when the foetus was female.

Differences across Generations

Both studies in Tamil Nadu held focus group discussions (FGDs) with younger and older women to ascertain whether there were any differences in the way they experienced abortion or their reasons for seeking it. Abortion in Tamil Nadu (Anandhi) by older women was considered to be shameful since such women sought abortion not to limit family size (because large families were accepted as a norm by their generation and not viewed as a burden or impediment to their standard of living) but in order to free themselves from childcare responsibilities. Since abortion was also seen as indicative of women's sexuality, pregnancy in older women was perceived to be the result of 'too much sexual desire'.

In contrast, younger women use abortion as a spacing method not only because it is permitted by law but also because notions of shame and honour among them are different from those of the previous generation: 'With the younger generation, it is not frequent pregnancy per se, that was once perceived as an expression of excessive female desire, but frequent childbirth, especially at the later stage of a woman's life, that is associated with the notion of shame.' Honour now lies in having fewer children and women are not ashamed of their sexuality.

The other Tamil Nadu study (Balasubramanian et al.), on the other hand, examined, separately, the abortion experience and the perceptions of women (as well as those of some husbands) below and above 35 years of age. Here, instead of caste or class differences, age had more to do with which women needed their husbands' consent for abortion. Instances of women going for abortion without explicit permission from their spouses were far more common among older women (11 out of 27 abortions) than among those below 35 years of age (4 out of 25 abortions).

The reasons for abortion cited by older and younger women in the two Tamil Nadu studies might appear to be contradictory at first glance. However, when older women report that they choose to undergo abortion 'to limit family size' or because they are embarrassed about being pregnant if their children are already teenagers or adults, or they are unable to support additional children, they are indicating, without articulating it, that their embarrassment at becoming pregnant beyond a certain age is also due to the fact that it being viewed as an expression of women's sexuality.

Selection of Provider

Given that the studies were carried out in relatively more developed states of the country (with several being located in peri-urban areas), it is not surprising that most women said they used the services of qualified private doctors/institutions or government facilities for abortion.

However, as married respondents pointed out, unmarried, separated and widowed women preferred, or were taken by family members to, informal providers because of their need to maintain confidentiality and secrecy.

Information about providers usually reaches women by word of mouth, from friends, relatives, paramedical workers or other community members. Advertisements in public places like buses or in newspapers are a more common source in urban areas. One Maharashtra study (Morankar et al.) found that 'Information [on abortion] is usually sought under the pretext that someone else needs it. Women gather this information from other women when walking to the river to wash clothes, while working in the fields, or while fetching water. Men get such information during gossip sessions with friends.'

Preference for Private Providers

The major determinants influencing the choice of provider by married women are the reputation of the provider, the vicinity, familiarity and the cost. Overall, private facilities are considered to be much better than those run by the government, and women cite a wide range of reasons to justify their use of them. This suggests that women and their families do weigh the alternatives before deciding where to go. Some of the reasons put forward by the women are:

- Abortion in a private facility takes much less time since all procedures are taken care of in one visit. Further, most private providers do not insist on a prolonged hospital stay. Some women in urban Gujarat (Barua) complained that in public hospitals 'a lot of time is wasted in waiting and going through formalities; these hospitals are not client-friendly and the quality of services is suspect'. This is supported by Maharashtra respondents (Radkar), according to whom the quality of care and the time needed to be spent at the provider's facility are major considerations in the selection of a provider.
- Private doctors have better facilities and equipment.
- Private providers are not in a hurry to discharge women after the procedure if they need to rest for an hour or so before going home; on the other hand, due to shortage of beds, public hospitals require women to leave as soon as possible.
- Women are treated with more respect and dignity by private doctors than by those working in government facilities.
- Private doctors are more likely to ensure confidentiality, which is why unmarried women prefer private facilities if they can afford them.
- Private providers are preferred by women who want to determine the sex of their foetus, and/or abort if the foetus is female. (The majority of women in Gujarat and Haryana know the towns where private doctors with nursing or maternity homes providing such services are located.)

However, when women wish to undergo sterilisation along with abortion, they prefer government hospitals, where acceptance of sterilisation means that the abortion does not cost them anything. The same holds true for women whose families are poor and cannot afford to pay for abortion services.

Women who choose to use the services of informal providers usually do so for termination of very early pregnancy or for treatment of delayed menstruation. They do not approach informal providers if abortion is sought for sex selection.

Cost Considerations

While it is true that private abortion services are expensive, visits to government hospitals are not cost-free. Women often have to pay for medicines separately and are sometimes required to make repeat visits before the abortion is performed. Also, completing the formalities required by government facilities is a time-consuming process, and delays in provision of services means that the abortion seeker and the accompanying person (women usually prefer to take someone with them when visiting large, impersonal facilities) have to spend long periods of time just waiting in the hospital. In poor families this often translates into a loss of the day's wages.

The cost of abortion services can vary, depending on the type of provider and the gestation period. Many women in the Andhra Pradesh study area, who had chosen to go to the government hospital for abortion because they were poor and believed that government services were free, discovered to their horror that government doctors charge an average of Rs 600 per abortion. But though not free, government hospitals are generally the cheapest. However, the urban Gujarat study indicated that although gynaecologists in the private sector are the most expensive and charge according to the duration of the pregnancy, the cost of the procedure varies between Rs 400 and Rs 600, which is not very different from what women in urban Andhra Pradesh pay. Interestingly, it is the NGO in Gujarat that charges much more.

Some women and their families calculate the cost of abortion, especially of a female foetus, in a somewhat novel fashion. This came up in the FGDs conducted in Gujarat (Visaria) with women during the course of the study. Women (and their families) compare the immediate cost of abortion (including money spent on the sex-determination test) with the expenditure that would have to be incurred on the girl's dowry as well as on different occasions after the girl's marriage.

Quality of Care

Information collected on the place and the provider of abortion, client–provider interactions, and clients' expectations and experiences gives us some indication of the quality of abortion care available. For instance, other than sonography for foetal sex determination, which is done strictly on the client's request, no preliminary tests are carried out before abortion in urban Gujarat. Providers admit that instead of conducting any physical or internal check-ups, they rely on the date of the missed period as reported by the client. Some providers do insist on a urine pregnancy test prior to pregnancy termination, but often clients get this done on their own before coming to the provider.

Further, despite the availability and knowledge of safer and relatively simple abortion methods, providers in urban Gujarat continue to use older techniques such as Dilation and Curettage (D&C). This is also the case in Tamil Nadu and Andhra, where three out of the four doctors at the government hospital use D&C even for first-trimester abortions. Convenience and providers' experience are the main factors governing the choice of method. While factors like erratic electrical supply make it difficult to use Electric Vacuum Aspiration (EVA), providers consider unsafe the use of Manual Vacuum Aspiration (MVA) beyond eight weeks of gestation. In fact, the few providers who do use MVA follow it up with a D&C to ensure that abortion is complete. In Ahmedabad, however, providers are aware of medical abortion and several have already used RU 486 (mifepristone) or have treated patients who have taken the drug elsewhere and then come to them. But the use of this method has not been specifically mentioned in the other studies.

Counselling

None of the studies show much evidence of pre- or post-procedure counselling. In urban Gujarat, for instance, women reported that they were rarely explained any details about the procedure. However, it is also true that women themselves are not interested in such information. Their main concern is to get the procedure over with and leave as soon as possible. Private providers are aware of clients' lack of interest, and also admit that they do not have dedicated staff or the incentive to counsel women on contraceptive use or on the consequences of abortion. Neither is there an audit system for counselling in hospitals. Providers in government hospital on the other hand, do not have much time to spend with clients and the counselling they do is limited to warning clients about the harmful consequences of repeat abortions.

Public hospitals, at least in areas covered by our studies, do not coerce clients into accepting contraception. This finding is borne out by providers in the tertiary hospital in urban Gujarat and the public hospital in Andhra Pradesh and the clients of both.

Though women in Andhra Pradesh seemed quite satisfied with the abortion services provided by the government hospital in terms of abortion procedures, medicines, and bed and toilet facilities, they were unhappy that food was not part of the service package and had to be provided by the family. However, what concerned them most was the low water supply, which they felt compromised the cleanliness of the hospital. Women in Tamil Nadu (Balasubramanian et al.) were also satisfied with the services available at the government facility, apart from those who experienced post-abortion complications.

However, there is some evidence that women's sense of dignity was compromised during their hospital stay. Although initially, most women in the Andhra study said that they had been treated with dignity and respect, on further probing many (15 out of 27) admitted that the hospital staff was rude to them because they were poor and could not afford private services.

The length of hospital stay usually depends on the procedure used for abortion and the period of gestation; the longer the gestation period, the longer the client is required to stay on in the facility. Although most hospitals provide women with information about danger signals and the need for follow-up visits and rest, poverty and domestic responsibilities often prevent women from taking time off to recuperate. In fact, some of them view abortion as a minor procedure compared to sterilisation, and do not feel that it warrants any post-procedure care.

In general, very few women in the areas covered by these studies reported serious post-abortion morbidity. It is possible that they confused lifetime morbidity episodes with post-abortion illnesses, which may not have been life-threatening and therefore easily forgotten. However, in Andhra Pradesh, where the study focused prospectively on this issue (and interviewed women immediately after abortion, and then at intervals of two weeks, two months and six months thereafter), 21 of the 27 women reported morbidity such as excessive bleeding, weakness, nausea, abdominal pain, and discomfort after abortion. In fact, 18 of them even sought medical care, though this may have been at the prompting of the auxiliary nurse midwives (ANMs) with whom the women were in frequent contact. While it is difficult to correlate this fact with medically significant morbidity, it does mean that women need care and support after abortion. In the Tamil Nadu study (Balasubramanian et al.), an almost equal number of young and older women (21 out of 34) said that they had experienced post-abortion problems like excessive bleeding, and lower abdominal and back pain.

Providers' Perceptions

Awareness of Abortion Laws

According to the findings from these studies, not all para-functionaries like ANMs are aware of the MTP Act. Some of the formally trained providers are informed in general terms, though not necessarily familiar with the various situations in which the Act is applicable. Even when they are, many insist that clients fulfill certain requirements that are not mandated in the Act. For instance, though providers know that the family's consent is not necessary, most insist on it in order to protect themselves. To preempt husbands from blaming them at a later stage, providers in Andhra Pradesh do not perform an abortion unless they obtain written authorisation from the husband. In urban Gujarat this demand is justified by the argument that abortion is a surgical procedure done under anaesthesia.

The study on sex selection in Gujarat (Visaria) indicates that service providers are aware of the PNDT Act, its ramifications and the consequences of aborting female foetuses. They appear, however, to be caught on the horns of a dilemma: on the one hand, they believe that the PNDT Act should be implemented strictly and that any person violating it should be punished; on the other hand, they conduct sex determination tests in violation of the Act because they sympathise with families that wish to determine not only their family size but also the sex composition of their children.

Registration, Certification and Reporting

Most providers view registration as a long and cumbersome procedure and equate the requisite reporting requirements with harassment. The Gujarat study (Barua) reveals that qualified doctors tend to shy away from registering as abortion providers because they are wary of the registration procedure and other legal formalities associated with it. Providers also admit that they do not record or report all the abortions they perform. While registered providers do report a few cases, unregistered providers do not maintain any records.

Providers' View of Abortion Seekers

Providers claim that most urban women who wish to limit family size generally seek abortion within the first eight weeks of pregnancy. Those who want to terminate pregnancy for spacing usually come between eight and 12 weeks. Providers also feel that some clients come to them for abortion after having undergone a sex determination test elsewhere, though it is difficult for them to determine which of their clients have done so. Since they view their job as essentially one of providing a service, providers feel that they have limited responsibility. Most providers, particularly in urban Gujarat, prefer to turn a blind eye to the issue and mind their own business, or presume that the abortion being sought is for the termination of unwanted pregnancy.

In Tamil Nadu (Anandhi), many providers reportedly feel that the stigma attaching to unmarried women seeking abortions is decreasing and many such women have started accessing abortion services early.

Challenges and Emerging Issues

As highlighted earlier, findings and leads from small and disparate micro-studies cannot be generalised to represent the situation in the country as a whole and need to be interpreted with caution and in context. Nevertheless, the studies in this volume do throw up some common patterns and themes, some of which are listed below:

The Link between the Unmet Need for Contraception and Abortion

Most women wanting to limit family size or space births seem to prefer abortion over temporary spacing methods like contraceptives, which they consider difficult to obtain and as having harmful side effects. This is especially the case in the two Tamil Nadu study areas, but similar reasons for not wanting to use spacing methods have been reported in all study areas.

Reliance on abortion for limiting or spacing children clearly indicates an unmet need for contraception among women. Family welfare programmes should address this issue and work towards not only expanding contraceptive choice but also ensuring that contraceptives are easily available. Providing women and men with information about the merits, limitations and possible side effects of different contraceptive methods would go a long way in helping them accept such methods. While it is encouraging to note that both public and private providers have stopped insisting on or coercing clients into accepting family planning after abortion, providers cannot absolve themselves from their duty to promote responsible family planning through appropriate counselling.

Son Preference

Preventing the birth of a female child or ensuring the birth of a male one, often under pressure from conjugal and extended families, is a major reason for abortion in most settings. While the use of 'modern' sex determination tests is more common in the western and northern parts of the country, studies in southern India also show that though women here rely on more traditional methods of predicting the sex of the foetus, their objective is the same: to prevent a female child from being born. While a campaign mode is increasingly used to address the issue of 'missing girls' and to advocate saving the daughters, it is important to assess whether these methods are able to bring about, in the short range, necessary changes in the behaviour of people, and, in the long range, social transformation.

Links between the PNDT and MTP Acts

Although the two legislations are independent of each other, our studies suggest that this distinction is hard to maintain in actual practice. The widespread campaign against sex determination has enhanced awareness of the PNDT Act among communities; knowledge of the legality of abortion services and of the MTP Act, however, is still inadequate. Under the MTP Act, abortion (on economic or social grounds) is one among the many rights that Indian women enjoy today. Yet there is some evidence that it is being equated with the ban on sex detection tests and with 'killing of girls'. Further, the PNDT Act is interpreted to mean that all abortions (whether sex-selective or not) have now become illegal. Surprisingly, even providers often link the provisions of the two acts. As our studies show, the most common reason for women to have an abortion is still linked to limiting and spacing their children (irrespective of sex composition), and unless we maintain a clear distinction between these two issues and understand the reasons underlying the PNDT Act, efforts to expand access to safe abortions are bound to receive a setback in the coming years.

The Need to Increase Awareness about the MTP Act

Women and their family members, particularly those who are likely to be involved in the decision-making process, need to be made aware about when, where and under what circumstances abortion can be legally availed of. Women should also be made aware that they have a right to ask for information and, if necessary, question the quality of care being provided to them. They would therefore need to be educated about what constitutes safe quality services. Service providers, too, need to be clear about the provisions of the Act and refrain from allowing their own apprehensions and/or moral concerns to cloud the issue.

Preference for Private Providers

Wherever private providers are available, women prefer to use their services if they can afford them. Women view private providers as being more qualified, as able to provide more efficient services speedily so that not too much time is spent waiting in the facility, and as more likely to maintain confidentiality. In the light of the current debate on the introduction of a user fee in public health care facilities, one would also need to determine both the quality of services and the image of whether there would be a concurrent improvement in public sector. A huge investment has been made and expenses incurred in creating and supporting a vast network of public health facilities in the country and, therefore, their effective and extensive use must remain a national priority. Also, the poor and marginal groups should continue to be able to afford to use public health facilities and treating patients with dignity must also be ensured.

Needs of Single, Widowed and Separated Women

Although the studies did not focus directly on unmarried adolescents, widows and separated women, there is sufficient evidence to show that pregnancy is considered a stigma for such women. The processes involved in their decision to abort are therefore quite different from those followed in the case of 'acceptable' pregnancies. Not surprisingly, such women receive very little, if any, support from family and community or from public sector facilities, and rely on private facilities.

The Role of Medical Technology

Despite the availability of safer options like Vacuum Aspiration, the continued use of D&C to perform abortions is another cause for concern. The recent legalisation of mifepristone in the country provides yet another option of a safe and effective technology that can increase access and expand choice. But since mifepristone was legalised after the studies were designed, they do not explore its implications in any systematic way. Some studies do, however, suggest that it is used by some practitioners and is preferred by some clients. Further, as our research in Ahmedabad suggests, mifepristone might also be available, in some settings, directly to women, over the counter (as indeed are most drugs in the country). All these issues require further exploration. The technology is known to be safe and effective and we need to understand how best to exploit its full potential in promoting safe abortions, while at the same time guarding against misuse that can stem from misinformation.

Quality of Care

While life-threatening morbidity from abortions has not emerged as a major issue of concern, women's experiences at health facilities as well as providers' own assessments show that quality of care, especially of counselling, is a neglected area. While high caseloads leave public sector facilities with very little time to provide pre- or post-abortion counselling, providers in the private sector tend to view it as unneces-sary or unwarranted. Women are often subjected to rudeness or judg-mental behaviour by providers, particularly in public facilities. All types of providers, therefore, would benefit from gender sensitivity training, the inculcation of non-judgmental attitudes and value clari-fication. It is time that family welfare programmes began recognising women and their individual needs as the focal point around which services should revolve.

Last, and of immense importance, is this: our studies indicate that partnerships between diverse groups of people drawn from different disciplines and with differing ideologies and positions are both pos-sible and productive. The collective process of integrating diverse viewpoints enhances a common understanding of the issue of unsafe abortions and, in the long run, is an essential step in progressing towards the common goal of making abortion an infrequently used but safe alternative for women faced with an unwanted pregnancy.

Notes

1. According to the latest figures available, the number of MTPs performed increased to 7.2 lakh in 2001. The number performed in facilities other than the institutions approved for MTP is believed to be even higher. See MOHFW 1999 and 2003.
2. The studies explored some or all of these issues in varying degrees based on the focus of the study. In some studies both providers and clients were interviewed; in some, women were interviewed without ascertaining if they had abortions. Barring one study based in Tamil Nadu, where sexuality issues were explored in focus group discussions (FGDs) with women regardless of their marital status, in all other studies only married women were interviewed. Even the findings on unmarried women reflect the views of married women and represent community attitudes or the interpretation of researchers rather than actual behaviour or practices.
3. A CD with all the studies can be obtained by writing to CEHAT, Bombay. For information on how to order the CD, the readers may check CEHAT's website: www.cehat.com.
4. The studies are cited by the state in which the fieldwork was carried out, along with the name of the principal investigator, in view of the fact that in three of the states (Gujarat, Maharashtra and Tamil Nadu), two studies each were carried out by two different investigators, who explored different issues.

5. The Tamil Nadu study carried out by Balasubramanian et al. in an area where the NGO has been focusing on increasing the awareness and use of spacing methods, such as condoms, among community members in the area of their operation by making them available in the clinic free of cost. Despite this, the study findings on contraception show that it is difficult to increase the acceptance of reversible spacing methods.
6. This is not unique to Tamil Nadu or to the study villages. There are other studies which also cite this as one reason for seeking abortion. For instance, see Ganatra 2000.

References

Bandewar, Sunita. 2000. 'Unsafe Abortion'. *Seminar* 489.

El Dawala, Aida Seif. 2001. 'Women's Wit over Men's: Trade-offs and Strategic Accommodations in Egyptian Women's Reproductive Lives', in Rosalind Petchesky and Karen Judd (eds), *Negotiating Reproductive Rights: Women's Perspectives Across Countries and Cultures*. London: Zed Books.

Ganatra, Bela. 2000. 'Abortion Research in India: What We Know and What We Need to Know', in Radhika Ramasubban and Shireen J. Jejeebhoy (eds), *Women's Reproductive Health in India*. New Delhi: Rawat Publications.

HealthWatch Trust. 1999. *The Community Needs-Based Reproductive and Child Health in India: Progress and Constraints*. Jaipur: HealthWatch Trust.

Johnston, Heidi. 1999. 'Abortion Practice in India: A Review of Literature'. Working Paper No. 1, Abortion Assessment Project—India, HealthWatch and CEHAT.

Khan, M. E., S. Barge and Nayan Kumar. 1994. 'Availability and Access to Abortion Services in India: Myth and Realities'. Working Paper. Baroda: CORT.

Khan, M. E., S. Rajagopal, S. Barge and N. Kumar. 1998. 'Situational Analysis of Medical Termination of Pregnancy Services in Gujarat, Maharashtra, Tamil Nadu and Uttar Pradesh'. Paper read at the International Workshop on Abortion Facilities and Post-Abortion Care and Operations Research, New York, 19–21 January.

Manushi. 2002. 'Legal But Not Available: The Paradox of Abortion in India'. January.

MOHFW (Ministry of Health and Family Welfare) 1971. *Manual for First Trimester Medical Termination of Pregnancy*. New Delhi: Government of India.

———. 1975. The Medical Termination of Pregnancy Rules. New Delhi: Government of India.

Varkey, P., P. P. Balakrishna, J. H. Prasad, S. Abraham and A. Joseph. 2000. 'The Reality of Unsafe Abortion in a Rural Community in South India'. *Reproductive Health Matters* 8 (6).

APPENDIX

Table 1.1: Eight qualitative studies: geographical coverage and objectives

Researcher, organisation and title of study (2004)	Geographical area	Study population/ respondents	Main focus of study
Anandhi, S., 'Women, Work and Abortion Practices: Kancheepuram District, Tamil Nadu', Chennai: Madras Institute of Development Studies	Four villages in Kancheepuram district of Tamil Nadu	Dalit women (married and unmarried) working in pharmaceutical companies; village functionaries and opinion leaders; abortion service providers	Abortion decision-making and practices, in the context of increasing employment of rural women in the industrial sector in peri-urban area
Barua, A. 'Abortion Care in Urban Slums: A Case Study from Ahmedabad', Ahmedabad: Foundation for Research in Health Systems	Two urban slums in Ahmedabad	Married women with an induced abortion experience; abortion service providers	Provider choice; women's perspective on quality of abortion care; provider perspectives on accessibility and quality of abortion care
Morankar, S.N., B. Mhaskar, V. Purohit, M. Patil and A. Kudale, 'Abortion in Rural Pune District: An Ethnographic Exploration', Pune, Maharashtra Association for Anthropological Sciences	Fourteen villages in Pune district, Maharashtra	Married women and men from the community; opinion leaders, service providers	Ethnographic exploration of community attitudes around abortion
Prakashamma, M., 'Post-Abortion Care in the Public Health System, Hyderabad: Academy for Nursing Studies	Three villages and selected public health facilities in Medam district, Andhra Pradesh	Women with a spontaneous or induced abortion; service providers: both doctors and mid-level providers (ANMs); facility assessment	Role of public health system in care for women during and after abortion (both spontaneous and induced)

(*Table 1.1 continued*)

(*Table 1.1 continued*)

Researcher, organisation and title of study (2004)	Geographical area	Study population/ respondents	Main focus of study
Radkar, A., 'Abortion in Rural Communities near Urban Areas: The Experience of Married Women', Pune: Independent Researcher	Villages near Pune, Maharashtra	Women in the 15–49 age group	Provider choice
Balasubramanian, P., T.K. Sundari Ravindran and U.S. Mishra, 'Processes and Factors Underlying Choice of Induced Abortions: Rural Tamil Nadu', Chengalpattu, Tamil Nadu: RUWSEC	98 hamlets from the RUWSEC project area in Kancheepuram district of Tamil Nadu	Low-income, socially marginalised couples (both wives and husbands)	Gender dynamics and abortion decision-making; inter-generational differences in abortion-seeking behaviour
Susheela, K. and K. Nagaraj, 'Socio-Economic and Medical Correlates of Pregnancy Wastage among the Poor: A Village in Coastal Karnataka', Chennai: Madras Institute of Development Studies	One village in the Udipi district, Karnataka	Woman *beedi* workers and agricultural workers	Estimate the extent of pregnancy wastage (including spontaneous and induced abortions) and associated socio-economic, cultural and medical factors
Visaria, L. 'Sex-Selective Abortion in the States of Gujarat and Haryana: Some Empirical Evidence', Ahmedabad: Gujarat Institute of Development Research	Six villages in Mehsana district, Gujarat; six villages in Kurukshetra district, Haryana	All currently married women in the age group 15–49; abortion service providers in Gujarat	Decision-making process and role of son preference in sex-selective abortions

II

Abortion Care in Urban Slums: The Case of Ahmedabad

Alka Barua

The World Health Organisation (WHO) estimates that of the 20 million unsafe abortions taking place each year, nearly 90 per cent are in the developing world. Of these, almost one-third occur in South Asia alone. According to the Government of India's family planning yearbook, 4,65,705 pregnancies were medically terminated in India during 1996–97. These, however, are recorded or legal abortions. It is estimated that several times this number are performed outside the legal system, often by unskilled providers, and are deemed unsafe.

In India, the Medical Termination of Pregnancy (MTP) Act of 1971 allows legal termination of pregnancies to women over 18 years of age—irrespective of marital status—as a health measure, as a humanitarian measure in case of sex crimes, as a eugenic measure and in the event of contraception failure. Abortions induced for these *specified reasons* and *conducted by recognised/registered service providers and centres* that meet the stringent criteria under the Act are deemed legal (Chhabra and Nuna 1993).

While the cumbersome recognition process under the Act is a major bottleneck in the provision of recognised or legal services, skewed distribution of recognised centres also serves to keep such services beyond the reach of women who seek them. This, perhaps, is one reason for the large numbers of illegal abortions. Even where available, recognised services are frequently not used. In urban areas, where physical accessibility to legal services is not an issue, factors such as the attitude of health care providers and the degree of privacy and confidentiality available (CEHAT 2001) are known to inhibit recourse to safe legal abortion. On the other hand, a large proportion of women undergo abortion to regulate family size which, as per the MTP Act, is illegal. Under these circumstances, women access any available centre that provides the services, even if that centre is illegal or unrecognised (Shelley et al. 2001). Reasons for low utilisation of approved, legal services are multiple, and span the entire range from seekers of abortion to service providers and their facilities. Thus the Act, though liberal, has not translated into availability of safe legal services for pregnant women who seek abortion (CEHAT 2001).

Women's organisations and critics of the Act argue that in a country like India, where national programmes covertly and openly encourage smaller families, exploitation of the Act for demographic purposes is inevitable (Gupte et al. 1997: 77–86). The committee responsible for drafting the Act had clearly stated that 'legalising abortions with a view of obtaining demographic results is unpractical and may even defeat the constructive and positive practice of family planning through contraception' (Ministry of Health 1966: 47, cited in CORT 1996). However, statistics indicate that abortion services are used primarily for spacing, limiting family size and having children of the desired sex.

In implementation, therefore, there appears to be a significant gap between intent and practice. Although the Act was passed to ensure women safe, legal medical services for pregnancy termination when required, ground reality indicates that for making good quality services available to women, the social and cultural context of utilisation as well as provision of services should form the cornerstone of the implementation process. Therefore, if we are to make services more socially appropriate and acceptable, and at the same time increase their accessibility, it is critical to take into account both the women's as well as providers' perspectives on

- the nature, distribution and quality of abortion services available, and the characteristics of and reasons for women seeking abortion services from approved or non-registered centres, and unqualified providers; and
- abortion-related morbidity and mortality.

It is to understand these two sets of perspectives that a study of selected abortion care providers and seekers was undertaken in two urban slums of Ahmedabad city in the state of Gujarat.

Abortion Care: The Current Scenario in India

There are a few studies undertaken in India on which women seek abortions and why they do so. While the reasons for abortion among unmarried girls and widows are obvious, adolescent married girls in rural Maharashtra chose abortion when their previous child was still too young and the older women because they did not want any more children (Ganatra and Hirve 2002: 76–85). In Patna, Bhubaneswar and Baroda, 67 per cent of the women who underwent abortions had achieved their desired family size and did not want additional children (CORT 1996). Some women felt that their last child was still too young, while others wanted to space the next child (Khan, Patel and Chandrashekhar 1990: 70–85).

Another reason, which earlier used to be covert but is now very visible, is the desire for male children. The sex ratio (females to 1,000 males) in Gujarat in the 0–6 age group has fallen to 878 from 928 (Government of India 2001). Even in progressive states like Maharashtra, one in six married women with a history of induced abortion in the previous 18 months unhesitatingly admitted that abortion had been carried out subsequent to a sex-determination test showing a female foetus (Ganatra and Hirve 2002: 76–86). What are the factors responsible for this state of affairs? Can we just attribute it to poor implementation of the MTP Act? Or is it lethargy on the part of the medical community to comply with legislative measures and medical ethics and/or their poor awareness of the Act's provisions that allow such abortions to go unchecked? Or is it the country's socio-cultural milieu that impels women to abort female foetuses (CEHAT 2001)?

The MTP Act does not permit induced abortions on demand. In a much-debated paragraph (8.25), the document on the ICPD's (International Conference on Population Development) Programme of Action (ICPD 1994) states: 'In no case should abortion be promoted as a method of family planning.' However, ignorant of the conditions stipulated under the MTP Act, a large number of women continue to undergo abortion to regulate family size (Ganatra and Hirve 2002: 76–85). The onus of judging the necessity for abortion rests with the medical practitioner, whose opinion is taken in good faith to reflect valid, legal indication. But there is little regulation and it is known that many practitioners regard all kinds of conditions as eligible for abortion, depending more on their personal beliefs than on stipulations of the law (*Manushi* 2002).

A study conducted in an urban hospital in Maharashtra reveals that the majority of the 195 women (84 per cent) who were part of the sample assumed that induced abortion is illegal in India, but more than half of them (56 per cent) also said that if need be, they would go ahead and have an abortion regardless of whether or not it is legal (Shelley et al. 2001). This disregard for legal requirements is clearly reflected in women seeking abortions after sex determination, though awareness about its illegality is almost universal. Women and their partners are not overly concerned about the legal indications for abortions specified under the Act; in their view termination of an 'unwanted' pregnancy is their right.

In the same study, 14 per cent of the wives, 18 per cent of their husbands, and 29 per cent of married men felt that women should be able to have an abortion if the foetus is female. Further, nearly 90 per cent of the same men and their wives knew where to go for a sex-determination test (Shelley et al. 2001). The significance of this needs to be underscored as it is the men who usually take the decision for abortion, either alone or jointly with their wives.

This is borne out by another study in urban Maharashtra where, while all couples reported having discussed the issue, the husband's consent was a major factor in the decision. Out of the 170 unwanted pregnancies, 34 of the 49 women who wanted an abortion had to first obtain their husband's consent (Shelley et al. 2001). Though no precise information is available on this issue, women's lack of autonomy in making decisions relating to abortions seems to be more pronounced in the case of abortions after sex determination as compared to abortions for other reasons (Ganatra and Hirve 2002: 76–85).

The process of decision-making takes before abortion takes a variable length of time. A study spanning six years of obstetric admissions in a hospital in Maharashtra reflected delays in accessing abortion. Of the 17 per cent admissions for abortions, 59 per cent were in the first trimester and 41 in the second trimester (Solapurkar et al. 1985: 46–52). The delay was particularly evident among adolescent married girls, who are more likely to have second trimester abortions.

It is usually the reason why women (or couples) decide to go in for abortion that determines the gestation period at which the pregnancy is terminated. For example, sex determination by amniocentesis is done after 18 weeks, by ultrasound after 13 weeks and by 'Chorionic Villi' sampling at around six to seven weeks. Of these, ultrasound is the most often used method for sex determination in rural areas. It is therefore not surprising that half the women in rural Maharashtra who opt for abortion after 12 weeks of pregnancy do so after sex determination.

The decision-making process determines not only *when* but also *where* abortions are sought. Earlier, women resorted to home remedies and the services of quacks. Recent studies show that only illiterate women (Varkey et al. 2000), women who do not have their husbands' support, or married adolescent girls who lack mobility and control over resources are more likely to use untrained and inexpensive health providers (Ganatra and Hirve 2002: 76–85). The rest go to qualified providers. However, not all these providers are recognised under the MTP Act and therefore the abortions performed by them are not 'legal'.

The government sector statistics on abortion in Gujarat show that MTP cases are either stagnant or are decreasing in spite of the increase in the number of registered MTP facilities. There are several explanations for why women go to qualified but unregistered providers. According to one study, only about 53 per cent of primary health centres (PHCs) and community health centres (CHCs) that were registered for providing abortion services in the state were actually offering the services. About 70–92 per cent of the facilities were not providing services because of lack of trained doctors and 14–31 per cent because of non-availability of required equipment (Khan et al. 1994).

Conversely, there are facilities that provide abortion services though they are not approved or registered. In nine *tehsils* of Maharashtra, for every registered abortion care facility (ACF), there were around three non-registered ACFs. Of the total, 56 per cent were not qualified under the MTP Act and only about 8 per cent of the qualified abortion providers were based in public health care facilities (Bandewar 2000: 39–43).

Qualification or registration under the MTP Act is a major obstacle in the provision of recognised services. The certification process requires installation of equipment and supplies for general anaesthesia and abdominal surgery, a guarantee that a trained provider and anaesthetist are available, site inspection and sequential recommendations by district and state health authorities (Iyengar and Iyengar 2002: 54–63).

Providers in rural areas who do only early abortions using Vacuum Aspiration (Iyengar and Iyengar 2002) perceive the clause relating to general anaesthesia and major surgical equipment as unwarranted, expensive and difficult to arrange. The Act exclusively addresses hospital-based provision of induced abortions and the emergence of medical methods (Population Council 1998: 257–59) makes these requirements appear excessive (Iyengar and Iyengar 2002: 54–63). The insistence by the Ministry of Health and Family Welfare (MOHFW) on the purchase of equipment with the Indian Standards Institute (ISI) mark produced by only one company in the country makes it difficult for the demand to be met (Khan et al. 1994).

The other problem is the stringent training criteria. Most training centres find the prescribed norm of 15 days of on-the-job training and practical experience of conducting at least 25 abortions impossible to meet. Further, in most states, only teaching hospitals carry out MTP training and their courses are not accessible to doctors in private service. This limits the number of legal abortion providers (Iyengar and Iyengar 2001: 54–63).

The registration process itself is fraught with problems and mired in red tape. In Rajasthan, a doctor's application was returned twice for re-submission with additional documents which had not been listed in the application guide (Iyengar and Iyengar 2001: 54–63). A survey of its members by the Federation of Obstetrician and Gynaecologist Society of India (FOGSI) revealed that while 29 per cent of centres did not have any problems, 13 per cent experienced delays ranging from one to seven years, 44 per cent had difficulties in navigating the recognition process, and 12 per cent were unaware of the need for obtaining recognition. Many FOGSI members applied for registration, but because of delays in approval, they continued to perform technically illegal services albeit under safe and hygienic conditions (Sheriar Committee 2001).

Study Design and Research Methodology

It is in the context of these findings that the conceptual framework (Figure 2.1) and the methodology[1] to be used for this study, which covers two urban slums in Ahmedabad, were developed.

Figure 2.1: Health-seeking behaviour for abortion

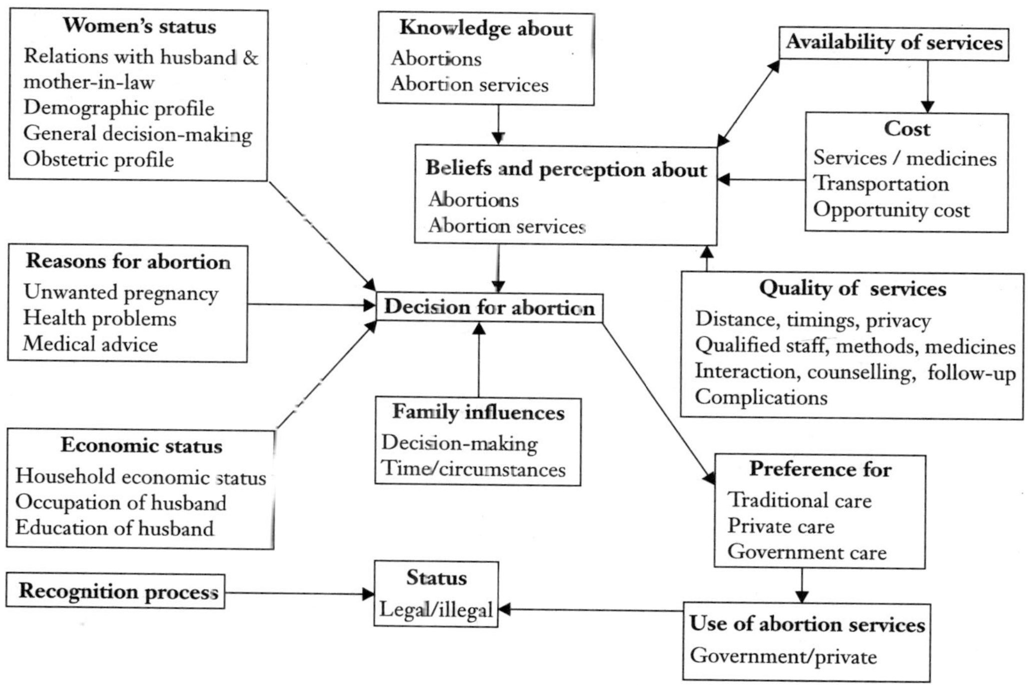

Location

Ahmedabad is the second largest city in western India with a population of about 42 lakh according to the 2001 Census of India. About 40 per cent of this population is located in slums. The population has a sex ratio of 889 girls for 1,000 boys and a literacy rate of 67 per cent. Health facilities to the city's slums are provided by a network of government and municipal tertiary care hospitals, municipal clinics, maternity homes and Urban Family Welfare Centres (UFWCs), as well as by private doctors. There are about 37 UFWCs, including five post-partum units.

Assuming that the affluent classes, with relatively more time and money at their disposal, would have little problem in accessing providers, we felt it more appropriate to concentrate our research in two urban slums.

SLUM–1

This slum is a ward within Ahmedabad municipal limits and, being very close to the city centre, enjoys very good connectivity with rest of the city. It has all basic amenities provided by the city municipal corporation. It has a population of about 70,000, constituted mainly by Patels, Thakores and Rajputs. The socio-economic condition of the residents is better than that of those in SLUM–2 and the houses are largely *pucca*.

Table 2.1: Slum characteristics

	Area	
Indicator	SLUM–1	SLUM–2
Location	Close to city centre	Outskirts
In corporation limits	Yes	No
Population	70,000	40,000
Predominant population	Patels, Thakores,Rajputs	Migrant tribals
Civic amenities	Available	Not available
Abortion services	*Dais*	*Dais*
	Gen. practitioners	Gen. practitioners
	Pvt. gynaecologists	Pvt. gynaecologists
	National NGO	
	Local NGO	
	CFPC	
	Tertiary care hosp.	

Health facilities are available in the form of a large tertiary care municipal hospital, a national-level non-government service facility which is also an approved abortion service centre, several private practitioners including *dai*s, and a Comprehensive Family Planning Centre (CFPC) run by a non-government organisation. While the tertiary care hospital is a full-fledged, well-equipped, multi-speciality service facility, the national NGO has facilities mainly for provision of antenatal, family planning, menstrual regulation, MTP, tubectomy and laparoscopy services; it does not, however, have any outreach services. The CFPC provides basic curative and preventive services mainly through its out-patient department (OPD), as well as outreach services through its cadre of female health workers. In addition, the doctors staffing the OPD refer cases for any surgical intervention, mainly tubectomy and MTP, either to the tertiary care hospital, the national-level NGO or to private gynaecologists' maternity homes.

SLUM–2

This slum is on the outskirts of the city and has a population of about 40,000. It is inhabited mainly by migrants from a tribal community of Udaipur district in the neighbouring state of Rajasthan. The houses in this slum are mostly *kachcha*/semi-pucca. Since the slum is outside the corporation limits, it does not have the amenities usually provided by the municipal corporation, but it does have a local *panchayat* that supplies water in some areas and runs a clinic along the lines of a PHC.

At the time of the study it had poor health facilities. It had neither a tertiary care hospital nor a national or a local NGO-run service facility. However, it did have clinics owned by two private gynaecologists in its close vicinity.

Since our objective was to understand the perspectives of abortion-service users as well as providers, and the effect of these along with the family dynamics of the users on their use of abortion services, we decided to use a qualitative methodology. The methods adopted therefore comprised in-depth interviews and focus group discussions (FGDs). However, flexibility about the order in which to use the two techniques was deliberately retained as the topic is sensitive. It was felt that women might not be very forthcoming in a group discussion, at least initially. Also, since individual perceptions, knowledge and practices relating to abortion service use were equally a part of our focus, we felt that one-to-one interviews would yield richer data. We therefore began the research with in-depth interviews. Once the investigators developed rapport with the women, FGDs were conducted to triangulate the findings that emerged from the interviews, as well as to determine the general trend of perceptions and practices.

In-depth Interviews and Focus Group Discussions

Loose, semi-structured interview field guides were designed for in-depth interviews with women and abortion-care providers. These field guides were formulated based on the research questions developed from our conceptual framework and were finalised after pre-testing and getting feedback from our investigators and consultants. Though we were not working with a well-delineated construct, we preferred to leave the interview guides semi-structured as we felt that this would provide clarity and focus to our research.

Since we were not attempting to study prevalence, morbidity and mortality rates, we held in-depth interviews with a purposively selected sample of 18 abortion-service providers and 60 women users in the two slums. Because our choice of providers depended on the information supplied by key informants and women who had availed of abortion services within two years prior to the commencement of the study, and they did not mention any unqualified providers, they were not identified for the study and private providers were interviewed, since their services were reported to be more frequently used. Similarly, though the government tertiary hospital is not located in either of the slums, women did report using the services there. We therefore decided to include medical officers from that hospital in our sample. Thus, we finally ended up interviewing two gynaecologists from the tertiary-care hospital, a medical officer each from the national- and local-level NGO, two private gynaecologists, one qualified general practitioner and two nurses in SLUM–1, and two private gynaecologists, one qualified general practitioner and two dais in SLUM–2.

Access to health providers was not a problem at all. They were quite forthcoming in talking about their understanding of the stipulations contained in the MTP Act and its actual implementation. They did not hesitate to voice their views, even when these conflicted with the stipulations of the Act.

The 60 women, 30 from each slum, were selected based on their having availed of abortion services within two years prior to the commencement of our research. But when we asked key informants to help us identify them, we deliberately excluded service providers, as the ethics of medical practice do not allow revelation of specific services used by clients. We also used the snowballing technique to identify women for interviews. Accessing women in SLUM–2 was not difficult, as the women in this area, who are mainly migrants from Rajasthan, looked forward to any initiative which they thought might at a later date help them with their problems. Still, there was no need to offer them any incentives to obtain their consent, which they gave readily, and their response remained good till the end of our research.

Both the women users and the providers were interviewed at a time and place specified by them. In cases where information on all our questions was not forthcoming in one sitting, another interview was scheduled. However, this was rarely necessary. As far as possible, the interviews were completed in one sitting, as the respondents found repeated contacts inconvenient and were unwilling to give more days for the interviews.

FGDs were planned with the NGO staff, key informants and community women in the reproductive age group. However, given their heterogeneity, and the fact that there were very few of them, meant that we were unable to conduct FGDs with NGO staff and key informants. In the end, we held FGDs with only two groups of community women in the reproductive age group from each of the slums. The discussions covered our research questions as well as the local terminology for abortion (both spontaneous and induced) and the methods used for induced abortions.

Fieldwork

The four investigators selected to do the fieldwork were young college graduates with some research experience. They came from urban backgrounds and could speak the local language. Before commencing the fieldwork, experts were invited to provide them with intensive training in research methodology, perspective building and information on technical details relating to abortion.

Training sessions for the investigators and supervisors were held in January 2002 and included information on conception, abortions, the MTP Act, sex determination, communicative skills and vocabulary listing. The interviewers were also given training in the field.

In all, 18 service providers and 62 women (30 and 32 SLUM–1 and SLUM–2 respectively) had been interviewed, though interviews with two women had to be discarded as their history of abortion was not very clear despite repeated checks.

Problems Encountered

Given the sensitive nature of the study, we did encounter a few unanticipated and some anticipated problems, and addressed them in the course of the study without compromising the design, objectives or quality of data. For instance:

- There were problems when the fieldwork started, because of the communal tension in the city. This not only cut drastically into the time available to us for research, it also resulted in our having to replace one of the selected slums with another site with similar characteristics.
- We had decided to include in our sample only women who had accessed abortion services in the last two years before commencement of the study. However, due to the curtailment of the study period and with a view to covering the sample agreed upon, we decided to increase the reference period to five years.
- Unqualified providers had to be dropped from the sample as not a single one was reported to have been accessed by the women interviewed. Similarly, general practitioners, nurses and dais were included only as referral service providers since this was their reported role.
- FGDs were planned with the staff of the NGO providing/facilitating these services, as well as with key informants. But the NGO working in the area did not have enough workers of the same cadre to make an FGD worthwhile. The number of key informants was also too small.
- Access to women was a little difficult in SLUM–1 since they were a little circumspect and did not open up to the interviewers very easily. To get around this problem, we took the help of the local NGO which has been running a clinic in the area for the last two decades. Its fieldworkers accompanied the investigators and introduced them to the women, and this

greatly eased our entry into the community. After that, most women in this area had no hesitation in admitting that they had undergone abortion and that too after sex determination, even though they were aware that it was against the law.

- Although not a single woman in either area refused to be interviewed, the investigators realised, within the first couple of days, that it might not be possible to arrange a second interview with the same woman. They therefore conducted the interviews in teams of two and, as far as possible, elicited all the required information in one sitting.
- Access to the medical officer from the municipal tertiary-care hospital followed a very strict protocol and it took the research team two months to get clearance from the superintendent of the hospital.

Ensuring Ethical Standards

Research in sensitive subjects usually requires the interviewer to obtain the written consent of respondents and express a guarantee of confidentiality. However, in our experience, any mention of written consent becomes a major obstacle since women are generally not prepared to sign any written statement. But as long as they know the purpose of the study and are certain that their identities will remain confidential, they are quite prepared to give their oral consent. We therefore not only gave informants detailed information about what our research meant to achieve, but also the option of not participating or even quitting midway if that was what they wanted. At the same time we made it clear that no specific benefit would be accruing to them if they decided to participate. Confidentiality of the data collected and anonymity of the respondents were assured and data were collected only with their informed consent. While quoting the respondents, their names have been changed to ensure anonymity.

Service providers, both registered and non-registered, were not used at any stage as key informants to identify abortion seekers, keeping in view the ethics of medical practice. Confidentiality of information, relating to service provision, obtained from them was strictly maintained.

Though key informants did list a few unmarried and single women who had opted to abort an unwanted pregnancy, they were not included in our sample. It is important for such women to keep their abortion a secret and we did not wish to draw attention to them by actively seeking them out for an interview. We were similarly concerned about compromising the confidentiality of married women who had undergone abortion without the family's knowledge. Luckily, we did not come across a single case where abortion had been done without some family support.

Findings from Interviews of Women

Profile of Women

As mentioned earlier, a total of 62 women—30 from SLUM–1 and 32 from SLUM–2—were interviewed. More than half the interviewed women were in the 25–30 age group. Only about a third of them had got married after the legal age of marriage, i.e., 18 years. More than half the women in the sample were literate. More than one-third or (23) reported three or more living children. Only six women reported having no living child. In all, the women reported 92 induced and 5 spontaneous abortions.

While this was the overall picture, the women in SLUM–2 differed from those selected in SLUM–1 in terms of certain characteristics.

Table 2.2: Characteristics of Women

Indicator	Category	Number
		62
Current age	<=20	6
	21–24	10
	25–30	35
	31–34	8
	35+	3
Age at marriage	<18	40
	>18	22
Education	Illiterate	28
	Literate	34
Living children	0	6
	1	8
	2	25
	3+	23
Abortions	1	42
	2	13
	3+	8

The women in SLUM–2 were comparatively younger and the majority of them, i.e., 8 out of 10, had married before completing 18 years. More women (about two-thirds) in SLUM–2 were illiterate, but had some form of employment. All the six women who had no living children were from this slum.

The respondent women from SLUM–1, on the other hand, had at least one living child. This slum also reported a higher number of abortions and more repeat abortions. Of the 92 abortions reported, 30 women in SLUM–1 accounted for 50 (1.67 abortions per woman) while 32 women in SLUM–2 were responsible for 42 (1.31 abortion per woman).

Reasons for Induced Abortions

Though 92 abortions were reported, the information pertaining to service use presented here covers only 62, i.e., the latest abortion per woman in the five-year reference period before the study.

More than half of the total abortions (34) in the last five years were for limiting family size or spacing children.

Table 2.3: Reasons for induced abortions

Reasons	Total women
	N = 62
Family planning	34
Health problems	18
Sex determination	10

College-educated 30-year-old Jaya from SLUM–1 said: 'I already had two children and was on Mala D. Once or twice I forgot to take the pills and I missed my periods. I realised that I must be pregnant and went with my *nanand* [husband's sister] to Dr M's hospital for an abortion....'

Eighteen abortions were consequent to medical advice. These were more common in SLUM–2, which reported as many as 15 of these. All abortions based on medical advice were reportedly due to health risks faced by the woman or the foetus.

Jiyaben, an illiterate daily-wage labourer from SLUM–2, said:

> In the beginning of the fifth month, when I was in the toilet, I had a suffocating sensation and felt as if something fell down from

my body. I then started bleeding. My mother and brother immediately took me to a private doctor in an autorickshaw. The doctor examined me and said that perhaps I had started losing the baby and advised *'andar saaf-sufi karvi padshe'* [the inside of the uterus needs to be cleaned]. My relatives agreed and I had to get the abortion done.

Since almost all these pregnancies were 'wanted', the women consulted gynaecologists and made all attempts to salvage the pregnancies before getting them terminated. Some women also reported being unconvinced by the doctors' advice to terminate for medical reasons and sought second opinions.

Ten of the abortions (of which eight were from SLUM–1) were after sex determination and confirmation of female foetuses. These abortions were usually conducted after sonographies, generally around 12–16 weeks of pregnancy. A few were performed after 16 weeks and the women did not see anything wrong with this.

Deepika, a woman from SLUM–1, said:

I became pregnant for the second time when my daughter was one and a half years old. I went to a private doctor after the third month for a sex determination test, since I knew that that is when it is done. The doctor did a sonography and said it was a girl. But he did not write this down as it is illegal. My husband and I did not want another girl and decided on abortion. I had my abortion at the same clinic.

There were some rare cases where the reason for abortion was cited as 'family dispute' or as a way to teach an 'erring' husband or the husband's family a lesson. As one of the women said:

My mother-in-law and husband have been harassing and beating me since my marriage. Once, when I was about four months pregnant, my husband, who was drunk at the time, beat me up. There and then I decided to abort the baby. The doctor did a sonography on his own and said that it was a male foetus, so maybe I would like to continue with the pregnancy. But I was very clear in my mind. I got the abortion done without telling anyone except a close friend.

Decision-making for Induced Abortions

Seventeen women whose pregnancies were terminated on medical advice said that the decision for abortion had been made by the doctor. About a fourth of the women in the sample claimed that the decision was made either by family members or the couples themselves. A fifth (12) said that it was their own decision and only four said that they had been asked by their husbands to terminate the pregnancy.

Table 2.4: Decision-making for induced abortions

Decision maker	Total women
	N = 62
Doctor	17
Family members	15
Couple	14
Wife	12
Husband	4

Family members seemed to have played a major role in decision-making in SLUM–1 (10 out of 15). In this context, it must be pointed out that more women belonged to joint families and there were more terminations after sex determination in this slum. However, there was no obvious evidence of the women being coerced into abortion (except for one woman who was forced to abort though she wanted to continue with the pregnancy).

Most (15) of the abortions based on medical advice were from SLUM–2. Also, more women (8 out of 12) from this slum said that the abortion was their own decision. This was especially true in the case of the slum's nuclear families, in which wives played a significant role in deciding whether the pregnancy should be continued or not. This slum also had more women who were employed.

Services Used

Facility

The majority of abortions took place in private hospitals (48) or in the NGO-run hospital (12); only one each was conducted in the government and municipal tertiary-care hospitals. All abortions were performed by qualified gynaecologists.

Table 2.5: Service facilities used

Indicator		SLUM–1	SLUM–2
Provider	Private hospitals	16	32
	Government hospitals	2	0
	NGOs	12	0
Reason for preference	Reputation	Yes	Yes
	Vicinity	No	Yes
	Familiarity	No	Yes
	Cost	Yes	Yes
	Confidentiality	Yes	No

The major determinants in the choice of provider were reputation, vicinity, familiarity and cost of services. Women thought twice about using the government tertiary-care hospitals where, according to them, a lot of time is wasted in waiting and completing the paperwork. Also, these hospitals are not client-friendly and the quality of service they provide is suspect. The general feeling was that any facility that provides free service is not very good.

In SLUM–1, women who had had multiple abortions and/or had resorted to abortion after sex-determination tests said that they had gone to different clinics for each episode in order to maintain secrecy. Confidentiality is thus a major consideration when choosing a provider. Women in this slum either directly approached the well-known local or national-level NGO facility, or consulted the NGO outreach health workers, who referred them either to these facilities or to the tertiary-care hospital in the area. Some of the women went to a specific NGO-run clinic which they had seen advertised on hoardings, walls, buses, etc.

In SLUM–2, all the abortions were conducted at private gynaecologists' clinics, as these were the only facilities available. The preference for a particular provider depended on the clinic's proximity and the client's familiarity with the provider. Recommendations made by family members or friends who had used a particular facility earlier also had a bearing on choice. The main reason for women's reluctance to use the services of the government tertiary hospital was the excessive time spent in completing the requisite formalities.

Services Received

Women judged the quality of services and care received in terms of explanations given to them before the procedure, the conduct of preliminary tests or examinations, the insistence on the husband's consent, post-procedural advice, follow-up and complications, and their own satisfaction with the services.

Table 2.6: Method of abortion

Indicator	SLUM–1	SLUM–2
Do not know	9	16
By 'machine'	8	8
Curetting	2	2
Two stage	10	6

More than a third of the women said that they did not know anything about the method used for their abortion. It appears that not a single woman was told by the doctor exactly what would be done. No explanations were given either to the woman or the accompanying person. In this context it is important to note that the women themselves did not seem to be particularly interested in knowing anything about the method or procedural details either. Neetu, who is literate, said:

> I do not know what the doctor did after I became unconscious. The doctor must have used some machine for abortion. I did not ask anything and the doctor did not volunteer any information. I am unaware about the legality of abortion and different kinds of method to terminate pregnancy. That does not concern me.

Women did not report any pre-procedural tests other than sonography for foetal sex determination. In many cases, they consulted the doctor only after confirming their pregnancy through a urine test at a private pathological laboratory. Very few mentioned vaginal examination for confirmation of pregnancy. In fact, Bharati, a literate, employed woman from SLUM–2, recounted a harrowing experience that could perhaps have been avoided had she been thoroughly examined and investigated:

> The day after the abortion I developed severe abdominal pain. When I consulted the doctor the next day, she said that it was natural after abortion. She gave me some medicines and advised rest. Even after resting and taking the medicines, I did not get relief. My periods, too, did not resume. My husband and I went back to

> the doctor. This time she did a sonography and said, 'During the abortion the foetus leaked into the tube, because of which there is now a danger to your health.' She told me that this was a very serious problem and that I would have to undergo an operation, which would cost me Rs 16,000.

Though the doctors do not lay any particular stress on pre-procedural investigations or tests, when it comes to obtaining consent for abortion, many women reported that doctors insist not only on theirs, but also on that of the accompanying person(s).

All women reported that doctors do give post-operative advice, but it is no more substantial than prescribing painkillers and rest. However, women found even this advice difficult to follow due to pressures of household work or the need to rejoin their jobs. Very few were advised contraceptive use and only about a third of the women reported being users of any type of contraception. One woman who had undergone six abortions was still a non-user at the time of the interview. There have also been instances where, even when the accompanying person was the husband, the doctors did not advise the couple to use condoms. Despite these lapses, however, most women expressed satisfaction with the services they received.

While both slums yielded very similar data, more women from SLUM–2 were ignorant about the abortion procedure, and more women from SLUM–1 had undergone sex-determination tests and subsequent abortion.

Cost

Of the women who could recall the cost, the majority said that they had paid between Rs 400 and Rs 600 for the abortion. There did not appear to be any standard cost for abortion in the area. Despite advertising the cost of abortion as Rs 150, even the local NGO was charging different women different amounts. When two women, who accessed the NGO's service delivery centre after reading the advertisement, questioned the amount they were being charged, they were told that Rs 150 was only the basic cost, to which other costs were added as and when other tests, procedures or medicines were required. The cost also varied depending on the stage of pregnancy at which abortion was sought and the type of method used.

In SLUM–1, especially in joint families, where abortions took place with the family's consent, the expenses were borne by the in-laws. In SLUM–2, poor socio-economic conditions and the high cost of abortion did not deter women from having abortions in private facilities. Somehow or the other, these women managed to scrape up the amount needed. Over 40 per cent of the women had paid for the abortion from their own personal savings; some had borrowed money from employers, friends, neighbours or relatives, or had pawned their jewellery.

During the FGD in SLUM–2, women said that their in-laws were often against the couples' decision to abort. They therefore had to conceal the abortion from the in-laws, which is why they could not get any monetary help from them. In such situations, a considerable number of these women went to their natal homes to get the abortion done, and their parents paid for all abortion-related expenses.

Provider Perspectives

Provider/Facility Profile

In keeping with their mandate, the two tertiary-care hospitals offer all curative, preventive and specialist services. The NGOs and private gynaecologists offer obstetric and gynaecological curative and preventive services. The general practitioners provide minor curative services, immunisation and other preventive services, while the nurses and dais handle only antenatal care and deliveries.

The local NGO reported performing the highest number (between 150 and 200) of abortions per month. The national NGO reported 100 to 200 cases, while each of the two tertiary hospitals provided abortion services for 75 to 100 cases per month. The private gynaecologists handled 20 to 30 abortion cases per month. General practitioners said that 20 to 40 women came to them for abortions every month, while the nurse and dais reported only one or two cases. The general practitioners, nurses and dais, however, referred the cases which came to them to gynaecologists at private or NGO-run clinics, or to tertiary-care hospitals.

While the tertiary hospitals and the national NGO are approved centres for abortion, and though the local NGO's status in this regard is still unclear, the other facilities are not certified. However, some private gynaecologists did claim that they had applied for certification

Table 2.7: Characteristics of service facilities/providers

	Government tertiary	Municipal tertiary	National NGO	Local NGO	Private gynae.	General practitioner	Nurse/dai
Services provided	ALL Curative Preventive Specialist	ALL Curative Preventive Specialist	OB/GYN[a] Curative Preventive	OB/GYN Curative Preventive	OB/GYN Curative Preventive	ALL Curative	ANC[b] Delivery
Recognised for MTP	Yes	Yes	Yes	?	Not all	No	No
Special training	No	No	No	No	No	No	No
Reported MTP case-load	75–100/ month	75–100/ month	100–200/ month	150–200/ month	20–30/ month	20–40/ month	1–2/ month

Notes: [a] OB/GYN: Obstetrician/Gynaecologist.
[b] ANC: Ante-natal care.

two years ago and were still awaiting approval. None of the providers in any of the centres have received any special training to provide abortion-related services.

Profile of Abortion Seekers

According to the medical officers in the tertiary hospitals, the majority of women seeking services from their facility are illiterate, while the education level of women seeking services from the other facilities is variable. Except for private gynaecologists, all other providers reported that their clients come from a poor socio-economic background. While most providers said that both married and unmarried women from the age group 15–45 years seek abortion, the two NGOs reported a younger age profile, of 20–30 years. The tertiary municipal hospital doctor confessed that they actively discourage unmarried women from coming to them for abortions, and in the recent past had (unofficially) also turned them away in order to avoid any subsequent problems with their relatives.

Over 75 per cent of all abortions are sought in the first trimester, with two-thirds being within the first eight weeks. The dais reported that the women who come to them are generally under 21 and unmarried, and 60 per cent of them come early in the first trimester. All service providers confirmed the trend of using termination of pregnancy as a family-planning method. According to most private providers, those who want to limit family size undergo abortion as soon as they miss their periods, i.e., within eight weeks, while those terminating pregnancy for spacing have abortions between 8 and 12 weeks. As Dr P., the gynaecologist at the tertiary-care hospital, said:

> In my experience, multiparous women seek induced abortions either because the last child is still very young or because they do not want more children. In such cases even the husbands and in-laws support termination of pregnancy. Generally, 80 per cent of such women come for induced abortion within 6–8 weeks of pregnancy. Among the 20 per cent who come late in the second trimester, at around 14–16 weeks, the delay is usually the result of late decision, money problems, or unawareness about pregnancy due to lactational amenorrhoea….

With the exception of the municipal tertiary hospital, all providers mentioned that though they did not have any documentary evidence, they were certain that many of the abortions that they had conducted were after sex determination. They claimed it was difficult for service providers to ascertain whether the woman coming for the abortion of an 'unwanted' pregnancy had undergone sex determination elsewhere. In their view, their services were mainly sought for termination of 'unwanted pregnancies', in which case providers' responsibility is limited to merely providing the service. The gynaecologist from the government tertiary hospital explained further:

> All pregnancies are regarded as 'wanted' by service providers; it is the women who have to decide whether they want the pregnancy or not. The client's opinion has to be followed by providers. If a couple comes after sex determination, it is their decision. However, according to me, aborting a female foetus is not wrong. Women should be organised to elevate their status—banning such abortions will not work. In fact, aborting the female foetus is an indicator of women's liberation. The girl is not subjected to ill-treatment and does not become the victim of discrimination after birth.

One reason for seeking abortions, reported by all providers but not mentioned by women for obvious reasons, is premarital or extramarital pregnancies. A private gynaecologist explained the differences in abortion-seeking by unmarried girls from different socio-economic backgrounds:

> In many communities, the betrothal of girls and boys takes place at a very young age. The girl lives with her parents, but both girl and boy are allowed to go around together. They invariably end up having a physical relationship. Though the community permits their going out together, it does not approve of pregnancies before formal marriage. So these girls come for termination. The community knows that these things happen, but the attempt is to keep it concealed ....

While abortions are sought across all caste and community groups, the municipal hospital and the two NGOs reported a high percentage of seekers from minority communities, possibly because the facilities are located closer to the minority localities and also because the residents of these localities are from a poorer background.

In the context of decision-making for abortion, providers confirmed that the decision is usually made either together by the couple or by the woman herself. Dr Y., a lady gynaecologist in SLUM–2, said:

> The decision for MTP is usually that of the woman or her husband/partner. The mothers-in-law are kept in the dark as this is a conservative community and has a strong belief that children are God's gift and one should not try to limit their number. Also, the mothers-in-law in this community are very domineering, and insist that their daughters-in-law should have at least two sons.

Pre-Abortion Services

Providers admitted that pre-abortion services mainly comprise a physical examination and enquiries about medical and obstetric history. They do not do any internal check-ups or ask for further investigations, as these tend to put off the women. Instead, they depend on the history of amenorrhoea, a positive urine test or the sonography report, the woman's consent and, in the case of anticipated problems, the presence and consent of relatives or accompanying persons. Except for the government tertiary hospital, none of the other providers felt that pre-abortion services are warranted or mandatory. The medical officer at the government tertiary hospital was the sole exception who said that at least a blood group test needs to be done, as women who are Rh-negative require an anti-D injection even after abortion.

When specifically questioned about why they insist on the consent of people other than the woman when it is not mandatory under the Act, the medical officer at the national-level NGO said:

> Every surgical procedure, however minor, has the potential of becoming complicated. We do not insist on the consent of the accompanying person, but we do want someone from the family to be around. The consent of this person is for surgical procedure under anaesthesia, not for the abortion itself.

The providers also felt that the women themselves are not particularly concerned about issues like consent or privacy. They therefore make no special arrangements for maintaining privacy.

Abortion Methods and Processes

There is unanimity amongst the providers regarding the methods 'recommended' for abortions at different stages of pregnancy. They mentioned that Manual Vacuum Aspiration (MVA) is recommended for pregnancies under six weeks, and Electric Vacuum Aspiration (EVA)—usually under local anaesthesia—for 7–12 week pregnancies. For late first trimester and second trimester pregnancies, i.e., at 14–20 weeks, the recommended procedures are all two-stage. The first stage comprises a prostaglandin injection, per-vaginal Laminaria tent insertion, per-cervical instillation of 150 cc of ethacridine lactate using Foley's catheter, or local application of prostaglandin/cerviprim jelly to ripen/dilate the cervix. This is followed by a pitocin/sintocin drip to induce expulsion of the products of conception, or a Dilatation and Evacuation or Curettage (DE/DC) process, again under local but sometimes under general anaesthesia. For the rare abortions performed beyond 20 weeks, the recommended method is either intra-amniotic prostaglandin (PGF12) injection and, in rare cases, hysterectomy.

Though these methods are recommended as suitable, providers pointed out that their actual use depends on factors other than just the gestation period. For example, some providers, particularly those in the private sector, do not use the EVA, as the electricity supply in the area where they practise is uncertain. Again, some do not recommend the MVA or EVA beyond eight weeks because, according to them, it is at this time that bones begin to develop in the foetus, which makes aspiration difficult. One private doctor said:

> The 12–14 week window is a problem period. During this period, it is too late to use the methods used in earlier stages of pregnancy, and too early to use the methods used at later stages. I ask my clients to wait for 14 weeks to be over before I do the abortion.

In addition, providers also have their own personal preferences regarding the methods to be used. According to one private male gynaecologist:

> I use only the D&E method. I prefer to see what I do, so I also use the laparoscopic method. I do not recommend RU 486 for the same reason. But my Jain clients prefer the medical method for termination of pregnancy; in such cases I prescribe RU 486.

Whatever their views on the methods used, all providers described a more or less similar pattern and route of service use for married and unmarried women. According to a private gynaecologist:

> Married women usually want to terminate the pregnancy to delay the first childbirth, space the next childbirth, get rid of a female foetus, or for career reasons. In Gujarat, many women who get married to non-resident Indians also get it done because they fear that their visas might be rejected. Some women, despite being literate and aware, do try traditional methods like consuming 'hot' foods or primolute/epiforte tablets. When they do not get withdrawal bleeding, they get their urine tested and also try RU 486, a pill that is now available over the counter in some shops.
>
> Unmarried girls, on the other hand, come for termination of illegitimate pregnancy, or for visa and career reasons. They usually come alone or with their mother or close friend; it is very rare for the partner to accompany them. Usually, the rest of the family is kept in the dark. They come a little late, at least a month after the due date of the period. They, too, first try out 'hot' foods or over-the-counter medicines. When these fail, they consult the local nurse or general practitioner (GP). They are then referred to a gynaecologist. Gynaecologists at government hospitals conduct an 'inquisition', but we in the private sector do not. We just provide the service and discharge the girls as soon as possible, keeping in mind the social repercussions of in-door admission.

Post-Abortion Care

The duration of women's stay in the hospital usually depends on the period of gestation and the method used for abortion. Typically, the

Table 2.8: Hospital stay

Period of gestation	Hospital stay
<8 weeks	<1/2 hour
9–12 weeks	2–3 hours
13 weeks	Half a day
14–16 weeks	Full day
>16 weeks	2–3 days

duration increases exponentially with the period of gestation. From less than half-an-hour for less-than-eight weeks' gestation, it goes up to 2–3 days for over 16 weeks' gestation.

Post-abortion care mainly comprises a tetanus toxoid injection, antibiotics, anti-inflammatory pills and painkillers. Two private gynaecologists also mentioned giving women Mala D. They do not ask the women to come for follow-up visits if there are no complications. Counselling is limited to explaining the possibility of post-abortion sterility to primiparas, and the consequences of repeat abortions to frequent users of abortions. Though the providers, particularly those in tertiary hospitals, insisted that they believe in contraceptive counselling since termination is most often used for family planning reasons, one also admitted:

> Most providers in government hospitals do not have much time to spend with the client, so counselling is not effective. And private hospitals do not have dedicated staff or incentives to do contraceptive or consequence-related counselling. Further, hospitals do not have any system to audit counselling and its effect.

Cost

The cost of abortion usually varies, depending on the type of provider, the gestation period and the method used. The medical officers at the tertiary hospitals quoted the lowest charge. Being government-run, these hospitals are expected to provide free services but, as the medical officers acknowledged, women do have to bear some costs: they have to pay for the medicines which, when not in stock at the hospital, need to be purchased from outside.

Table 2.9: Cost

Facility	Cost in rupees
Nurse	500–700
General practitioners	700–1500
Private gynaecologists	1st trimester: 750–1500
	2nd trimester: 2500–5000
Local NGO	1st trimester: 350–400
	2nd trimester: 1500–2000
National NGO	1st trimester: 400
	2nd trimester: 800
Tertiary hospitals	Free–300

The private gynaecologists quoted the highest charge. The local NGO advertised abortion services at Rs 150, but admitted that the total cost could even go up to 15 times that, thus corroborating what the women had said in their interviews.

Providers hold very strong and divergent views on the issue of cost. The medical officer at one of the tertiary hospitals was vehemently against abortion being offered as a free service. He said: 'It should not be done free of cost, except for Below Poverty Line (BPL) families. Otherwise people do not use contraception since they feel that whenever they do not want a pregnancy, there is an easy remedy available.' His counterpart at the municipal tertiary hospital was of a contrary view. According to him: 'Abortions should be part of the family planning programme and be offered totally free of cost. It should be accepted as a family planning method.'

Private gynaecologists, however, seemed very much against any standardisation or regulation of cost. One of them categorically stated: 'Cost cannot be advertised correctly nor can it be regulated. It depends on the gestation, the methods used and the risks taken by the provider.' They also feel that since women are willing to spend the money, there is no reason for anyone, including the government, to interfere in what they charge.

Quality of Services

Most providers feel that, by and large, most women are satisfied with their services; about a third of them even had another abortion within the year. Though women usually prefer to use a different facility for their next abortion, this is not always the case. But two providers, who were more candid, also said that women really have no option and therefore, despite all the problems they might face, have to be satisfied with whatever services they receive. None of the providers mentioned having come across any instance of death or sterility due to abortion during their careers. But they did sometimes witness cases of incomplete abortion, spotting or bleeding and, very occasionally, a woman with a pelvic infection, abdominal pain or perforation as a consequence of abortion. These complications, according to them, are bound to occur when services are not freely available and women are unaware of the availability of qualified providers.

Reactions to Abortion

Providers claimed that most women do not feel any permanent remorse after terminating a pregnancy. According to private gynaecologists, a few suffer from something called '*smashan vairagya*' (temporary remorse). To quote one of them:

> Women's initial feeling is not good. They do not like what they have done. They have what we call a *shamshan vairagya* feeling. They say that they have committed a *paap* [sin]. But they soon forget about it and 20–30 per cent come back for a repeat abortion. The married ones have become fairly hardened. They come back to the same doctor repeatedly. But unmarried girls who have repeat abortions go to different providers.

Not all providers are happy with having to provide abortion services. Two mentioned conscience problems, but also stated that they had no option but to provide such services for economic reasons. They also spoke about the problems they have with the authorities as well as with the families of some women who seek abortion without their knowledge.

According to a private gynaecologist, who has discontinued providing abortion service:

> The MTP Act does not permit abortions on demand and rightly so. I do not conduct abortions any more. All my clients are educated and from the upper class. I do not want to correct their mistakes. I always encourage contraceptive use. They should avoid the situation in the first place.

Views on Available Services and the MTP Act

The universal view is that abortion services should be widely available but that very few providers in the private sector actually have the technical approval for providing such services. The entire training and approval procedure is unrealistic and needs to be revised. Training is unnecessary and impractical for private doctors. The certification process involves administrative delays and is tedious. The primary visit by the approving authority to the centre is usually a year after the application is submitted and costs about Rs 800 to Rs 1,000. But after that there is no follow-up action despite repeated submissions. Private providers also said that the professional body of obstetricians and gynaecologists has presented their problems to the appropriate authorities, but has yet to receive a reply.

Since they find it difficult to refuse women the service, they feel that abortion should be included in the government's family planning programme because, in any case, the services are being used primarily for family-planning reasons. There is also no need to standardise the requirements and procedures. They feel that the MTP Act is open to interpretation and the government should therefore trust the qualified allopathic providers, i.e., the gynaecologists, to do the right thing. They are equally insistent that the consent of accompanying persons must be taken for surgical procedures and women activists should not view this as an attempt to undermine women's autonomy.

The paperwork, too, needs to be rationalised. Record maintenance should be limited to terminations after sex determination or suspicion of sex determination. They feel that accountability for any wrongdoing should not stop with the provider but should go right up to the top, i.e., the concerned government department or appropriate authority. Given the absence of safeguards for doctors and the increasing use of the Consumer Protection Act (CPA), it should come as no surprise if the medical lobby has attempted to ensure that either the services are not easily available or that no doctors are punished. They also feel that the accountability of providers should be restricted to technical mistakes. They should not be hauled up for having provided the services in contravention of the Act. According to one of them:

> The Act allows women to undergo abortion as many times as they wish. This is not good; it should not be so liberal. The implementation of the Act is poor, as there is a lack of accountability, which should be there at all levels—from the lowest cadre to the Health Minister. Qualified providers like me should be protected against legal hassles. Also, there should be proper selection of the health provider. The prevalent view of training paramedics is untenable. Who will be accountable for any problems? With the Consumer Protection Act, even legal services will soon be unavailable.

Conclusions

Our data show that awareness about the possibility of terminating an unwanted pregnancy is universal and high, as is awareness about the availability of services. A substantial number of the women interviewed viewed abortions as a method to control family size and space children. They either did not know that this is not within the legal mandate of the MTP Act, or, if they did, did they did not seem particularly concerned about it. Most, however, were certainly aware that termination of pregnancy after sex determination is illegal. While the decision for abortion to regulate family size was not necessarily with the knowledge or consent of the elders in the family, abortion after sex determination was usually a family decision, often made with the active participation of the women themselves. We also found that abortion after sex determination was more common among better-off and educated women, perhaps because sonography itself is an expensive proposition for most. However, this observation may not stand statistical scrutiny, as our sample was small and largely purposive.

The majority of women in our two study areas took the decision to abort within the first eight weeks of pregnancy. They also admitted to trying out over-the-counter medicines like epiforte/primolute for withdrawal bleeding to rule out delayed periods. This practice extended across all educational and economic classes. Once the tablets failed to yield the desired result, women went to qualified gynaecologists, either directly or through referrals by general practitioners or local dais. Not a single woman reported going to quacks or dais for abortion or what they called 'curetting'. Awareness about the need to go to qualified gynaecologists was thus high and their services were availed irrespective of their cost and the women's status.

Women accessed gynaecologists who would admit them, conduct the abortion and discharge them on the same day. Pre-abortion investigations and examinations were perfunctory and, in the absence of complications, post-abortion follow-ups were non-existent. Counselling was not seen as a critical element of the service either by the women or the providers. The process seemed to be predominantly demand-driven, with the women dictating some of the terms such as hospital stay and post-abortion care, with a total disregard for medical norms or requirements. These were also some of the reasons why private services were preferred. Privacy, confidentiality and, to some extent, cost were often quoted as reasons for preferring private over government facilities. Our study seems to indicate that the reputation and flexibility of private providers to meet the demands of women and their families in complete contravention of the MTP Act also play a sizeable role.

The providers corroborated most of the information reported by women except with regard to two critical issues. First, they claimed that they do not do sex-determination tests and if the woman had it done elsewhere, there was no way for them to ascertain this. And second, that they usually do a complete physical examination and counselling before actually conducting the abortion. The providers, mainly private gynaecologists, also spoke of the constraints under which they worked. The undue delays in the certification process meant that the facilities of most providers who were interviewed were not 'approved' centres and, by virtue of this, they were forced to provide services which, though essentially safe, were deemed illegal. In their view, the unrealistic requirements and impractical stipulations for provision of services made proper implementation of the Act practically impossible. They likened the authorities' deliberate disregard of the use of abortion for family planning purposes to an ostrich burying its head in the sand.

To conclude, in view of the changing social scenario wherein women are increasingly using abortion to terminate pregnancies for reasons other than those mentioned in the Act, and given that over-the-counter medical abortion pills are freely available, the Act needs to be revised to ensure that it is in consonance with the field realities. On their part, professional bodies of providers, particularly gynaecologists, need to come up with measures to handle the laxity of providers in abiding by the medical code of ethics while terminating pregnancies after sex determination. Thus, policymakers and service providers need to work together to make the Act more realistic and easy to implement.

Notes

We place on record our thanks to Dr Rekha Bhatt, Consultant Gynaecologist, and Dr M. H. Shah, Consultant, FRHS, without whose support and guidance this study would not have been possible.

1. Data were collected on various key factors and variables that were relevant in the context of our conceptual framework. Additional background information on women as well as service providers was collected wherever deemed necessary to get a holistic picture of the dynamics involved in

accessing abortion services. For example, providers' views were sought on a range of topics such as prevalence and frequency of induced abortions, profile of women seekers, reasons for induced abortions, process of decision-making, steps taken by women before actual use, pre-abortion services offered at the facility, methods of abortion, cost, stay, post abortion counselling, care, follow-up, experiences with use/provision of services, legality of abortion and the MTP Act. A preliminary list of research questions based on the framework was made with the objective of making the theoretical assumptions more explicit. The main aim, however, was to come up with the methodology to be adopted and make the data collection more focused.

References

Bandewar, Sunita. 2000. 'Unsafe Abortion'. *Seminar* 489.

CEHAT. 2001. *Abortions in India: Health Panorama*. Compiled by Sunita Bandewar, Rajeshwari Ramani and A. Ashraf. Mumbai: Cehat.

CORT (Centre for Operations Research and Training). 1996. *Situation Analysis of Medical Termination of Pregnancy (MTP) Services in Bihar*. Monograph. Baroda: CORT.

Chhabra, R. and S. C. Nuna. 1993. *Abortion in India: An Overview*. New Delhi: Ford Foundation.

Ganatra, B. R. and Siddhi Hirve. 2002. 'Induced Abortions Among Adolescent Women in Rural Maharashtra, India'. *Reproductive Health Matters* 10 (19): 76–85.

Government of India. 2001. *Census of India, 2001*. New Delhi: Registrar General of India.

Gupte, Manisha, Sunita Bandewar and Hemlata Pisal. 1997. 'Abortion Needs of Women in India: A Case Study of Rural Maharashtra'. *Reproductive Health Matters* 9: Special issue on 'Abortion: The Unfinished Business'.

ICPD. 1994. Programme of Action. New York: UNICPD Secratariat. (International Conference on Population Development).

Iyengar, K. and S. D. Iyengar. 2002. 'Elective Abortion as a Primary Health Service in Rural India: Experience with Manual Vacuum Aspiration'. *Reproductive Health Matters* 10 (19).

Khan, M. E., Bella Patel and R. Chandrashekhar. 1990. 'A Study of MTP Acceptors and their Subsequent Contraceptive Use'. *Journal of Family Welfare* 36 (3).

Khan, M. E., S. Barge and Nayan Kumar. 1994. 'Availability and Access to Abortion Services in India: Myth and Realities'. Working Paper. Baroda: CORT.

Manushi. 2002. 'Legal But Not Available: The Paradox of Abortion in India'. January.

Population Council. 1998. 'Medical Methods of Early Abortion in Developing Countries'. *Contraception* 58.

Shelley, C., Elul Batya, S. Ambardekar, A. Leonard and K. Coyaji. 2001. 'Husbands, Wives and Legal Abortion in India'. Unpublished paper.

Sheriar, N. K., MTP Committee. 2001. 'Navigating the MTP Act in Clinical Practice'. *Journal of Obstetrics and Gynaecology*. Available from http://www.journal–obgyn-India.com/issue_nov_dec2001.

Solapurkar, M. L. and R. N. Sangam. 1985. 'Has the MTP Act in India Proved Beneficial?' *Journal of Family Welfare* 31–3.

Varkey, P., P. P. Balakrishna, J. H. Prasad, S. Abraham and A. Joseph. 2000. 'The Reality of Unsafe Abortion in a Rural Community in South India'. *Reproductive Health Matters* 8 (6).

III

Women, Work and Abortion Practices in Tamil Nadu

S. Anandhi

> Abortion is a necessary, though far from sufficient, condition of women's essential right and need, not only for bodily health and self-determination, but also for control over their work, their sexuality, and their relations with others—including existing children. From this perspective, abortion conducted under safe, affordable, and stigma-free conditions is neither a necessary evil nor a matter of private choice. Rather, it is a positive benefit that society has an obligation to provide to all who seek it, just as it provides education and health benefits.
>
> (Petchesky 1986: 387)

Much of the literature on abortion in India focuses primarily on aspects such as the quality of abortion care and services and post-abortion complications. Critiques of the MTP (Medical Termination of Pregnancy) Act are also available.[1] However, there is virtually no study that locates abortion in the larger context of production, reproduction and sexuality.

As far as Tamil Nadu is concerned, there have been a few quantitative surveys on the incidence of abortion, conducted mainly in the context of fertility decline. Most of them document how abortion is used as a method of contraception in order to achieve desired demographic objectives.[2] But even these, while analysing the 'structural' factors that have led to the utilisation of abortion as a method of birth or population control, fail to pay attention to either the 'personal' factors involved or the process through which women arrive at the decision to abort.

Further, such studies do not take into account how these 'structural factors' translate into actual personal-level processes of reproductive choice/non-choice for and by women. A reformulation of the issue of abortion in these terms would conceptualise women not as passive victims of medical and state policies of reproductive control, but as active—though not always entirely free—agents in reworking their reproductive interests. In other words, even while their choice and resistance are conditioned by 'external structural' factors, women have to be recovered as active agents of their fertility and reproductive choices, however circumscribed their agency.

Our emphasis on women's agency, however, is not to minimise or undermine the fact that women's decision to abort and their experience of abortion are simultaneously controlled and mediated by larger institutions (the state, medical institutions, patriarchal families) and by structural conditions and processes (socio-economic transitions and the sexual division of labour). As Rosalind Petchesky argues, women's access to material resources in the form of landownership and employment outside the domestic sphere does effectively change their conception of reproductive control, as also the structures of knowledge about fertility control among them (Petchesky 1986: 7). For instance, work conditions might force women to choose abortion as an alternative to losing their jobs. Similarly, access to industrial work and the new collectivity of women might generate an alternative knowledge system about abortion practices. Besides, the very meaning of abortion derives 'from the specific historical and political context in which it occurs and the circumstances (class, marital status, employment conditions) of the woman involved' (*ibid.*: 9). Abortion as women's choice or as a symbol of their reproductive freedom is always entangled with various patriarchal structures and social conditions. Therefore, even while our emphasis is on women's consciousness and agency in the practice of abortion, it is not possible to abstract the concept of the 'right to choose' or 'reproductive right' from the social and material conditions under which the choices are made.

Abortion in Tamil Nadu: Two Scenarios

From the early 1980s, Tamil Nadu has been witnessing a sharp decline in the fertility rate, essentially due to a strategy of family limitation, especially among the younger age group, which largely seems to have followed terminal methods like abortion and sterilisation.

As K. Nagaraj points out, fertility decline in Tamil Nadu has not been accompanied by factors such as the increase in the age of marriage or in longer intervals between births. Instead, this decline has been achieved by 'bunching' births around shorter birth intervals, with a high proportion of pregnancies-at-risk and high levels of pregnancy wastage (Nagaraj 2002).

Significantly, rapid fertility decline has also been made possible by the near-universal knowledge of at least one method of contraception among married women in Tamil Nadu, as is shown by the *National Family Health Survey* conducted in 1998–99 (IIPS 2001). Although the extent of women's knowledge about modern methods of contraception is significantly higher than that of traditional methods, they seem to know more about sterilisation and clinical abortions. According to the survey, while the contraceptive-use rate was 52 percent, sterilisation accounted for 87 per cent of the total prevalence of contraception.

At 11.4 per cent, the incidence of abortion—i.e., abortion as a percentage of pregnancies—is the highest in Tamil Nadu compared to the all-India figure of 6.1 per cent (Nagaraj 2002).[3] In particular, the induced-abortion rate for Tamil Nadu is as high as 5.2 per cent, while the all-India rate is only 1.7 per cent.[4] The total number of reported abortions in Tamil Nadu is 42,364, with 73.8 per cent of them occurring among married women of below 30 years of age. (A study on abortion in Kerala, too, notes that over a period of time an increased proportion of abortions was carried out among younger women, i.e., two-thirds of the abortions were among women below 30 [Rajan et al. 2000: 76]). All this points to the fact that abortion plays a big role in reproductive control and choice in Tamil Nadu. It also indicates that abortion is widely practised by married women as a birth-control or birth-spacing method. As many studies have already argued, the state's fertility-control programme has always promoted abortion along with sterilisation as an important method of population control.

Another aspect worth considering is the manner in which the practice of abortion by unmarried young girls has changed production relations and women's employment in various industries. An important feature of the recent economic transformation in Tamil Nadu has been the employment of an increasing number of women in informal-sector industries. In contrast, men are unable to find regular jobs in the growing industrial sector. The consequent reversal of gender roles, by which men no longer perform the function of 'provider', has been a significant factor in changing women's reproductive relations and widening their access to abortion. On the one hand, the unmarried young women's status as earner/provider has led to increased surveillance of and control over their sexuality by the men in their families[5] and the employment of new notions of sexual morality and social dishonour associated with practices like abortion. On the other, their enhanced mobility and the very act of earning has enabled them to negotiate the disempowering conditions of their sexuality. The practice of abortion by unmarried working girls is thus affected by this specific condition of production and reproduction relations.

It is against this general background that we attempted to understand the practice of abortion among married and unmarried women in a region where the recent transformation of the local economy is drawing more and more women into industrial employment. In the case of married women we focused on how they negotiate 'structural factors', such as the state's policy of population control, the imposition of family-planning methods by medical institutions and patriarchal family relations through their personal 'choice' of abortion. In other words, this study analyses a) how married women negotiate and rework their 'reproductive interest'[6] through abortion; and b) what reasons other than birth spacing they advance for having abortions (e.g., women might link their abortion to childcare responsibility, son preference, marital violence, conditions of work, etc.). Simultaneously, by retrieving women's own perspectives and reasons for abortion, we tried to identify and understand the social and cultural conditions and values that facilitate and/or constrain women's choice of abortion.

In the case of unmarried women, especially young working girls, we explored how specific production relations that deny women labour rights and economic security produce the material bases for exercising (or not) their reproductive rights.[7] More specifically, we examined how unmarried young women's location in production mediates their relations of reproduction. While women's location in production helped us to explore structural factors, their action in the domain of reproduction gave us an understanding of 'personal' factors and their interconnectedness with 'structural' factors.

The Setting

The study was carried out in four villages in Kancheepuram district, which adjoins as well as forms part of the Chennai city agglomeration. The region is being swiftly transformed from an agrarian into an industrial economy, changing the occupational profile of its population.[8] In 1985, an industrial estate meant exclusively for small- and medium-scale pharmaceutical units was started in this region and about 50 production units, employing about 3,000 women workers from neighbouring villages, were established. In addition, export-oriented garment and leather units have also been set up along with software and chemical units, which absorb a rising proportion of unskilled workers. A significant aspect of pharmaceutical units is their recruitment of large numbers of young unmarried women, many of whom are employed as daily or contract labourers on a temporary basis. They receive a very low wage, ranging from Rs 21 to Rs 35 a day, without any other benefits, not even a medical allowance.

This area was chosen because of the high reported incidence of abortion among young women. A recent study (1996–97) of women's health in two blocks of the region indicated that out of 4,507 married women surveyed, 67 per cent had undergone induced abortions in hospitals, 19 per cent had undergone induced abortions through indigenous methods, 10 per cent had used 'injection' and 4 per cent had taken oral tablets.[9] Apparently, the incidence of unmarried young women accessing abortion facilities in private clinics is increasing, although data for this are not easily available.

Research Design and Methodology

Since our research involved mapping women's perceptions and their experience of abortion, we adopted a qualitative survey method. The field researchers were trained in different types of qualitative research, caste, gender and production relations in the study villages, issues of abortion and the need to obtain the informed consent of women participating in the study. A local ethics committee was formed consisting of senior researchers and academics working on reproductive health issues and experts trained in carrying out field surveys.

Since the primary focus of our research was women who work in pharmaceutical companies, we approached about 23 pharmaceutical units located in the industrial estate for a list of women working in their units, along with some details about their age, salary and the village(s) to which they belonged. But because of the 'unorganised' nature of these industries, which employ men and women mostly as contract or daily wage labourers, it was easy for many of them to deny us access to such information on the grounds that they did not maintain records for temporary employees. Even among those who did provide us with the requisite names, some furnished faulty information about salaries and so on, as they were apprehensive about our motives for wanting a workers' list.

We therefore informally interviewed the secretary of the Pharma association, who provided us with information about the villages from where a large number of women came to work in different companies on the industrial estate. Based on this, we selected four villages, which were located within 6 kms from the estate. We enumerated a total of 1,789 households with a 9,566 population of which 47 per cent were Dalits. Within each village, we selected only Dalit women as participants, not only because of their dominance in these villages but also because the Dalit women comprised the largest group employed by the companies.

Abortion is a sensitive issue that is even now shrouded in secrecy, especially among unmarried young girls. We therefore decided to obtain first-level information—from different groups of women who interact closely with women living in our study area about women who had undergone abortion and the possible reasons for its increasing rate, especially in these villages. We began by contacting the village health nurses (VHNs) for the four study villages to obtain information about a) the role that they play in these villages and their perceptions about abortion and family planning, and b) women's reproductive practices in their area of work. Our next batch of key informants comprised elected women representatives from the local panchayats. They introduced the researchers to the birth attendants in each of the four villages, from whom we gathered information about private clinics and unregistered doctors who provide abortion services to unmarried women.

With the help of ward members, we were able to prepare a population profile for each of the four villages, as well as a list of women who work in different pharmaceutical companies, along with details such as their age, marital status, family background and salary scale.

We used two qualitative survey methods to collect data:

Focus Group Discussions (FGDs)

FGDs were organised in all four villages, among women of varying age groups, to determine the differences in their views on abortion. Two FGDs were held in each village, with elderly women aged between 45 and 65 and with middle-aged women in the 25–45 age group. We were able to hold FGDs (one per village) with unmarried young women (those who work for pharmaceutical companies and are between 17 and 22 years old) in only two villages.[10] Each FGD had six to eight participants.

The discussions with elderly women, most of whom were married (though some were widows), centred around their experience and knowledge of abortion and the changes that had come about in the practice of reproductive control, particularly those that they had witnessed after women began to work in pharmaceutical companies. We also spoke about issues like decision-making within the family *vis à vis* fertility regulation and women's control over the family economy.

Our discussions with middle-aged married women focused on their perceptions of the linkage between women's work and fertility control, mainly their reading of the changes that had occurred in women's work and reproductive practices. Our talks centred around their perceptions of practice of abortion, myths relating to abortion, the methods used, sex selection and their knowledge of family-planning methods. We also discussed how, apart from their own families, different agencies, such as hospitals, the pharmaceutical companies and village panchayats, intervened in and regulated their reproductive practices.

The FGDs with unmarried girls working in pharmaceutical companies focused on the conditions and nature of their work and their experience of it, their roles and responsibilities, their roles in decision-making within the family and their views on female sexuality and reproductive health. While abortion was also included in the discussions, researchers consciously avoided talking about individual experiences of abortion.

In-depth Interviews

Three categories of in-depth interviews were conducted: one, with married and unmarried young women in the 16–30 age group who were working in pharmaceutical companies and had not undergone abortion; with married women who had undergone abortion and among whom some were working in the companies; and three, with young women who were now married but had undergone pre-marital abortion (this group of women were identified through FGDs with older and middle-aged married women and also through our key informants).

The fourth category of in-depth interviews, which were informal and unstructured, was conducted with key informants, such as service providers. These included three registered and two unregistered private doctors, the VHNs working in the four study villages, birth attendants in two of the study villages, women panchayat leaders and women's *sangam* activists. The doctors were our main source for information on the status of abortion practice, especially among working young girls who are unmarried, and the changes these doctors had observed in the lives of those women, particularly in respect to their attitudes towards abortion. The VHNs, birth attendants and women panchayat leaders provided us with detailed information about the sexual relations of young unmarried girls and the abortion practices in the villages where they work.

Table 3.1: Sample survey

FGDs	In-depth interviews				
Elderly, middle-aged and unmarried (FGDs 10 × 6 = 60)	key informants	Unmarried working women	Married working women	Married non-working women	Married abortion cases
60	15	50	20	20	10

Ethical Concerns

Given the sensitive nature of our research, we informed the study participants of the aims and objectives of the research and sought their informed consent after assuring confidentiality and apprising them for their right to decide whether or not they wished to participate in interviews and discussions. However, we could only obtain their oral consent, as participants were unwilling to give anything in writing.

Utmost care has been exercised to retain the women's voices and views, although for the sake of preserving confidentiality, we have withheld the names of the women and of the villages.

Admitedly, it was not possible to conduct interviews of unmarried young girls on their experience of abortion, because of the social stigma and dishonour attached to premarital sexual relationships. We therefore had to base our analysis of their sexuality and abortion practices on the observations/perceptions provided to us by other women.

The next two sections present an analysis of our findings. The first deals with the views expressed by three generations of married women on sexuality, fertility control and abortion. It details the changes that have occurred in people's perception of abortion, and analyses how women negotiate certain social and cultural values and constitute their agency *vis à vis* abortion.

The second section deals mainly with unmarried working women and abortion. While the first part of this section maps out in detail the conditions of work and production relations in the pharmaceutical companies, which forms the context for the analysis of abortion practices among unmarried working women, the second traces the link between women's work in the companies and the practice of abortion by young unmarried girls, through an analysis of different narratives of their sexuality and experience of abortion.

Three Generations of Married Women

As stated earlier, in this section we focus on how married women negotiate certain social and cultural conditions to constitute their own agency in abortion. We also discuss in detail women's changing perceptions with regard to abortion and sexuality; how women arrive at the decision of abortion; and in what way *that process* exemplifies women's sense of reproductive entitlement.

Sexuality, Shame and Abortion

While discussing their experience and perception of abortion, younger women in the study villages unanimously agreed that even before legislation, abortion was as widely practised as it is now. They also remarked that in those days, despite the fact that abortion was illegal, women did not feel guilty or sad about aborting the foetus since doing so was not considered a sin. What is different now is the manner in which abortion is linked to the question of female sexuality, honour and shame. Earlier, it had hardly anything to do with the public notion of limiting family size. According to these women, birth control had more to do with individual women's desire to do away with childcare responsibilities since they were already burdened with domestic chores as well as outside work. Abortion in such cases was not related to informed notions of family size, since a large family with many children was considered to be a credit to the women. Narrating her experience, a 65-year-old woman stated:

> In those days, it was not considered a shame to have many children. It was a shame only if you had an abortion. Unlike childbirth, pregnancy was always associated with female sexual desire. Having an abortion meant that a woman was exposing her sexual activities and was bound to be condemned for it. So, we were scared of abortion not for health reasons but for public condemnation of our sexuality. It is only for this reason that we had to keep it a secret. Nowadays, it is a shame only if you have many children. Abortion is no longer shameful.

Echoing the same sentiment, another elderly woman said that in her time secrecy had nothing to do with abortion but everything to do with sexuality. According to her, it was honour and shame that influenced their decision to abort. In this context, the method chosen was usually indicative of the woman's social status and the degree of her desperation to get rid of the foetus.

> My aunt had 11 children and she aborted twice using the normal method which most married women of those days used. They mixed black cumin seed powder with palm sugar and rolled it into a ball. They would take this everyday until the foetus dissolved or came out. Nobody felt guilty about getting rid of the foetus and women were healthy and normal after the abortion. But some preparations of abortion medicines claimed the lives of women. In our village, a widow who conceived felt ashamed about it and she prepared a spurious pickle containing *chitramoolam* roots and shards of glass. When she consumed this mixture, the glass pierced her intestine and killed her.

Even the second generation of (middle-aged) women, though exposed to the state's family-planning propaganda, did not consider abortion as a method of contraception or spacing. Frequent childbirth was not yet considered a burden or an impediment to the standard of living. But frequent pregnancies—especially during the later stage of married life—were still considered an expression of female sexual desire and therefore a matter of shame and dishonour for the woman concerned. The following narration by a forty-five-year-old pregnant woman illustrates how women's status within the family defined women's 'choice' and need for abortion:

> I have not had a family-planning operation. I delivered five children and after every delivery the doctor would advise me to have the operation. But I never went for it. It is only now that I feel ashamed about being continuously pregnant because my husband's first wife's daughter is also pregnant and she already has another child. Instead of being a grandmother, I am still delivering babies along with her. I tried to abort twice but I did not go to the hospital. I tried all the local methods: ate papaya and drank *gingili* water. Nothing happened. Then I took an injection from a local doctor. By then it was too late. People make fun of me and say that I have too much sexual desire. It is embarrassing for me. That is why I went for abortion. I do not mind having children. What harm have they done?

In contrast, the younger generation of married women seem to be using abortion as a spacing method, not only because the state has popularised it but also because of the change that has come about in the associated notions of shame and honour, partly due to the state's agenda of population control. For the younger generation, it is not frequent pregnancy that is an expression of excessive female desire, but frequent childbirth alone, especially during the later stages of women's lives, which is considered shameful. Today, therefore, a married woman can talk openly about her frequent pregnancies and her desire to abort for the sake of a limited family without feeling ashamed of her sexuality. Loss of honour is now associated with an early marriage and with limited but successive childbirths (even if there are frequent pregnancies, the use of abortion as a spacing method is considered normal) immediately after the marriage. No doubt, the availability of abortion services along with sterilisation in hospitals has enabled women to assimilate the family-planning logic into what they consider as reasons for seeking abortion. However, even within this logic of fertility control, how women reason out their choice for abortion, and what other factors are involved in this decision, are important issues that we explore in the following sections.

Beliefs, Myths and Abortion

Women's decision to abort is often a process of accommodating the pressures of cultural values and beliefs. Therefore, abortion as a felt need grows out of prevailing cultural constraints as a means to negotiate social reality. For instance, in the study villages, almost all the women were very clear that induced abortion is inevitable if a woman conceives in the Tamil month of *Adi*, which is considered bad for the mother as well as for the maternal uncle of the child. If they conceive in this month, young married women opt for abortion even if it is their first conception. This belief in the ill effects of having sex and conceiving in the month of Adi is quite prevalent in Tamil Nadu.

Consulting the local priest (*samiyar*) or persons who are 'possessed' seems to be quite a normal practice among women in the study villages. Women take the risk of aborting the foetus in the second trimester or even later if the priest warns them about a possible threat from the newborn child to the family men. A 21-year-old married woman told us about how, following the advice of a priest, she was forced to abort:

> When my first child was just one and a half months old and I was still breastfeeding him, I conceived again. I wanted to abort the second child and tried to do so with the help of some tablets purchased from a chemist. When this did not work, I gave up. At that time my husband and my mother-in-law were against the abortion. So I did not tell them about my efforts to get rid of the foetus. During the seventh month of pregnancy, I developed high blood pressure. My husband and my mother-in-law took me to the local priest who advised me to abort the baby immediately. He felt that baby was possessed by a ghost and that it could harm the male members of the family. So my husband insisted on the abortion. You might not believe this, but the abortion took place automatically. When we reached the hospital the baby was found dead in the womb.

Similarly, women go back on their decision to abort because they have been advised to do so by a 'possessed' person, especially if the latter predicts that the child is of the male sex. As a 25-year-old woman told us:

> When I conceived my third child, I did not want to have it. So I went to a local doctor and got some tablets for abortion. I consumed

> a lot of them. In the meanwhile, I also approached a woman in the village who was said to be possessed (*sami adi*) and asked her what I should do about the child. As you know, we respect the words of possessed persons as they voice God's opinion. The 'god' told me that I should not abort the child since it was male. That very day I stopped taking abortion tablets. I did deliver a male child.

Son Preference

Like elsewhere in the country, preference for male children and therefore sex-selective abortions are quite common in the study villages. Yet the women here do not avail of the new technology to detect the sex of the foetus.[11] Instead, they prefer to rely on local methods, which are largely myth-based. For instance, women in all study villages stated that they always looked for circular marks on their girl child's bottom (one near the anus and one above that). If there are two circles, then the next child is bound to be a girl! Even though some women admitted that their own experience had proved the belief to be false, most seemed to be guided by it when taking the decision to abort. Doctors in private clinics confirmed the existence of this local belief and its role in abortion. For instance, a doctor from a popular abortion clinic informed us that most of her clients asked for abortion based on their observation of circular marks on the girl child.

> Most women who seek abortion complain to me about the problem of having girl children frequently. They do not want a girl child, especially if the first one is already a girl. Usually they guess the sex of the second child by looking at the girl child's bottom. If she has more than one circle or curve, then the second child is bound to be a female. I do believe in it. It is only in a few instances that this belief has failed.

In many cases, son preference has been the deciding factor for abortion. Women prefer to undergo sterilisation only after a male child is born. If there is already a male child, they do not hesitate to abort the second child even if its sex has been 'predicted' as male. This is especially the case if the first one is still at the nursing stage. As many of the women informed us, it is to provide special care and attention to the first male child that they opt for abortion.[12]

Decision-making

Respondents listed domestic violence related to alcoholism and suspicion about female sexuality as the most common reasons for their opting to abort. In other words, married women often perceive abortion as a means to negotiate domestic violence. For instance, a 35-year-old married woman stated:

> My husband is a drunkard and does not bring any money home. He only loves to sleep with me (have sex). After I conceive, he ignores me or physically abuses me. Or he pretends to be concentrating on some work. When the child is born, he denies paternity by saying that he is not the 'real' father. Since I have experienced all this twice, I decided to go for an abortion. There is no other way I could have handled the situation. In any case, when they [the children] are born I have to provide them with food while he goes around disclaiming his fatherhood.

Similarly, a 38-year-old woman told us how happy and relaxed she felt after aborting her fourth pregnancy:

> When I conceived again after three girl children, I was afraid that this one might also be a girl. Even that did not bother me as much as my husband's obscene remarks about my sexuality. For this reason, every time I got pregnant I tried to commit suicide. This time I decided to abort the foetus. But the doctor advised me against an abortion, as it was too late to have it. So I threatened the doctor, saying that I would commit suicide right inside the hospital if she did not perform the abortion. Only then did she agree to abort the foetus, which turned out to be a male child. Still, I was happy with the abortion, as this time my husband could not suspect the child and me.

As we can see from these narrations, while the act of abortion does reflect women's self-determination to deal with specific oppressive conditions, it does not necessarily indicate women's freedom of choice. In the study villages, the onus for childcare and supporting the family is often exclusively on the women and abortion is one way to cope with the situation. The choice to abort is also related to their perception that sterilisation weakens the body whereas abortion does not lead to any health problems.

A 29-year-old married woman stated that she consciously made the decision to abort twice because she is the main earner in the family:

> I have been working in the company for the past 13 years. My husband is a coolie with no regular income. After the first two children, I have had two abortions. Only three years back, along with the second abortion, I had the family-planning operation. I did not feel bad about having abortions and there has been no health problem after that. I took about a week's rest after the abortions and got back to work. There is no one to take care of the children at home but if I do not work, my family will starve.

Thus it is clear that women without power exercise their choice to abort only under restrictive social and material conditions. However, though opting for abortion rather than sterilisation seems to be a conscious choice that women make, this choice is entangled with several other issues that need further exploration. For example, while they choose abortion as a method of fertility control, they seem to resist the idea of 'family planning'.[13]

Despite the availability of good abortion facilities in the government hospitals, women seem reluctant to use them, mainly because of the aggressive attitude of the medical personnel working there. Explaining why she chose to have her abortion in a private clinic, a 25-year-old woman stated:

> I went to a private clinic for the abortion of my second pregnancy. They charged me Rs 1,000. I refused to go to the government hospital because there too they demand this much money through various means. They force us to have sterilisation or use some contraceptives after the abortion. Only if we agree to this do they consent to perform the abortion. Many women do not go there precisely because of these reasons.

Women in all the study villages consistently and vehemently argued against going to abortion facilities at government hospitals. Not only were they against making the availability of abortion services contingent on sterilisation, they also strongly resented the disrespectful, inhuman and abusive treatment meted out to them by the medical personnel, whom they accused of being caste- and gender-biased. Voicing concern about the abusive treatment women receive in government hospitals, a 36-year-old woman remarked:

> When we go to the hospital for delivery, we are not allowed to express our pain. The doctors not only scold us but also pass rude remarks about our body and about our pregnancy. They shout at us, saying, 'You could enjoy sex and not feel the pain of penetration but come here and scream about pain.' If we ask for abortion, they say things like: 'You can lift your legs for your husband (i.e., you enjoy sex) without saying no and now you want an abortion.'

The women's narratives clearly and quite eloquently establish not only the alienating and insensitive nature of the medical services available, but also the women's awareness of their reproductive entitlements, such as their right to abortion without the imposition of any conditions or abuse of their sexuality. However, the desire to have non-coercive, humane medical services does not mean that women totally boycott government hospitals that force them into 'family planning'. In fact, many young married women, who cannot afford costly private clinics, continue to use the abortion facilities offered by government hospitals.

So far, the burden of our argument has been that, despite the state's promotion of abortion as a method of family limitation, women have not just 'substituted' it for contraception but have consciously sought abortion for various other reasons. Women's decision to abort seems to be linked to various factors like responsibility for childcare, marital conflicts, son preference, astrological beliefs, and resistance to the sexual morality imposed upon them by the medical world. 'Choosing' abortion is thus a way of negotiating with these factors. Though the logic of family limitation through abortion, as promoted by the state's population policy, might also play some role, how women arrive at the decision to abort is based less on received notions of family planning or birth control than on the social and cultural conditions/relations that define their lives.

Women, Work and Abortion

In order to understand how a particular form of production relation and its associated work culture produces a specific socialisation process among working women, especially young unmarried girls, it is necessary to map the production process, the work culture and conditions of work that operate in the pharmaceutical companies *as perceived by women themselves*. This is important, because the relation between women's work and women's sense of 'reproductive entitlement' is exceedingly complex.[14] In other words, we analyse how the social relations of reproduction of young unmarried women are shaped by the culture and conditions of their work and how women who work in pharmaceutical companies negotiate the harsh realities of work through their relations of reproduction, which include their practice of abortion.

Women as Workers

As noted earlier, pharmaceutical companies recruit young unmarried girls in large numbers, along with a few young married women. They are mostly employed as contract labourers. Some companies recruit only unmarried young girls, who are dismissed as soon as they get married. Explaining why they recruit only unmarried girls, the secretary of the pharmaceutical companies association said:

> Only young unmarried girls without any family responsibilities can spend so many hours at the company. Young women are physically better fit for arduous work. They lose their physical strength and energy once they get married and have children. We cannot afford to give them maternity or sick leave. Moreover, what we care about is efficiency and concentration at work, for which we train them. In any case, they are like machines, with little brains. So if you mould them at a young age, they become as efficient as machines and work for as many hours as we want them to work.

The observation of a 22-year-old woman worker about how women are perceived within these companies corroborates the secretary's comments: 'Our company prefers only unmarried girls and makes them work like machines. In fact, women workers are often referred to as machines....we are not allowed to talk to each other and are expected to work like machines from morning to evening.' Commenting on the company's demand for unmarried women, a 20-year-old woman said: 'Today a boy and his parents had come to fix a marriage alliance with me, but I refused as I will be dismissed from work the moment I get married. Then who will look after my family?'

The few men in these units are employed as supervisors, chemists or machine operators. The companies seem to deliberately avoid recruiting men from nearby villages, as they do not want to risk any collective opposition or protest against their work culture. For instance, a 60-year-old woman noted:

> There is not a single man from this village recruited for company work. They are afraid if the men come to know of how the girls are exploited, they might mobilise the entire village to uproot the companies from here. That is why you see the young fellows here, though quite well educated and willing to work in the companies, roaming the streets without any jobs.

Almost all the companies recruit girls from the age of thirteen and they are made to work from 8.30 a. m. to 5.30 p. m., with just a half-hour break for lunch. The salary is paid either as a daily wage ranging from Rs 18 to Rs 30, or as a monthly wage of up to Rs 1,500. Overtime work, which is usually an extra two to three hours, fetches the girls an additional Rs 2 to Rs 4 per hour, though some units pay an hourly rate of upto Rs 10. Since many of the girls have to commute to work, the companies deduct van and tea charges from their salaries, which leaves them with only Rs 600 to Rs 800 per month. In order to save the money that would be spent on commuting, many girls, even from far-off villages, prefer to walk to work. Given their poor economic condition due to the non-availability of agricultural work or other forms of employment for the men in the family, most parents take their daughters out from school and send them to work in these companies despite the meagre salaries they receive.

The units are very strict about timings and if workers are late even by a few minutes, the day's salary is cut. Most companies do not give their workers medical coverage, despite the fact that the working conditions in these units place the workers in close proximity to various chemical-related health hazards. As a 28-year-old married working woman noted:

> They [the companies] do not bother to give us medical allowance or to meet our medical expenses. Three months ago, a young girl

> in our company met with an accident while operating a machine. It was a major accident—her hand got caught in the machine and was mutilated. Her medical expenses amounted to something like Rs 5,000, but they paid her just one month's salary and, instead of giving her medical leave or even leave without pay, they dismissed her, stating that she could no longer work with a maimed hand.

Very few companies offer an annual bonus; in fact, in most companies contract workers are denied a bonus. The usual tactic used is to dismiss them just before the bonus is given. Some companies routinely offer workers six-month contracts, which are then renewed after a break in order to avoid making the jobs permanent.

The companies seem to follow an arbitrary employment policy, offering permanent jobs and other benefits to some but denying them to others, even if they have been working in the company for many years. A 28-year-old married woman commented:

> I have been working in this particular company for the past eight years and before this I worked in another company for two and a half years. I am doing all the work that they require me to do: right from bottle washing to lifting heavy cartons. But they have not made me permanent, nor have they made any provision for a PF [Provided Fund]. But a girl who is known to be having an affair with a supervisor has been made permanent despite the fact that her fingers got twisted in the lab and she is hardly able to do any work.

Even having a permanent status does not empower the girls to bargain for a better salary, better working conditions or even medical benefits. It merely ensures job continuity. As a 34-year-old permanent employee of one of the companies stated:

> In this company even those who are permanent employees do not raise the issue of low salaries, although they participate in meetings with the employers. In these meetings, only issues relating to increase in production, efficiency of the labourers and how to meet the competition from other companies are talked about. There is never a word about labour welfare or any discussion about workers' benefits.

The Production Process

Women workers in pharmaceutical companies are engaged in a variety of work, which can be broadly identified as batch taking, mixing, liquid or powder filling, blister packing, strip packing, bottle washing and packing, fixing of labels, and loading and stacking medicine-filled cartons.[15] Jobs like mixing the ingredients specified by chemists for the preparation of drugs, sieving the powder as well as broken pieces of capsules and tablets, filling them into or packing them as strips, filling liquids into bottles and bottle washing are all done exclusively by women workers. As soon as they enter the company, the supervisors divide them into various groups and allot each group specific tasks for the day. Each worker in the group has to complete the target set for her, otherwise she loses her job.

Usually, illiterate women workers and new entrants are assigned with washing bottles, which is a very demanding and backbreaking job. A 17-year-old girl, who has now left the company, described it thus:

> When my cousin and I joined this company, we were given the job of washing bottles. It was only later on, after looking at my educational qualifications, that they shifted me to another section. Bottle washing is a horrible job. We have to lift thousands of bottles in a sack, carry them to the wash area without breaking them and then wash them all. It takes the entire day and sometimes even more than the usual working hours to wash, dry and dump them in the packing section. My cousin used to complain of itching and blisters on her hand and I myself once sustained a serious injury due to a broken glass bottle. Other women in our section used to complain of continuous backaches since we had to crouch on the floor for long hours.

Other women complained about the unreasonable targets set for filling bottles with tablets or liquids and for packing the filled bottles in boxes. They also complained about how they have to keep pace with the machines, especially in the packaging section. However, most women regard these jobs as considerably less demanding when compared to the lifting and loading of heavy boxes, which also has targets.

We can gauge the nature of work in these companies from the description given by an 18-year-old girl:

> I do jobs like sticking labels, and packing, lifting and loading heavy cartons. Only women do these jobs. The men are there, but they do not lift weights. We also have to load and unload sacks of sugar and other heavy boxes from the van. They weigh at least 100 kg each, and four women are needed to lift one box. So many of them have to be loaded and unloaded per day…. They have a target for each day. If we cannot meet the target, they abuse us saying: 'You do not have any brain, you are useless', etc. Even the liquid tank has to be cleaned only by women. If we do not wash that properly, they ask us if we are eating shit or food and make us wash it repeatedly. The men only run the machines. If there is no machine work to be done, they sit around and chat and laugh. Nobody questions them or controls them. Only we are scolded for everything. Women suffer so much in these companies.

Conditions of Work: Regulating Female Sexuality

It is not just the targets, heavy workload and health hazards that swamp the women workers. Any lapse on their part leads not only to dismissal but also to physical and sexual abuse, especially of young unmarried girls, by male supervisors and chemists. Describing the attitude of the supervisors, a 17-year-old girl said:

> The supervisors always dominate us. We are not supposed to question them. We are not allowed to rest but have to work continuously, without any break and without showing our tiredness. If we are slow or if we appear to be sluggish, they abuse us, using terms like 'street dogs', 'lazy bums', 'wasteland' or 'dirty pigs'; sometimes they ask us if we are eating food or shit. They always address us as 'brainless ones', 'machines' and 'lazy bums'. Earlier, when we made even a minor error, they hit us on our heads. This has stopped now, as it led to some women being seriously injured.

The power that chemists and supervisors wield invariably expresses itself in the sexual abuse of young unmarried girls and in regulating female sexuality in general. While narrating her encounters with chemists and supervisors, a 27-year-old married woman noted:

We have never seen the owner or the director of the company. Only the chemists scold us and order us around every time we are a little slow with our work. I have often had altercations with the supervisors as they abuse us in bad language. I was bold enough to question them. There was one supervisor who used to misbehave with the girls and even sexually abuse them. I objected to his behaviour, as did many other girls. When the management finally learned of our objections, they removed him from the job. Not that they were concerned about us. They felt he was disruptive and that the girls could not work because of him.

For many young unmarried girls, fulfilling the sexual demands of supervisors and chemists seems to be the only way of escaping physical and verbal abuse and easing their harsh working conditions. A 23-year-old unmarried girl described how the supervisors in her company favour young unmarried girls who give in to their sexual demands:

They [the supervisors] do not value work experience. Even new recruits, if able to entice the supervisor, get paid well without having to do much work, because it is he who decides the quantity and quality of work that each worker has to put in. No one, including the manager, questions the authority of the supervisor.... One supervisor of our company only employs girls who attract him and he is well known for dismissing those who do not fulfill his desires. We are afraid of him. Only the married women have the guts to stand up to him. This is the reason why I am losing interest in the work.

Similarly, another 37-year-old woman talked about how sexual exploitation by supervisors is rampant in her company and what it has done to women workers:

In our company, a young supervisor has a sexual relationship with an elder woman and so overlooks the mistakes she makes. Now he has given employment to her daughter. This lady goes to the extent of purchasing vegetables, etc., for him from her salary. All the supervisors in this company are like that; there is no exception. Another girl in our company was seduced and raped by a supervisor. But she was under the illusion that he would marry her. He refused and

> even denied having sexual relations with her. She had to undergo an abortion and she is very sick. Now she refuses to marry anybody and has also left the job.

The power and authority vested in the supervisors is such that, even in cases of rape and sexual exploitation that come to the notice of the management, it is the girls and not the perpetrators who are punished and risk losing their jobs if the issue becomes public knowledge.

It is not only sexual exploitation by supervisors that affects young women workers, but also the rules and norms set by the companies to regulate female sexuality. One such rule, in almost all the companies, is that no woman worker is allowed to talk to any male worker other than the male supervisors. They are assigned the duty of monitoring the behaviour of women workers, especially the young unmarried ones. If they are found in violation of this rule, they are immediately dismissed. As is evident even from the earlier narrations, the supervisors enjoy enormous powers and can easily manipulate the rules in their favour. This account by a woman worker gives us a sense of how these rules are misused by the supervisors:

> In our company, a fellow male worker jokingly pulled a girl's coat to ask her to wash the tray. They know each other but there is no love affair between them. On seeing this, the supervisor informed the manager, who dismissed both of them from work. They tell us that male-female relationships always lead to wrongdoings. They have even displayed this rule on a board that has been placed at the entrance of the industry. Since the companies view male-female relationships as causing unnecessary interference in work, monitoring young girls' behaviour with men has become as essential as monitoring their efficiency at work.

Speaking about her company, a 20-year-old unmarried worker said:

> There is a general rule in the company that women and men should not talk to each other. There are three supervisors just to monitor our behaviour. Even in the extreme situation of an accident, fellow workers are not allowed to talk to each other. They are very strict about love affairs between workers. If they get to know about any, they dismiss the woman worker at once. If there is a love marriage

> between the workers, they allow the boy to continue working but dismiss the girl. At the time of recruitment, they always advise us against love affairs. If some workers share a friendship, they deliberately separate them by placing them in different work groups.

Some companies also regulate the clothes that women workers wear. Further, they monitor their social activity, even that which occurs outside the company. In addition to regulating the social life of their workers, some companies strictly prohibit the entry of married women into their workforce. Those that do employ married women dismiss them as soon they come to know that they are pregnant. In this context, it is important to analyse how women workers, especially the young unmarried ones, negotiate these conditions at work. For it is in resisting and negotiating the work conditions that unmarried women workers seem have exercised their 'choice' in reproductive control.

Negotiating Work and Sexuality

For many young unmarried women, there is no escape from the harsh working conditions. Often, they are the sole breadwinners. They cannot, therefore, afford to leave their jobs. Instead they are compelled to negotiate the conditions of their place of work. The following narration by an 18-year-old girl sums up the dilemma and tensions that unmarried girls share about the workplace and earning their livelihood:

> Only we are scolded for everything. Women suffer so much in these companies. The money they give us [Rs 600] is not enough even for our daily meals. I give the entire amount to my mother and she takes care of our needs. We have no option, so we work in these wretched companies. I don't like to work in the company but my parents will not let me leave. They scold me if I do not go there. If I go there, the supervisors scold me for little things. I cannot escape this daily ordeal. If you were not sitting with me to chat, I would be made to fetch water and do household work too. My sister, who goes to school, is not allowed to do any household work. I am burdened with company work and household work. I cannot rest after a long day's work. I do not like either of the places.

> My parents are not arranging my marriage, as there is no money. I do not know what I am going to do.

On the other hand, some young girls felt that working in the company enables them to escape household work and also the family's control over their mobility. For instance, a 17-year-old girl said:

> We do not feel so great working in the company. But the company is better because unlike our mothers we do not have to toil under the sun. Besides I like going out to work because I can dress up well. If I were at home I would not have been allowed to dress up like this.

However, most of them felt that the rules set by the companies favour only the supervisors and work against the interest of the workers. The reaction of an 18-year-old girl illustrates their desire for breaking the rules:

> We slog in the company like cattle and they treat us like machines. Why should only the supervisors have fun? We are not asking for any facilities or allowances. But why should we not be allowed to socialise with our fellow workers?

Many of them find ways to violate some of these rules. A woman worker said that since her company is very strict about male-female socialisation within the workplace, the girls speak to the men through masks, which are given to them as protective gear. The supervisors cannot make out whether they are speaking to each other or to the men. The women also use sign language to communicate and, during lunchtime, tease each other about their affairs. A 17-year-old mentioned that since her company employs only unmarried girls, those working with her have lovers but do not get married to them immediately as they are likely to lose their jobs after marriage. A twenty-eight-year-old married woman commented on how unmarried girls utilise the few minutes of break from work:

> A major pastime of unmarried girls in the company is to talk about love affairs. The ten-minute break we get for tea is spent by them talking about their partners. They even forego their tea for the sake of chatting. Only married women like us drink tea.

Narrating how unmarried girls violate company norms, a middle-aged woman observed:

> When I worked in the company, many young girls used to have love affairs. The company people did not get to know of this, as the girls would deliberately choose to form relationships only with men from other companies. They would spend time with each other on the way to work and while returning home. Some of them got married, but most of them were deserted.

Even married women violate the rules and norms that regulate their sexuality. For instance, a young married woman told us how, in order to get work for a few months, she violated the company norms:

> When I sought a job in one of these companies, I did not reveal that I was married, or that I was pregnant. My husband also worked in the same company but they did not know about this. Co-workers always help each other in these matters. Be it a love affair or pregnancy, they will not talk about it to the managers or supervisors. Since they gave me an apron and a thick coat, I was able hide my bulging stomach. Even though we girls know how strict the management is about marriage and pregnancy, we constantly defy these rules. Otherwise we won't be able to earn. Of course, despite our condition, we had to lift heavy weights and do all the jobs required of us. If we didn't, we would lose the job.

As we can see, such secrecy resorted to by married/pregnant women involves health risks, but it is the only way they can get around the rigid demands of the company. In addition to breaking rules relating to socialisation, many young girls seem to negotiate the burden of their work by allowing themselves to be sexually exploited.[16] Explaining how this takes place, an 18-year-old girl stated:

> All this does not take place inside the company as they are very strict about rules and we can't even talk to the men. But the girls and supervisors or chemists fix their meetings elsewhere and even stay out. We know of many such cases. All of them don't get married. In fact, we know of no instance where a marriage has taken place between a supervisor and any girl who works there. Abortion is bound to take place. We know about it. What else can we do?

> Not that all girls do this sort of thing. Supervisors are the main culprits and they should be blamed for all this.

Even though the majority of women feel that supervisors sexually exploit unmarried women, some think that working girls negotiate their unequal relationship in the workplace through sexual involvement with supervisors and managers and it is they who use private clinics for abortions. Narrating the case of a young girl who had recently had an abortion, a 19-year-old fellow worker from the same village observed:

> She comes from a poor family who is dependent on her salary. She is involved with a supervisor who is married and has no intention of marrying her. She has had at least two abortions. The benefit that she gets for all this is that she has been made a permanent employee. She has even taken one month's leave, which none of us is allowed to do and she does not put in that much work because of her sexual relationship with the supervisor.

Unmarried Working Women and Abortion

There are two aspects that are clearly discernible in our discussion on women's work and the regulation of their sexuality. One: the unmarried girls both participate in sexual relationships and comply with sexual exploitation by their male superiors in order to negotiate their harsh working conditions. Two: their engagement in sexual relationships is a way of resisting the regulation of their sexuality by the companies and protesting against the increasing restrictions placed upon them by their families. As some of the narratives show, abortion emerges as an important indicator of both these trends (compliance and/or resistance). Their experience of abortion is also mediated by the notions of sexuality that prevail within their families, especially in the context of their enhanced status as wage earners and providers. In this section we will show how the incidence of abortion among unmarried working girls is linked to women's work, social status and sense of sexuality and reproductive control. Since we could not obtain personal narratives from them, our analysis is based on interviews with doctors and women of different age groups.

Almost all those we interviewed, including the working women, said that there has been an increase in the rate of abortion among unmarried girls after they started working for the companies.[17] According to two doctors from private clinics located at a 5-km. distance from the companies, about six to seven unmarried working girls, employed mainly in the pharmaceutical companies, seek abortion services in their clinics every month.[18] As a doctor reported:

> I started this clinic nine years ago and from then I have seen an increase in the number of unmarried girls coming for abortion. Mainly, it is the girls working in the pharmaceutical companies who come to me for abortion. They are mostly 17 or 18 years old and come with their mothers or with their friends. Some come with their partners.

Similarly, another doctor in a private clinic reported that the girls who come to her for abortions are mostly between 18 and 22 and an overwhelming number of them are unmarried. She also observed that before the establishment of the companies, there used to be hardly two or three cases of abortion among unmarried girls. This number has now increased to about 10 a month. An unregistered doctor, who is well known for her abortion services and runs a private clinic located at a distance of 15 km. from the companies, noted:

> Earlier, very few unmarried girls, mainly agricultural labourers, used to come to me for abortion after being raped by either the landowners or the upper-caste men of the village. In recent years, however, a lot of young unmarried women—mostly between 18 and 22—employed by the companies have started coming to me for abortion. I don't keep a record of all those who have come here, but I recognise them when they come again.

Older women in these villages have come to recognise abortion among unmarried girls who work in the companies as becoming common and accept it as normal.

Family, Sexuality and the Secrecy of Abortion

As has been pointed out earlier, with a large number of young unmarried girls being pushed to work in the informal industrial sector, combined with the demand for dowry and the lack of employment for young men, new forms of control over female sexuality have emerged within the family. Simultaneously, there has also emerged resistance to these new forms of control—resistance that is visible in the attempts by unmarried working women to regulate their sexuality. In other words, the changing social conditions are also enabling working girls to rework their strategies and their sense of reproductive entitlements within the restrictions imposed by their families and the companies in which they work. During an FGD, an elderly woman said:

> Earlier, the caste panchayat would be called to arbitrate love affairs. They either separated the lovers or ordered their wedding. If a girl became pregnant, she was allowed to deliver the baby and the girl's family looked after both of them until they found a boy for her to marry. There was no taboo attached to those who gave birth to a child before marriage. There was community support even for those who made the mistake. Nowadays, girls are not afraid of their parents. They themselves decide on their marriage. Even if a girl's mother agrees to the wedding, either the brother or the father creates problems. The girl's brother or the uncle keeps vigil over her when she goes out to work, especially if she is travelling by bus. To escape this, the girl goes to some secret place with her lover and, if anything happens, she goes straight to the clinic [for an abortion]. Where is the need for panchayats now? In any case, panchayat decisions are not binding on these people, as the lovers of these girls are from outside the village.

It is not only surveillance by men but also the new social norms that have emerged within Dalit families that force young girls to work out their own strategies to negotiate social norms. In the words of a 20-year-old working girl:

> The girls who go to the company work very hard and at the same time manage to roam around with their boyfriends. At home, they say they are doing overtime work and then go off somewhere else to have fun. Usually, the parents do not know anything about the salary scale. They accept whatever the girl brings home, as they are in need of money. A lot of girls from my village have had abortions and everybody knows about it.

It is evident that poor Dalit families have become dependent on the earnings of young unmarried girls. In a sense, this authorises, if not empowers, these girls to make reproductive decisions. The self-assertion of unmarried girls on reproductive and sexual matters becomes very obvious when we consider how knowledgeable they are about abortion and the decisions they make relating to it. Commenting on how young unmarried girls in her village handle the situation of abortion, a 21-year-old working woman said:

> I have been working in the company for the past three years and I know exactly how the girls deal with issues like abortion. They are very secretive about these things. If we sense something and ask them about it, the girls do not tell the truth but say that have a fever or bodyache or some such illness. They go for an abortion either with their mothers or their partners. After two days, they resume work as though nothing has happened. The girls know everything about abortion and where to get it done. The mothers or partners just accompany them.

In the same vein, a birth attendant from one of the study villages remarked:

> These days, if unmarried girls have any problem with their lovers, the first thing they do is to get an abortion. They don't mind if they have to spend more than what they earn to do this. After all, it is their decision.

Knowledge about pregnancy and where to obtain an abortion is widely prevalent among unmarried girls, but they demonstrate virtually no knowledge about contraception and contraceptive methods. However, we found that, despite their having frequent abortions, they could not describe the methods used for those abortions. Many of them also said that they do not see abortion as a sin or mistake; rather, they consider it to be an inevitable part of sexual relations. The private doctors whom we interviewed corroborated this finding. One of them, who works in a private clinic located very close to the industrial estate, remarked:

> The unmarried girls very rarely come to me for irregular menstruation or other reproductive problems. They know that they are pregnant and very casually ask for an abortion. I have never noticed

inhibition or reluctance in them when they ask for an abortion. It has become a matter-of-fact issue for them.

However, even though unmarried girls now take this reproductive decision themselves, it is a decision that is enmeshed within new forms of social control and values that were hitherto unknown to the Dalit community. For instance, pregnancy and motherhood among unmarried girls is no longer acceptable; instead, family honour, and therefore the need for maintaining secrecy on issues like abortion, has become more important than even the girl's life. The following story illustrates this point:

> Last year, one girl in this village died after trying to abort her foetus. She was going around with a chemist from the company, and conceived. When she was five months' pregnant, he promised to marry her and her family knew about this. But her mother insisted that she abort and forced her to consume some tablets.[19] Perhaps she took an overdose, but it resulted in her death. At the last minute they took her to the Chengalpattu hospital but she died there. The post-mortem revealed a five-month-old foetus. Since she was unmarried, it had become important for her family to abort the foetus in order to save the family's honour. Her sister, who also works in a company, might have found it difficult to get a groom if the sister had delivered the baby.

It is evident from this that unwanted pregnancy or abortion is seen in the context of strengthening patriarchal values about sexuality, despite the changing circumstances related to young girls' positions as sole income earners. New cultural norms and patterns, or the new social relations, have emerged as a result which effectively control female sexuality and ultimately limit the 'choice' and 'free will' of women.

In most cases abortion is a fallout of the failure to contract marriages with 'outsiders'. An 18-year-old working girl contended that abortion has to be kept secret since the girls are not in a position to negotiate prevailing social values and hierarchies. She remarked:

> If a girl becomes pregnant [before marriage], no one questions the partner, since he is from outside the village. Marriage might not be possible with that person because the caste or economic status

> of the boy is different from that of the girl. Often the boy is the boss in the company. So she goes with her parents to an abortion clinic. It is a secret matter. Very few in the village get to know about it.

Since secrecy is important to those who undergo abortions, they have to choose clinics or doctors who will not divulge details about them, particularly to persons who belong to the same community or village. Therefore, despite the exorbitant charges levied by private clinics,[20] girls prefer to use them in order to 'save the family honour'. Some of them explained why they do not avail of government facilities:

> We would never go to a government hospital to have an abortion, where the functionaries misbehave even with married women who need an abortion. The doctors make obscene remarks about women's sexual behaviour. With unmarried women, they take even more liberties and scold and ridicule them. That is why most of us go only to private clinics, where the doctors are more understanding and keep our visit a secret. All we need is money for the abortion. But even to the private doctors, the girls do not provide all the details. Abortion is not a problem. But if the girl happens to marry somebody else, he should not harass her with past events.

We may conclude from the various narrations in this section that women's work in the informal sector, such as in the pharmaceutical industry, might have enhanced their status within the family as main income earners or as providers, but it has not empowered them as decision-makers in the domain of reproduction and sexuality. An unmarried woman's decision to abort does not signify her autonomy or free choice but emerges as an act of 'strategic accommodation'[21] or as a combination of both complicity and resistance.

Conclusion

As we have stated in the section on married women and abortion, other studies have concluded that women use abortion only as a birth-spacing method. In our study villages, however, women across generations seem to reject the idea of abortion as a method of limiting family size. This comes out clearly in their reluctance to use or perceive abortion as a 'family-planning method' and in their avoidance of sterilisation. Instead, women seem to view abortion as their reproductive entitlement: this is made explicit in their perception of abortion as a necessary tool to negotiate domestic violence and other oppressive social conditions. Their refusal to accept the disrespectful and sexually abusive abortion services offered by government hospitals clearly reflects women's assertion of their reproductive interests.

Young unmarried working women use their sense of reproductive entitlement to negotiate harsh working conditions and the increasing control over their sexuality in the workplace and at home. But, as Petchesky and Judd note: 'Having a sense of entitlement may be very distant from the ability to act on it effectively' (Petchesky and Judd 2001: 317). While abortion by unmarried girls might signify subtle sexual and reproductive strategies or even a 'counter-hegemonic morality', it simultaneously also signifies women's lack of control over the oppressive conditions of work and other social realities (*ibid.*).

What is significant about the escalating rate of abortion among unmarried young women is that it coincides with their increasing employment in the industrial sector.[22] The high incidence of abortion among them might appear as a conscious reproductive choice emerging from their role as providers in the family. Unfortunately, it is only a means of negotiating the disempowering conditions of their work and production relations. Abortion among unmarried girls, especially in the context of our study, is largely associated with the increasing visibility of women's sexuality outside the family and their view that the circumstances leading to abortion are not of their own making. It has also got to do with the changed consciousness among young unmarried women about their economic self-sufficiency (the fact that they have abortions in private clinics that are quite expensive) and their association of abortion with normal reproductive conditions. To some extent, the legalisation of abortion, combined with the increasing control of their sexuality, has also contributed to this trend. However, this is not to say that there was no abortion among unmarried women before abortion was made legal. Our claim is that in the past, when their monetary contribution to the family was insignificant and when their mobility was largely limited to just their village, unmarried women were denied the power to negotiate sexuality on their own terms. Besides, there was no stigma attached to unmarried motherhood, which was culturally acceptable.

As Upendra Baxi has argued, the unorganised sector is the 'the constitutive place of violation' that not only denies labour rights but produces the material bases for the denial of reproductive rights (Baxi 2000). It forces women to choose between the latter and the need to earn a livelihood. Given this, we would argue that labour and reproductive interests are mutually inclusive and should form part of labour legislations as well as of reproductive health policies. Therefore, the 'structural factors' that we talked about in the beginning of this chapter need to be taken into account when dealing with reproductive rights. For instance, in the absence of labour rights, such as the right to equal wages, enabling work conditions and the right to unionise—all of which directly impinge on reproductive rights liberal laws that encourage abortion and provide good abortion facilities might undermine women's reproductive rights.[23] This is because, as Baxi has argued, reproductive rights entail, among other things, respect for the right to reproductive self-determination and elimination of discrimination in the conditions of work and in health care (Baxi 2002). Thus, for marginalised poor women to achieve reproductive rights would require changes not merely in the quality and availability of health services but also in the structural conditions and state policies that promote gender-biased economic and social systems.

Notes

1. The Medical Termination of Pregnancy Act, which was passed in 1971, legalised abortion by making abortion services available through registered doctors in government and private clinics. The Act came into force in 1972. For details on how abortion came to be legalised in India, see Jesani and Iyer 1993 and Menon 2002.
2. See Nagaraj 2002 and IIPS 2001.
3. According to the NFHS data for 1992–93, the incidence of abortion in Tamil Nadu was 11.3 per cent and the all-India rate was 5.8 per cent.
4. The same trend could be noticed in 1992–93. As per the NFHS data for this period, spontaneous abortions accounted for 7.0 per cent compared to 4.5 per cent for all of India, while induced abortions in Tamil Nadu stood at 4.3 per cent as against the all-India rate of 1.3 per cent. Although our study has not dealt with the incidence of spontaneous abortion and its implication for women's reproductive rights, the high rate of spontaneous abortions in Tamil Nadu, especially in the age group of 15–19 years (17.5 per cent), point to the fact that abortion has a marked presence in fertility control in the state.

5. For detailed discussions on the increasing control over female sexuality as an effect of women's employment see Anandhi, Jeyaranjan and Krishnan 2002.
6. I have borrowed this term from Upendra Baxi, who explains reproductive interest as one that involves reproductive security, reproductive sexuality, reproductive health, reproductive equality and reproductive decision-making. It could also connote any one of the above. See Baxi 2000.
7. For a general debate on reproductive rights, see Baxi 2000; for the debate on situating abortion in the context of rights, see Menon 2002.
8. For details on the economic transition of the district in general and women's employment in particular, see Jeyaranjan and Swaminathan 2001.
9. Unpublished study carried out by RUWSEC (Rural Women's Social Education Centre).
10. The difficulties in bringing together young unmarried working girls for FGDs were manifold. First, given the nature of their work, which takes up most of their time, they were not available for discussions. Second, even on Sundays, when they were somewhat free, they had to seek their parents' or brothers' permission to come out of their house to chat about issues like sexuality and abortion—issues that unmarried young women are not expected to talk about in public. Third, the precarious nature of their employment made them very apprehensive about openly discussing their work conditions, leave alone issues of sexual exploitation and sexual relations.
11. One may note here that, in Tamil Nadu, unlike in other parts of the country, preference for a male child plays an insignificant role in abortion. The National Family Health Survey (1998–99) indicates that 82 per cent of women who wanted a child said that the sex of the child does not matter and 46 per cent who wanted another child said the same thing. Only 9.6 per cent stated that they wanted more sons than daughters.
12. This is not unique to Tamil Nadu or to the study villages. There are several studies that refer to this phenomenon. For instance, see Ganatra 2000: 201.
13. Women of all three generations across the study villages strongly opposed forced sterilisation and the state's propaganda on family planning. The older women constantly recollected the target era of the 1970s, when their men too had to undergo vasectomies. They also mentioned how that memory of forced family planning has made them oppose even 'voluntary' family planning today. The middle-aged women spoke of the era of incentives, when men and women were not forced, but were lured by material benefits. They therefore viewed family planning as a welfare programme and, apart from being attracted to the incentives it offered, did not consider family limitation as having much importance in their lives. Many of them were also critical of the programme as they felt that incentive-based sterilisation only brought more women under

the fertility-control programme but did not benefit them since the programme was implemented at the cost of women's health. Even the third generation of women, who are voluntarily opting for sterilisation, told us that abortion should not be linked to the idea of 'family planning'. According to them, since they undergo abortion not for family limitation but for other reasons, family planning (*kudumba kattupadu*) means only sterilisation, or what they call 'operation', and not abortion. Across generations, many women stated that sexual abstinence was their most common and frequently used form of contraception.

14. I have borrowed this term from Petchesky, who explains that the sense of entitlement is what women *feel* (emphasis mine) that they are permitted to do or *feel* that they have a right to do within a specific social context of norms and relationships, which are also continuously changing and contested. In reality, this sense of entitlement, as she argues, may remain unrecognised and unfulfilled. See Petchesky and Judd 2001: 13.
15. For details on the nature of work in pharmaceutical companies, see Jeyaranjan and Swaminathan 2001.
16. It may be relevant here to cite Petschcsky's analysis of teenage sexuality. She notes: 'For adolescents, sexuality, pregnancy, and abortion are densely mediated by agendas other than what they appear; they become the terrain for negotiating gender, child and adulthood, and gender-specific class and race' (Petschcsky 1986: 207).
17. For details on different methods used for termination of pregnancy among unmarried girls, see Ganatra 2000.
18. The increasing number of abortion seekers among young unmarried women, and the lack of authentic data on the issue, are matters of grave concern to feminist scholars and activists. See, for instance, Ramachandran 1999.
19. We consulted a private doctor to ascertain the possible cause of the unmarried girl's death. In the doctor's opinion, the girl's mother might have administered either a heavy dose of anti-malarial tablets or RU 486. According to her, the latter could also cause death in a woman with a low haemoglobin count (say, 7) along with the delay in taking the decision to abort.
20. Usually, private clinics charge Rs 1,000 for an abortion in the first trimester and a further Rs 100 or Rs 200 for each month of pregnancy over the three-month period. The cost is higher for unmarried girls. This is an exorbitant rate considering the poor economic condition of Dalit families and the extremely low income of industrial workers. In most cases, the girl herself or her parents have to meet the abortion expenses. A similar trend exists in other parts of the country as well. In this context, see Gupta et al. 1997.
21. I have borrowed this term from an Egyptian study of women's reproductive lives. It is a useful analytical tool to understand how unmarried

girls who work in the companies comply with the discriminatory and sexually exploitative work culture, against their own wishes, for the sake of deriving some strategic benefits like income, and some freedom and mobility. At the same time, they constantly complain and regret the situation they are in. Here, we can see 'accommodation' interacting with 'resistance'. For a detailed discussion on 'strategic accommodation' see El Dawala and Aida Seif 2001

22. We have no quantitative data on the increase of abortion among unmarried women. Our argument is based on the views expressed by medical personnel and the people in the study villages.
23. In another context, critiquing the abortion laws in India, Malini Karkal comments that in India, liberal laws like MTP are closely linked to the national family-planning programme which encourages good abortion facilities and abortion care. But this would only lead to an increase in the number of abortions with an adverse effect on women's reproductive rights and choices. See Karkal 1999.

References

Anandhi, S., J. Jeyaranjan and Rajan Krishnan. 2002. 'Work, Caste and Competing Masculinities: Notes from a Tamil Village'. *Economic and Political Weekly* XXXVII (43), 26 October.

Baxi, Upendra. 2000. 'Gender and Reproductive Rights in India: Problems and Prospects for the New Millennium'. UNFPA Lecture, 6 September (mimeo.), New Delhi.

———. 2002. 'Sense and Sensibility'. *Seminar* 511, March.

El Dawala and Aida Seif. 2001. 'Women's Wit Over Men's: Trade-offs and Strategic Accommodations in Egyptian Women's Reproductive Lives', in Rosalind Petchesky and Karen Judd (eds), *Negotiating Reproductive Rights: Women's Perspectives Across Countries and Cultures.* London: Zed Books.

Ganatra, Bela. 2000. 'Abortion Research in India: What We Know and What We Need to Know', in Radhika Ramasubban and Shireen J. Jejeebhoy (eds), *Women's Reproductive Health in India.* New Delhi: Rawat Publications.

Gupta, Manisha, Sunita Bandewar and Hemlata Patel. 1997. 'Abortion Needs of Women in India: A Case Study of Rural Maharashtra'. *Reproductive Health Matters* 9, May.

IIPS (International Institute of Population Sciences). 2001. *National Family Health Survey, India 1998–99: Tamil Nadu.* Mumbai: International Institute of Population Sciences.

Jejeebhoy, Shireen J. 2000. 'Adolescent Sexual and Reproductive Behaviour: A Review of the Evidence from India', in Radhika Ramasubban and Shireen J. Jejeebhoy (eds), *Women's Reproductive Health in India.* New Delhi: Rawat Publications.

Jesani, Amar and Aditi Iyer. 1993. 'Women and Abortion'. *Economic and Political Weekly*, 27 November.

Jeyaranjan, J. and Padmini Swaminathan. 2001. 'The "Cost" of Work: Social Transformation and Perceptions of Health in a Region in Transition: A Study of Chengalpattu, Tamil Nadu'. Unpublished paper, CEHAT, Mumbai.

Karkal, Malini. 1999. Abortion Laws and the Abortion Situation in India. *Issues in Reproductive and Genetic Engineering* 4 (3).

Menon, Nivedita. 2002. 'Abortion: When Pro-Choice is Anti-Women', in Nivedita Menon, *Elusive Woman: Law and the Feminist Subject*. New Delhi: Manuscript submitted to Permanent Black.

Nagaraj, K. 2002. *Fertility Decline in Tamil Nadu—Social Capillarity in Action?* Chennai: Madras Institute of Development Studies.

Petchesky, Rosalind Pollack. 1986. *Abortion and Woman's Choice: The State, Sexuality and Reproductive Freedom*. London: Verso.

Petchesky, Rosalind P. and Karen Judd (eds). 2001. *Negotiating Reproductive Rights: Women's Perspectives Across Countries and Cultures*. London: Zed Books.

Rajan, Irudaya S., U. S. Misra and T. K. Vimala. 2000. 'Role of Abortion in the Fertility Transition in Kerala'. *Demography India* 29 (1).

Ramachandran, Vimala. 1999. 'Shying Away from Sexuality: Government Reproductive Health Programme'. *Voices for Change* 3 (1), April.

Ramasubban, Radhika and Shireen J. Jejeebhoy (eds). 2000. *Women's Reproductive Health in India*. New Delhi: Rawat Publications.

IV

Abortion among Married Women

Anjali Radkar

The International Conference of Population and Development (ICPD) iterated an important goal when it stated that 'every pregnancy should be intended' (Tsui et al. 1997). Determining the extent of unwanted pregnancies that end up in induced abortions therefore would be of great value from several vantage points.

Unfortunately, abortion is still one of those issues in women's lives that is buried in silence. In a country like India, women's health is given very low priority and their lack of control over family resources denies them access to health care in general and abortion in particular. In addition to being considered dangerous to women's health, abortion is also deemed to be socially unacceptable.

Studies in many developed and developing countries show that, even where abortion is legal, women are reluctant to talk about it (Bart and Hill 1996). In India, its incidence is always under-reported, perhaps because of the guilt or the moral stigma associated with it. Some studies estimate the extent of under-reporting to be about 50 per cent (Tiwari 1994). Research has also shown that the ratio of illegal to legal abortions is highly skewed—there are many more illegal abortions than legal ones (Chhabra and Nuna 1994; Jesani and Iyer 1993). Because of illegal abortions, there are between 15,000 and 20,000 abortion-related deaths in the country every year, mainly among married, multiparous women (Chhabra and Nuna 1994). But even generally, deaths due to induced abortion are quite high; for example, in Maharashtra in 1995, 17.6 per cent of maternal mortalities were due to induced abortion (Bandewar 2002). It is therefore evident that legalisation of abortion is a necessary but not sufficient condition for reducing the number of unsafe abortions.

Abortion was liberalised in India after the 1971 Medical Termination of Pregnancy (MTP) Act came into effect on 1 April 1972, according to which a pregnancy may be terminated within 20 weeks of gestation. Before 1972, abortion was permitted only if it was necessary to save the life of the woman. Now, it is also allowed on grounds of preserving her mental or physical health, as well as in cases of pregnancy due to rape, incest or contraceptive failure. However, it is illegal if performed just because a woman (or some other person) requests it, or if it is sought only for social and/or economic reasons (United Nations 1993). The Indian government has also repeatedly emphasised that MTP should not be viewed as a method of family planning or of reducing the national birth rate.

A large proportion of abortions are now cited as falling under a special category that was almost non-existent at the time of the framing of the Act. This category is sex determination followed by abortion of the female foetus. In such cases, it is not the pregnancy but its outcome that is unwanted. The first sex-selective abortion was documented in India in the 1970s, with the advent of amniocentesis. Though chromosomal analysis of amniotic fluid was developed to diagnose sex-linked genetic disorders, it almost immediately began to be used in genetic clinics for determining the sex of the foetus, with the sole purpose of circumventing the birth of girls (Oomman and Ganatra 2002).

Despite the fact that it is now more than thirty years since MTP was legalised in India, women still fight shy of speaking about it. This has proved to be one of the major stumbling blocks in gathering information about the extent of foetal wastage in general and induced abortions in particular. There are a few clinic-based studies that provide some information about abortions, but since the sample used is very selective, it is difficult to extract information about the processes and patterns associated with abortion from this data. It is this lack of reliable data which necessitates research on abortion that can shed light on the pathways leading to abortion as well as on the associated underlying factors, including quality of care and cost.

Study Objectives, Research Design and Methodology

We chose to focus on two purposively selected villages on the fringe of Pune city. Though the living conditions of people there can be described as rural, they are employed in both agriculture-related and urban occupations. Because of easily available transportation facilities, commuting to nearby urban centres is easier, as is access to urban infrastructure. Unlike their rural counterparts in remote, interior parts of the region, women in these villages can quite easily access abortion services provided by various public and private health centres in the city.

The study objectives were:

- to determine the role women themselves play in decision-making about abortion;
- to determine the role their families play and the kind and extent of support, if any, they provide;
- to identify the various reasons why women choose to abort;
- to determine the extent to which sex determination tests are used for detection of female foetus;
- to examine the factors that influence women's choice of provider, the quality of care they get and the cost of abortion;
- to determine extent of contraceptive use after abortion;
- to study abortion-related trauma, if any;
- to explore men and village functionaries view abortion.

We started off by conducting houselisting in both villages in order to locate currently married women of reproductive ages (15–49 years) and then to identify those who had sought induced abortion at some time in their life. Apart from collecting background information, detailed pregnancy histories of women were collected. In addition, we obtained data on their attitude towards and awareness of the legal aspects of abortion and prenatal sex determination.

Women who had sought abortion were interviewed in depth in order to understand the why, where and how of abortion. In addition, village functionaries, opinion leaders and health personnel such as the *sarpanch* (headman), public and private doctors, auxillary nurse midwives (ANMs) and chemists were also interviewed. Apart from in-depth interviews with women who had sought abortion, five FGDs were conducted with women who had not sought abortion, in order to gauge their attitudes to and knowledge of issues surrounding abortion.

Women generally do not make decisions about abortion by themselves. Their husbands have a major say in the matter. We therefore felt it was necessary to learn something about men's perceptions of and attitudes to abortion. Accordingly, we conducted three FGDs with the men in both villages.

Since unmarried adolescent girls would also soon enter their reproductive stage, we conducted FGDs with them as well. We also conducted an FGD with adolescent boys in the hope that discussions with them would further add to our knowledge of abortion in the selected villages. In all, a total of 12 FGDs were conducted.

Ethical Concerns

- The informed consent of respondents was sought before starting the interviews.
- Since we were collecting information on a sensitive issue, care was taken to maintain privacy during the interviews.
- The names of the women and the content of the interviews were kept confidential.
- Provision was made to disseminate the findings of the study through meetings in both villages.

Findings

In all, 940 households were listed in the two study villages having a total population of 4,755, with sex-ratio (females per 1,000 males) of 887. (The 1991 Census reported the combined sex-ratio for these two villages as 906.) The sex-ratio of children below 6 years of age was 927. In all, 933 currently married women of reproductive ages were interviewed. The survey reported six female-selective abortions in the two villages. If we add these to the female child population, the child sex-ratio would have been 946, which is closer to the expected child sex-ratio in a country like India. The profile of the households and of individuals is shown in Table 4.1.

The percentage of pregnancies ending in abortion (spontaneous or induced) was 9.7 per cent in our study area, which was higher than the 7.2 per cent reported by NFHS–2 (see Table 4.2).

Women's Views on Abortion

Most women (90 per cent) in the study villages either did not approve of abortion (viewing it as sin or 'murder') or felt that it was justifiable

Table 4.1: Profile of study villages

Household characteristics	
Number of households	940
% nuclear household	60
% Hindus	95
% Buddhists	4
Dominant caste	Marathas
% with agriculture as main occupation	44
% with service as main income source	35
% in construction work and transport	15
% in agriculture labour	7
Individual characteristics	
Number of people enumerated	4,755
% male illiterate	13
% female illiterate	31
% male with more than 12 years of education	22
% female with more than 12 years of education	8
Average age at marriage of women	16.3 years
% women married before 18 years	69
Average no. of children born	2.52
Average no. of children surviving	2.35

Table 4.2: Percentage distribution of pregnancy outcomes

Pregnancy outcomes	Current study	NFHS–2 Maharashtra 1998–99
Live births	90.3	92.8
Spontaneous abortions	5.0	3.8
Induced abortions	2.9	1.9
Stillbirths	1.8	1.5
Total pregnancies	100.0	100.0
No. of currently married women in reproductive ages	933	

only in certain circumstances. Some of them (36 per cent) said if couples do not want a child, they should take precautions to prevent pregnancy. Only 4 per cent accepted abortion as a women's right.

According to 84 per cent of the women, the most probable cause for abortion was to avoid having 'a female child'. One in five women also indicated that abortion is used to limit family size. Women opt for sterilisation after undergoing abortion. Some 10 per cent felt that abortion is also used for spacing children. Surprisingly, very few respondents mentioned 'improper growth of child' or 'trouble to mother' as reasons for abortion. The women's responses quite clearly indicated that induced abortion was perceived as a method to eliminate a female child.

Though 47 per cent of the women knew that abortion is legal in India, only 37 per cent were aware of the provisions under the MTP Act, such as the reasons for which abortion is permitted and the period of gestation within which it is considered legal. However, they believed that the duration of pregnancy within which abortion is permissible is below five months.

As mentioned earlier, in order to better understand the process of abortion, detailed interviews were carried out with women who had undergone abortions. In cases of repeat abortions, we collected information for each abortion episode, since the reason, gestation period and conditions in which abortion was sought could differ. In all, data for 70 abortion episodes were collected from 65 women, of which three women reported having undergone two abortions each and one women reported three abortions. Two women had repeat abortions for medical reasons, while the other two used it as a method of spacing. All the abortions included in our study took place between 1985 and 2002, over a period of 17 years.

Characteristics of Women Seeking Abortion

Understanding the differentials in the proportion of women seeking abortion by their characteristics can shed light on the circumstances surrounding the reasons that lead to abortion (Bankole et al. 1999). Table 4.3 presents the background and demographic characteristics of abortion seekers in terms of educational level, occupation and standard of living. In 65 of the 70 episodes of abortion, the women were below 30 years of age; with the median age at abortion of 23 years. In 12 or 29 per cent of the cases, the age at abortion was 20 years or less. This is in line with the findings of hospital-based studies on abortion reported by Chhabra et al. (1988) and Solapurkar and Sangam (1985), which indicated that 27 to 30 per cent of the abortion seekers were of age 20 or less. The age of women seeking abortion shows an inverted 'U' pattern in the study area, similar to that described by Bankole et al. (1999). The reason for this is that, as they grew older, fewer women sought abortion as most of them were sterilised by then.

The proportion of educated women among abortion seekers was higher than among the entire population. Khan et al. (1990) and

Chhabra et al. (1988) also found the proportion of illiterate women among abortion seekers to be low. Confirming the findings of the ICMR (1989) study, our research revealed that the educational level of 12 per cent of the abortion seekers was above the SSC (Senior School Certificate) level, while the percentage of such women in the general population was just 8. Nearly 43 per cent of the abortion seekers were housewives, indicating they did not need to work for money. The others were mostly engaged in agriculture and allied activities, with a few being self-employed, running small shops or engaged in tailoring work. Further, 15 per cent of the abortion seekers enjoyed a 'high' standard of living as compared to 10 per cent in the general population. The profile of abortion seekers suggests that women were able to take and act upon a decision on abortion in the event of an unwanted pregnancy.

Table 4.3: Background of abortion seekers

Educational level	Number
Illiterate	13
Class I–IV	13
Class V–IX	20
SSC	11
Above SSC	8
Occupation	
Agriculture	25
Agricultural labour	2
Shop	4
Gardening	1
Self-employed	2
Tailoring	3
Housewife	28
Standard of living	
Low	5
Medium	49
High	11
Total of all categories	65

Further, 49 of the 70 abortions, or 70 per cent were of third- or fourth-order pregnancies, while only two were of the first order. Evidently, these women had, on an average, two surviving children at the time of abortion.

Pre-Abortion Considerations

Before a woman has an abortion, a number of factors are considered and decisions taken, at both the individual and family levels, to determine whether the pregnancy is wanted or not. Our research indicates that, even when pregnancy was not categorically unwanted, it was terminated because of certain specific reasons or situations. The obvious reasons for a pregnancy being unwanted ranged from the sex of the foetus, economic factors, contraceptive failure, wrong timing, etc.

'Unwanted' Pregnancy?

Our research revealed that not all pregnancies started out as being unwanted. Rather, certain circumstances during the course of pregnancy made them unwanted, such as the discovery that the foetus was female. Similarly, in lower-order pregnancies, the child was wanted but the timing was wrong. Sometimes, the question of being wanted or unwanted did not apply: pregnancy was discontinued for medical reasons.

Reasons for Abortion

The reason why a woman seeks abortion may differ from one abortion to another, depending on her socio-economic situation and the stage of life she is in at the time of seeking abortion. However, for most women, abortion means loss—loss of money and some loss of health. Our research revealed very clearly that the decision to abort was taken not just individually by the woman, but by the family as a whole.

When questioned about the reasons why they had sought abortion, women's responses varied. In several cases, the responses implied multiple reasons, suggesting that the decision to abort is a complex phenomenon (see Table 4.4). Nonetheless, in a large number of cases, abortion was used either for limiting family size or for spacing children. Other studies have also indicated these to be the overwhelming reasons for seeking abortion (Ganatra et al. 1999; ICMR 1989; and Khan et al. 1990). According to Bankole et al. (1998), the most commonly reported primary reasons for abortion in Asia are the desire to postpone and/or stop childbearing. Of the two, the latter appears to be more prevalent. This finding is consistent with the widespread preference for smaller families in most Asian countries and with the fact that more married than unmarried women undergo abortions.

Table 4.4: Reasons for abortion

Reason for abortion	Number
Spacing between children	17
Limiting family size	33
Female selective abortion	8
Contraceptive failure	4
Health risk to mother, including weakness	20
Economic reasons	3
Medical advice	11
Retarded/handicapped child	4
Already had a son	1
Pregnancy immediately after marriage	1
Twins	1

Note: Figures do not add up to 65 because some women reported multiple reasons for seeking abortion.

Of the 17 women who used abortion for spacing between children, the previous child of 11 of them was a male child. Women were concerned that their male child grow up well before they gave birth to another child. However, 8, i.e., 11.4 per cent women reported seeking abortion because the foetus was female, and they used ultrasound imaging for the purpose. Studies by Ganatra et al. (1999) and the VHAI (1999) show similar percentages: 16.8 and 10 per cent respectively.

A 30-year-old woman, who was educated up to Class IV and had four daughters, was threatened by her mother-in-law, who told her that if she did not produce a male child, the mother-in-law would get another wife for her son and throw her and her daughters out. So when the woman got pregnant for the fifth time, she went for a sex-determination test and, since the foetus was found to be female, decided to have it aborted, although she personally did not approve of sex-selective abortion.

The health of the mother was cited as another reason for abortion. This included problems during the early stages of pregnancy. Two women cited heart trouble and one a prolapsed uterus as reasons for abortion. Another five reported physical weakness. In three cases, women had had abortions for economic reasons. In one case, the woman said that she already had a son, while another woman said she did not want to have a baby immediately after marriage.

In addition to these reasons, women resorted to abortion because of unforeseen circumstances. For example, one woman had an abortion because her husband 'wanted to get married again'. In the woman's own words:

> My husband had relations with some woman and he wanted to get married to her. He would always tell me: 'You are dark. I don't like you.' When he knew that I was pregnant for the second time, he ordered me to have an abortion. When I refused, he said, 'I won't be responsible for whatever happens to you later', and walked off. So I got it done.

In another case of pregnancy eight years after sterilisation, the woman's husband and sister-in-law forcibly took her to the hospital for an abortion even though the woman wanted to continue the pregnancy, particularly because she had only two children. The abortion was followed by re-sterilisation. During an FGD, a young man described pregnancy after sterilisation failure as a calamity. 'What can we do if it rains heavily after the rice is cut and kept out?' he asked.

Contraceptive failure was cited as a reason for abortion by only four women. In three cases, pregnancy was due to Copper-T (Cu-T) failure, while in the fourth it was due to sterilisation failure. Ganatra et al. (1999) and Srinivasa et al. (1997) also found that 5 per cent of their study sample reported contraceptive failure as a reason for abortion.

Sex Selection

The 65 women who had had abortions were asked their views on sex-selection. While 16 of them were in favour of prenatal sex selection, 38 were against it, and 10 felt that it was justifiable if the woman already had a number of daughters. In FGDs women voiced similar views, reflecting the existence of son preference and the availability of facilities to conduct the test in the vicinity of their villages. Shah and Taneja (1991) have also pointed out that there is widespread acceptance of sex detection which is often followed by abortion.

Sex detection with amniocentesis is usually done at 16 to 20 weeks of pregnancy, whereas it is done at 13 to 14 weeks using ultrasound imaging. It is important to note that the accuracy of detection enhances with the increased duration of pregnancy. 'Chorionic villus' sampling is a more advanced test that can detect sex as early as 6 to 7 weeks of pregnancy, but it is generally used to detect genetic disorders in the foetus. When the embryo enters the uterus it is surrounded by chorionic villi which fit into the lining of the uterus. Scraping these villi—for sex detection—needs expertise, because if something goes wrong the risk of damaging the embryo is quite high. A private doctor, according to whom sex determination is rampant in urban areas, told us:

> It is good that the chorionic villi test is not conducted; otherwise the rate of abortion would increase very much—some women who are scared to have second trimester abortions after sex determination by ultrasound would opt for this.

In urban areas, ultrasound imaging is fast becoming an integral part of antenatal check-ups, conducted to determine whether the baby is normal. Since the women in our sample also preferred to go to the city for delivery, there is a distinct possibility that, apart from having routine check-ups, they also underwent ultrasound tests. Some women (19 out of 65) reported that they did undergo the test, of which eight admitted that they used it for sex detection. Another eight women underwent the test on medical advice. In the remaining cases the test was done either to confirm the pregnancy or to estimate the duration of gestation. After the test, nine mothers reported that they knew the sex of their foetus, which in eight cases was female.

However, one woman reported that she underwent amniocentesis solely for sex determination. She was 30 years old and already had two daughters. The family was educated and economically well off, and the husband appeared to be a supportive sort. The couple went to Mumbai for the test in 1992. When they discovered that she was carrying a female foetus, they decided on an abortion. Without informing her in-laws, she had the abortion in the fifth month of pregnancy, consequently suffering from post-abortion trauma. The in-laws were not very happy that she had aborted but they supported her. The woman herself had a very strong son preference; nonetheless she wondered: 'How many girls should one take out [abort]?'

We also discovered that two of the 65 women had undergone an ultrasound test during a previous pregnancy. They continued the pregnancy because the foetus was determined to be male. But the fact that 23 of the 65 women did not have any surviving son at the time of abortion is indicative of strong son preference. Sixteen women had one or more daughters and, for the rest, although it was the first pregnancy, they wanted to know the sex of the foetus.

Maharashtra has been witnessing a steady decrease in family size. In fact, even in villages, especially those on the urban fringe, family size is already limited to two children. Considering the preference for sons, there is always the temptation for those who have two or more surviving children and no son to resort to sex determination followed by abortion if the foetus is female. Even where women report undergoing abortion for reasons of spacing or limiting the family, contraceptive failure or 'problem to mother', it is possible, at least in some cases, that the desire for a son, though not explicitly stated, is the main reason for abortion.

A woman of 35 had three daughters in a row. The fourth time she conceived, she took a sex-detection test and aborted the female foetus in the fifth month. As this abortion led to some health problems, she did not undergo the test when she conceived again and delivered a fourth daughter. She said that the next time she conceives, she will take the test and, if it is female foetus, will get an abortion and a sterilisation at the same time.

Views on Sex Determination

In all the FGDs—with men, women and adolescent boys and girls—it very clearly surfaced that women who went in for sex determination followed it up with the abortion of the female foetus. Everyone seemed to know at least some women who had done this. The adjectives they used were '*raggad*' and '*chikar*', both indicating 'so many'. For them, sonography was used for sex detection in the same way as sterilisation was used for family planning. One woman said: '...These days, getting a sonography done is a fashion.' A similar view was expressed by another woman: '...Sonography has become a fad now.'

But we also came across a few cases where sex detection had failed. For example, a woman with three daughters underwent the test and was told that she was pregnant with a male foetus. She therefore continued the pregnancy but ended up delivering a daughter again. All the women in the village knew about this, and she was extremely embarrassed when they brought it up during the FGD. In a second case, a woman accompanied her pregnant sister, who already had one daughter, to the city for sex detection. At first the doctor, who was known to the woman, declined to do the test, but later performed it when the woman requested it repeatedly. The results indicated a female foetus, so the woman insisted that her sister abort the pregnancy. Again, the doctor was reluctant to perform the procedure as the pregnancy was already in an advanced stage, but in the end was persuaded by the woman to go ahead. When they learned that the baby had been a male child, they regretted their decision. After this episode the sister got pregnant again and delivered a daughter. She told the woman: 'Now I will never listen to you. If the time comes, I will get sterilised, even if I have only daughters.'

Sex selection was a topic on which everybody seemed to have fairly accurate information, and also on which everyone had an opinion. All women were in favour of sex detection in cases where a couple had daughters but no son. All felt that a son was a must. When the discussion veered towards whether sex detection was right or wrong, a 40-year-old woman exclaimed: 'Why do you blame our women? Did they know earlier that the sex of the child could be detected before birth? It is the doctors who told us about it.' When they were reminded that there were many things that doctors advise, particularly in terms of antenatal care or the health of the mother and children, which the women do not heed, the reply was: 'A person takes whatever she likes in the advice.'

However, an elected male member of the panchayat, who participated in the FGD, said: 'Sex detection may be a common practice in your city. In villages women don't even go for antenatal check-ups, leave alone the test and abortion.' As was evident here and also in our interviews with the *sarpanch* in the two villages, they took a politically correct stand, denying the occurrence of sex detection and abortion of the female foetus in their respective villages. Further, they said that abortion itself was very rare and, if it happened at all, it was only for 'valid' reasons.

Many women in the study area were aware of the fact that abortion of the female foetus is a punishable offence. At least one or two women in each FGD group were also aware of the declining sex-ratio and worried about its consequences in the long run, particularly that their 'sons will not get wives'. However, in all the interviews we conducted, we got the sense that most rural women regard *sansar* (married life) almost like a career and see producing a son as an indication of success;

having a son seems an important milestone, which they must all reach as quickly as they can.

Secrecy about Pregnancy

Information on the secrecy surrounding pregnancy is usually collected to get an idea of whether women feel guilty about their pregnancy or are embarrassed about letting others know about it. We found no indication of any secrecy relating to pregnancy, perhaps because all our respondents were currently married women. In all cases, the husband was aware of their wives' pregnancy and, for the majority of the women, the mother-in-law also knew about it.

Regarding abortion of the female foetus after sex detection, keeping the pregnancy hidden from other villagers is not possible. By the time the test is conducted, the pregnancy is already in an advanced stage (four to five months). In addition, it is usually women with daughters but no son who undergo such late abortions, so everyone in the village guesses that they are sex-selective abortions.

Decision-making and the Role of the Family

Making decisions about abortion is a dynamic process; we felt that it would be useful to find out with whom women discuss their pregnancy and who advises them to have an abortion. The role that women play in the decision-making process is also of interest whenever abortion is discussed. We found that the woman herself was involved in decision-making in 51 cases and the husband in 57 cases. In 49 out of 70 abortions, it was a joint decision by husband and wife. In four cases the mother-in-law was involved. The role of the husband in decision-making is thus much more important than that of the woman's.

When asked whether the women themselves had wanted the abortion, the answer was 'yes' for 54 episodes. In one case, since the abortion had been sought for economic reasons, the woman was confused about whether she had wanted it or not; in 15 cases, however, the women had not wanted abortion. Of these, 11 women had undergone termination of their pregnancy for medical reasons. In one case the husband had forced the woman to abort, and in another the in-laws had wanted a son. One woman cited sterilisation failure as the reason: 'I felt ashamed when I got pregnant after the sterilisation. So I had no other alternative but to terminate.' One woman who did not want abortion was compelled to seek it for economic reasons.

When, during our FGDs with men in the two villages, we asked them about the role that the woman's parents play in the issue, their unanimous response was 'no role'. As a rule, the woman's parents are not even informed, though sometimes after abortion women do go to their parents' home to rest. The men also emphasised that it is the usually the husband who takes the decision on abortion; more often than not, the women are just pressured into saying 'yes'. However, in case the couple has a large number of children, the woman *may* take the decision herself. As one man said: 'Women here have not progressed so much that they can take such a decision by themselves.'

It was clear that in both villages abortion was generally considered to be a couple's personal decision, though the family and people around did have a role to play. Family support, and someone from the family to accompany the woman to the clinic at the time of abortion, were also considered necessary.

In terms of family support, 50 women said that the husband had been supportive. In 18 cases, all the family members had been supportive, and in 12 cases, the support of parents-in-law was mentioned. However, from the women's responses we gathered that by 'support' they generally meant permission and approval. Most of them said: 'If they [family members, especially the mother-in-law and sister-in-law] don't approve of abortion, how can I get the required rest? Who will look after my children when I am away in the hospital?'

Similarly, without family support or approval, there would be no one to accompany them to the hospital at the time of abortion. In 52 cases, women reported that their husbands had accompanied them. Among these, in 24 instances, it was *only* the husband who accompanied them, but in the remaining 28 another family member was also present. In terms of other family members, we found that more often than not, it was mothers (16 cases) rather than mothers-in-law (8 cases) or any other relative who accompanied the woman.

Choice of Provider

It is common for women who find themselves saddled with an unwanted pregnancy to first try and abort it themselves. They usually try some home remedies to abort the foetus. These are actually induced abortions, though they are seldom reported as such. If they do not succeed in their first attempt, they consult a family member or friend and try again. Only if they fail again do they approach service providers. Of the 65 women in the study area who had undergone abortion, four admitted that they had tried home remedies. During our FGDs, women from both villages claimed to know methods like eating a whole papaya or jackfruit, or several bananas (Shrotri et al. 1980 reported a similar finding). A 50-year-old woman, the mother-in-law of two respondents who had undergone abortion, said:

> I had three sons and wanted no more. So the fourth time I ate a whole papaya twice, but nothing happened. Then I got headache tablets and had four at one time; still nothing happened. I think this was because our generation is constitutionally much stronger than today's women.

33-year-old woman reported a self-induced abortion that took place 14 years ago:

> I was menstruating at the time of my marriage. After the marriage I did not get my period. My husband did not like the idea of my getting pregnant immediately after marriage, and wanted me to terminate the pregnancy. I did not want to do that because—does any mother feel that she should not have a baby? I knew that if a woman takes Anacin tablets, she will get her menses. So in the third month I got five Anacin tablets from the chemist and consumed all of them together. I aborted and got my period. I did not tell anyone about this, not even the doctor.

After that she did not conceive again. She even went to Gujarat for treatment, but nothing happened. Her mother- and sister-in-law kept threatening to get a second wife for her husband. Her usual answer was: 'Why one, bring five.' But her husband supported her because he knew that it was on his insistence that she had sought abortion. She sadly related what happened when she returned from Gujarat:

> After the treatment in Gujarat I did not get my period for six months. I did not go to any doctor for a check-up. But I put on

weight so everybody thought that I was pregnant. My mother-and sister-in-law got me a green sari and arranged a function. After the function I got my period.

All the doctors we spoke to confirmed that women first try home remedies and only approach them for an abortion if they fail or suffer some serious consequences. A private doctor shared with us her knowledge of the methods women use to induce abortion, such as eating something they consider would destroy the foetus, hitting themselves on the stomach, jumping up and down, or making their children stand on their stomach. While these are all dangerous practices, even more dangerous is the insertion into the uterus of objects like sticks of *neem* and *babhali*, matchsticks, needles, safety pins or hairpins. When they finally come to the doctor, many of them say nothing about their attempts, which are discovered when metal pieces come out with the waste, though things like sticks might disintegrate and sometimes go unnoticed. In the process of evacuating and scraping, metal pieces can injure the uterus, as abortion is often a blind procedure. Women do not understand the extent of risk they take by inserting objects into the uterus.

Clearly, then, it is when all home and traditional remedies fail that the decision to seek abortion from a formal provider is taken. Usually, women have their own notions about where to go, depending on whether they have conceived within or outside marriage. It is generally believed that women who get pregnant as a consequence of *bhangad* (an extramarital affair) tend to go in for unsafe abortions. This came across clearly during our FGDs with women and men. A 46-year-old man said: 'There are cases, we know. They cannot go to the doctor openly so they have to go to quacks.... They do all this secretly. Whatever information we have is hearsay, so we cannot investigate whether women suffered any health problems afterwards.' Obversely, for married women secrecy is not so important. 'Why should women feel ashamed to go to a doctor if the pregnancy is within marriage?'

At the same time, there was general agreement among women in FGDs: 'Now everybody goes to the doctor. The villages are not backward. People are educated and can afford to go to the doctor....' People may visit traditional healers for other health problems. If women go to traditional healer for abortion, it is to keep the visit hidden. However, they all insisted that there was no healer in the vicinity who practised abortion. This may well have been true as women in both villages do have access to safe abortion services because of their proximity to an urban centre. In a city, anonymity—which is what most women, especially those in extramarital relationships, want—is also not a problem.

Not only do the women have easy access to all Pune hospitals, they also have access to the health facilities provided by the government for rural areas, such as the sub-centre (SC) or the primary health centre (PHC) and the rural hospital (RH). While government centres charge a nominal fee for the abortion procedure, women (and those accompanying them) do have to spend an appreciable amount of time waiting. In the process they sometimes end up losing an entire day's work. They also have to pay for the medicines prescribed. In financial terms, therefore, the women did not find much difference in cost between urban private health facilities and government centres. They also felt that doctors in private centres are more careful and, unlike government hospitals, have better equipment and facilities. In addition, their time is not wasted because doctors in the private sector are usually in a hurry to finish their work. On the whole, therefore, women preferred to use private abortion facilities.

In order to get more information on providers, we asked the 65 women to list the abortion facilities and providers they had used. They reported a large number of providers; 45 in all. Of these, 32 had private clinics, 12 worked in public facilities (seven government or municipal hospitals and five trust hospitals) and one had an abortion clinic. Of the 70 abortions, 41 were conducted in private clinics, 15 in government or municipal hospitals, eight in trust hospitals and six in the abortion clinic.

Women thus have a wide range of facilities from which to choose one that would suit their needs. When we asked them about why they had chosen a particular provider over another, 31 women said that they had preferred a particular doctor or hospital because of their good reputation and 13 said that they had known the particular doctor for a long time. The reputation of the concerned provider or facility thus carried a lot of weight in the selection. In 14 cases, women chose certain providers because they levied lower charges, while in 13 cases women chose hospitals or clinics that were closest to their homes. In some cases, where the company in which the husband worked reimbursed medical expenses, the choice depended on the facility with which the company had an arrangement.

There also appeared to be some link between the period of gestation and the choice of provider. For instance, we found that half of the first trimester and three-fourths of the second trimester abortions were conducted in private clinics. Where the PHC or RH is concerned, it was usually the government servants working in the villages who took women there. Visits to both these facilities were strongly associated with sterilisation; 14 of the 33 women who sought abortion and sterilisation at the same time visited either the government health facility or the trust hospital, which functioned more or less like a government hospital and charged a comparatively lower fee than private clinics. The women were unanimous in their belief that if performed in safe conditions, abortion poses little risk to their health.

The Abortion Experience

Duration of Gestation

All the women in our sample showed awareness that second trimester abortions carry risks and are comparatively more hazardous for the health of the women. Of the 70 abortions, 46 reportedly took place in the first trimester (66 per cent), of which 23 were carried out before the woman had completed two months of pregnancy. Likewise, 23 abortions were performed in the second trimester. The mean duration of gestation was 12.4 weeks. In this context it is important to note that the duration of pregnancy is directly related to the reason for abortion. Those who want to have a sex-determination test and then abort have to complete 16 to 20 weeks, which is when ultrasound imaging can detect the sex of the foetus. On the other hand, those who opt for abortion for reasons of spacing or limiting family size can seek abortion immediately after the pregnancy is confirmed.

The duration of gestation also impacts women's perception of abortion. If the abortion takes place in the first 12 weeks or three months of pregnancy, they refer to it as *'divyatale'*, i.e., they do not consider it to be an abortion. Since the foetus is unformed until then, having an abortion in this period is not considered a 'killing' or a 'sin'. Because of this perception, it is likely that a few women may not have reported the abortion if it was conducted early, because they may not view it as an abortion. They consider it an abortion only after organs are formed.

Quality of Care

Women's concerns and priorities while seeking abortion care are different from those in other health-seeking situations. Factors like 'confidentiality', 'quick service and return' and 'not wanting husband's signature' are given higher priority than safety and quality of care (Ganatra et al. 1999; Gupte et al. 1997). Since, in the lives of 61 of our respondents, abortion represented a one-time procedure rather than a repeated experience, we assumed that they would remember the services they received at the time of abortion. However, it is possible that they were reluctant to talk about it if the experience had not been a happy one; it is also possible that they might not have expected too much from the health facilities in any case; or perhaps the experience had become one of minor importance in their lives and they no longer felt strongly about it. Whatever the reason, it was difficult to gauge the quality of care they received from the accounts they gave us.

We collected information about the behaviour of doctors and other hospital staff from the 29 women who did not seek abortion in private health facilities. Of the 20 who responded, only one described the behaviour of the doctor as 'very bad'; the paramedics' behaviour, on the other hand, was described as 'bad' in three cases. We also asked them about the competency of the staff, the cleanliness of the hospital and the general quality of the services provided. Staff competence was reported as 'bad' in only two cases, whereas cleanliness and services were reported as 'very bad' in only one case. In three instances, the response was 'neutral', but in all other cases the women responded positively.

As mentioned earlier, one woman (35 years old) suffered from Cu-T failure and became pregnant. Because she was using a CU-T, her pregnancy went unnoticed for four months. When it was realised that she was pregnant, the ANM from the SC had her admitted to the government hospital in the city. The woman had to spend a week in the hospital, where she was paid no proper attention. No one spoke to her or, despite repeated enquiries, gave her any information regarding her health status. The hospital was also extremely dirty. After the abortion was performed, no one came to ask how she was feeling, even though she had developed complications. The family finally had her transferred to a private hospital, where she received better treatment and survived. She is still grateful to the private doctor. While we were interviewing her, she said: 'The poor should die at home and the rich in private hospitals, but nobody should go to a government hospital.'

Women related horrendous accounts about their experiences at the PHC, which had advertised its abortion facilities very widely. To list a few:

> We went there after reading the advertisement. Nurses in the centre beat the women and shouted at them. We could hear the sound of beating and shouting even outside.

> They don't allow patients to wait there even for half an hour after the procedure. They want us to vacate the bed after five minutes. My husband had gone out after the abortion. The nurse told me: 'You find him and just go.' I told her that I was getting *chakkars* [giddiness], but she did not pay any attention.

Surprisingly, a woman who had gone to the PHC for an abortion followed by sterilisation did not seem unhappy. She said: 'Why do we criticise the facilities in government hospitals? They give us services. We get cured. What else do we want from them? Of course there were mosquitoes, but don't we have mosquitoes in our homes?'

Number of Visits and Stay in Hospital

When one decides to have an abortion, one customarily makes at least three visits to the hospital/clinic. The first one is for confirmation of pregnancy and blood and urine testing, the second is for the actual abortion procedure, and the third is a post-abortion visit. Data on the number of times women went to the hospital reveals that in 37 instances women just went there to get the abortion done. They did not have to make any other visit. The remaining 33 women, however, had made multiple visits.

When the abortion procedure is conducted properly, women are not required to stay in the hospital overnight. In 39 cases, women reported that they returned home the same evening after the abortion was carried out. However, in cases where the abortion was immediately followed by sterilisation, women had to stay on in the hospital.

So did the women who had sought abortion on medical grounds or, as in the Cu-T-failure case, had suffered complications after abortion.

In both villages women had no clue about the methods generally used for performing abortions, not even about the procedures used for their own abortion.

Contraceptive Use after Abortion

In their studies, Ganatra et al. (1999) and Gupte et al. (1997) have mentioned that public abortion services are generally not accepted because of their insistence on contraceptive use immediately after abortion. However, since all the women in our sample were currently married and were terminating an unwanted pregnancy, they did not have any objection to accepting contraception. In 38 cases, contraception was accepted immediately after abortion (condom: 3, oral pills: 8, intra-uterine device (IUD): 2, female sterilisation: 23, vasectomy: 1, and safe period: 1; of the 24 sterilisation cases, 12 were conducted in private hospitals and 12 in government hospitals). One woman underwent a hysterectomy. Of the four women who cited contraceptive failure (three IUDs and one sterilisation) as their reason for abortion, only two had started using contraception. The woman who reported sterilisation failure got herself re-sterilised immediately after the abortion, and one opted for condoms.

Contraception as Condition for Abortion

Only two women claimed that they had been coerced into accepting contraception. In seven cases, the doctor had suggested contraceptive use and in three cases the women themselves felt that it was necessary. Of the two cases where contraceptive use was made mandatory, one occurred in a low-cost trust hospital and the other in a private hospital. Both abortions were during the first trimester, which indicates that the decision to abort was taken immediately after pregnancy was detected. The reason for abortion in both cases was 'completed the desired family size'. Both women had two surviving children, including one son. All these factors suggest that the two women had used some form of contraception even earlier. The woman in the trust hospital got herself sterilised, while the one in the private clinic opted for a Cu-T.

Husband's Consent

When women go to a hospital for abortion, they are often asked to get the signature of the husband as an indication of the latter's consent. This has become a vexing issue in the context of women's reproductive rights. Research has shown that the husband's consent is demanded despite the fact that it is not a legal requirement (Gupte et al. 1997; Khan et al. 1996). Our own study indicates that in 62 of the 70 cases we covered, women were asked to get their husband's signature before abortion. In most instances (52), the husband had accompanied the woman and could therefore give his signature on the spot. Although a relative's consent is required for surgical procedures, and the husband certainly qualifies as a relative, not a single woman in our study area knew that his signature was not mandatory for abortion. But because it is generally demanded, they all felt that it was a legal requirement.

When we discussed this issue with a private doctor in the city, she said:

> It is safer to have the signature of the husband—or another responsible relative, especially when a woman comes for abortion without the husband's knowledge. Because later he can come to the hospital and make a *tamasha* [drama]. Who is going to face all that afterwards? We have our work....

Cost of Abortion

We cannot obtain a holistic understanding of abortion without taking into account the cost of the procedure. Sometimes, when ready cash is not available, women cannot afford to have an abortion. They therefore continue with the pregnancy and end up having an unwanted child. The cost of abortion includes travel expenses, expenses on medicines and the doctor's fees. Only 39 women in our sample could put a figure to the cost, which varied sharply (Rs 50 to Rs 10,000) from woman to woman.

The woman who paid Rs 10,000 had sought abortion in a public hospital after conceiving due to Cu-T failure. She had complications and, since she did not receive adequate care, was moved to a private facility where she had to spend a huge amount. So even though women opt for public services because of their low cost, they sometimes end up paying much more.

The most frequently reported figure was Rs 3,000. While the overall median cost for abortion worked out to Rs 2,500; it was Rs 3,000 for the private facilities and Rs 1,500 for the public facilities and the abortion centre. The differential in the median cost for abortion in the first trimester (Rs 1,500) and the second (Rs 2,500) is significant.

However, since the abortions that we covered were lifetime abortions and were spread over 17 years—from 1985 to 2002—the data on costs should be interpreted cautiously. Five abortions were sought during 1985–92, 10 during 1993–95, 12 between 1996 and 1999, and 10 from 2000 to 2002. The median costs for the four-time periods were Rs 1,000, Rs 1,750, Rs 3,000 and Rs 2,750 respectively. Like all other costs, the cost of abortion has also increased over time.

The cost of abortion also depends on the duration of gestation and, possibly, the reason for abortion. As Gupte et al. (1997) mention, if the abortion is not legal within the frame of the Act, then women have to pay more. Also, such abortions are usually performed in the private sector. This was confirmed by a young woman of 26 who said during an FGD: 'You throw more money and get anything done in private.'

Of the 39 abortions for which the cost was reported, 13 were second-trimester abortions. In 11 cases the women had to spend over Rs 1,000, while in six cases the cost was over Rs 3,000. Since ultrasound imaging and amniocentesis are both second-trimester tests, abortions performed after them are usually risky. For six of the eight women who had aborted their female foetus, the cost varied between Rs 2,000 and Rs 5,000. Women know that sex-selective abortion is illegal, so they are ready to pay the high charges if the services meet their needs and quality requirements (Ganatra 2000).

In order to learn a little more about the spending capacity of rural people in relation to abortion, we probed this issue in the FGDs. Most participants claimed that the cost of abortion was not very high and well within the householders' capacity to pay. But we did receive two rather peculiar answers:

> Get a loan and celebrate the festival.

> Abortion is like celebrating Diwali—a festival of lights.

We can conclude, therefore, that abortion was perceived as a necessary evil as far as cost is concerned: whether affordable or not, if an abortion is needed then money has to be spent.

Post-Abortion

Side Effects

As mentioned earlier, if not performed carefully, abortion, especially in the second trimester, can prove to be a risky procedure and women can end up facing problems like haemorrhage or perforation of the uterus. There is also the possibility of secondary sterility and ectopic pregnancy. Unfortunately, most of the women (49) in our study area seemed unaware of these potential risks. Some women (14) said that they knew about these risks, but could not explain what they knew: one said 'bleeding', another said 'weakness' and one just said '*tras*' (trouble) if gestation is at an advanced stage. Three women spoke of 'pain in the waist' and 'backache', while another said that she knew 'all about the trouble': 'When I was waiting in the hospital for abortion, I read all the posters on the wall.' None of them really had any idea of how much trauma an abortion can cause if something goes wrong.

When we asked them about health problems after abortion, 56 women said that they hadn't had any. However, 14 did admit to some problems: four reported 'heavy bleeding' and five 'pain in the waist'. A 32-year-old woman reported that a month after the abortion she started bleeding so heavily that, wherever she sat, the floor would become red.

Two women spoke of 'weakness', while another two claimed to have suffered severe problems for which they had to be hospitalised and, as they explained, 'just managed to survive'. One reported respiratory problems due to an allergic reaction to a drug that was administered during the procedure. This 39-year-old woman had gone to a city hospital to have her abortion. Just before the procedure, she was given an injection to which she had a severe reaction. She lost her vision, 'got *chakkar*s' (giddiness) and then lost consciousness. There was no provision in the hospital to treat her so she was referred to another hospital where she was admitted into its intensive care unit. After this life-threatening experience, she concluded that the decision to abort was a wrong one and that the trauma she suffered was visited on her as a punishment.

It was clear, however, that even though most women did not know the exact nature of the potential risks, they did have some vague sense that abortion does or can cause some form of health problem. One said: 'Abortion *mhanje dehachi kharabi* (abortion means spoiling the body)', while another woman remarked: 'Fruit falls down only when it ripens. Abortion is like plucking the raw fruit from the tree. It is of no use to anybody…not to the tree at least. How will it come out without trouble?'

Feelings and Reactions

Women's post-abortion reactions are generally complex. The two most commonly expressed reactions were that they 'felt bad' (38 women) and that they had 'no feelings' (23 women). Thirteen women said that they had felt 'relief' after abortion. Eight said that they had suffered 'extreme' grief. Almost all of them spoke of the experience as something that they 'had to do…there was no other way'. Three women labelled abortion as murder, whereas one felt that it was a criminal act. On the whole, however, their feelings vacillated between grief and relief:

> I used to cry continuously. Not even eat anything. I was in a really bad state. (23-year-old woman, abortion for female foeticide)

> I had nausea and vomiting all through the pregnancy. I thought I couldn't sustain it this time. Our life is more important after all. (32-year-old woman, abortion for limiting family)

> It was a great relief. Abortion and childbirth are a cross that women have to bear. (27-year-old woman, abortion for limiting family)

> I did not want an abortion, but could not do anything. I was angry with the doctor. He made the mistake and I had to pay for it. I had to kill my own child. (35-year-old woman, pregnancy with Cu-T)

> Felt bad about the abortion, but was happy that another daughter had not come. (34-year-old woman, abortion for female foeticide)

> I killed my child to save my life. (30-year-old woman, abortion because of prolapsed uterus)

Family Support and Rest after Abortion

Traditionally, women in this area rest for at least five weeks after childbirth. Whether women rest after abortion, or are at least advised to do so, was another issue probed in this study. In 63 cases, women reported that they had been advised rest. In 48 cases, the women followed this advice, in 15 they did not. In the remaining cases, no such advice was given. When the procedure was performed successfully, women reported that they rested for a day or two or they did 'light' housework while others in the house did the 'fetching of water' and the 'cooking'. Almost all of them said that since they had to work in the field—where they lifted and carried heavy loads—they could not afford to take more than a couple of days off. A large number of women, especially from joint families, said they had received support from their mothers- or sisters-in-law. This support was both emotional and physical, such as in terms of sharing housework.

Information on when sexual relations are resumed after abortion can indirectly indicate how supportive the husband is. According to 59 women, this period varied from 6 to 90 days. Most of them (49) reported one month and more.

Pregnancies after Abortion

One-third of our respondents, i.e., 24 women said that they had conceived again after abortion. Of these, 19 had live births, one had a spontaneous abortion and four had induced abortions. Two women were pregnant at the time of interview. This shows that every time a woman has an abortion, it is not necessarily the pregnancy that is unwanted. It is perhaps the timing of the pregnancy or its outcome that is unfavourable.

Repeat Abortions

Four of the women in our sample admitted to undergoing more than one abortion—three of them twice and one thrice. The woman who had three abortions was the second wife of a man who had three children by his first wife. The woman's first two abortions were medically indicated. Then she delivered a son. When she conceived yet again, she felt that the family size needed to be limited and sought abortion for the third time. In the case of the other woman, too, the abortions were medically indicated because she had a heart problem. However, she did manage to deliver a son between her two abortions. Irrespective of their health problems, in both cases the women ensured that they had a son before opting for sterilisation. In the other cases, each of the two women already had children—two sons in the case of one woman, and a son and a daughter in the case of the other. Both sought abortion because their last child was still too young for them to opt for sterilisation. However, they did get sterilised after their second abortion.

Except for temporary weakness and pain, none of the four seemed to be aware of any other problems or consequences associated with repeated abortions. In the FGDs, most women reported weakness and loss of blood. But the men were more precise. One man said: 'It is like a small delivery. It is a loss of her body. Women get emaciated. They lose their glow.' In all the FGDs with them, men unanimously said it was all right to have one abortion. According to them, women should not go for it again and again as it could be dangerous for their health.

Perceptions about Legality of Abortion

Although it is now more than thirty years since abortion was legalised in India, awareness of its legality is still not universal. Of the 65 women who had undergone abortion, 24 did not know whether it was legal or illegal. They were not even aware of the issue; however, 41 women did know that abortion was legal, but they did not know the grounds for its legality. Six mentioned that it was allowed only if the foetus was deformed and two said that it was legal if medically advised. However, seven of them were aware that abortion after sex determination was not legally permissible.

There was similar lack of awareness about the permitted period of gestation. When 20 of them said three months and 16 said four months, it seemed like they were guessing based on their own pregnancy and childbirth experiences. Despite living in such close proximity to an urban area, the women knew very little about the provisions of the MTP Act.

One woman who already had two daughters underwent a sex-detection test when she conceived for the third time. When the third child was also determined to be a daughter, the husband insisted that she abort the pregnancy. Immediately after the abortion, she got herself sterilised. After relating this to us, she asked: 'Will somebody come and arrest me now because I have undergone sex-selective abortion?' Thus, while some awareness about the illegality of female foeticide had trickled down to them, details of the MTP Act had not. As our FGDs revealed, knowledge of the Act was relatively more precise among adolescent boys and girls (though even they were not aware of all its nuances) than among grown men and women.

Conclusions and Ways Forward

As our data clearly show, women, at least in our two study villages, do play a role in decision-making *vis à vis* abortion. It is also clear that the majority of husbands are supportive of them. In most cases, pregnancy is not kept a secret and support from the family, especially the mother-in-law, is often sought. The degree of support the family provides also impacts on the decision to abort, which is taken after much thought because it takes a toll on the mother's health as well as on family finances. Most abortions are sought for spacing children or for limiting family size, though sometimes abortion is also preceded by prenatal sex determination. Other reasons for MTP include medical advice or a malformed foetus, the family's financial condition, contraceptive failure and, more rarely, the husband's desire to remarry.

Given the proximity of the study villages to the city of Pune, women were able to choose from a large range of providers and did not have to resort to the services of traditional healers or quacks. All of them chose to have safe abortions in either private or government health facilities, though this did not stop most of them from first trying out home-grown methods to get rid of the foetus. In this context it is important to point out that these women could seek safe abortions because they could access abortion facilities easily. Abortion services thus need to be made more widely available. This will make women feel less compelled to use unsafe and unhygienic services, particularly if the cost of abortion is also brought down.

The majority of abortions were during the first trimester, with a mean gestation period of 12.4 weeks. The most commonly reported cost of abortion was Rs 3,000, with the median cost in private clinics reported as Rs 3,000 and that in public facilities as Rs 1,500. Women paid more for sex-selective abortions which, being second-trimester and banned procedures, are conducted only in private hospitals or clinics.

Although about 90 per cent of the women had no complaints about their experience in government hospitals, none of them were overly enthusiastic about the doctors and staff working there or the facilities they provide. With regard to the abortion centre, women felt that it should be run by a lady doctor and have running water. They also said that the centre should have the necessary medicines readily available. It is clear from this that, apart from legally recognising abortion centres, care must be taken to ensure that they have the equipment necessary to conduct safe abortions, as well as to handle complications or emergencies. Similarly, there should be provision at such centres for some space where women can rest for a few hours—at least until the effects of anaesthesia wear off and women feel confident enough to go home.

We found that 24 of the 65 women who sought abortion were not aware that abortion is legal in India. Also, while they did know that abortion of the female foetus is a punishable offence, they did not know that sex detection itself is illegal and banned. Further, even those who did know that abortion is legal were not aware of the reasons for which it is permitted, nor do they know of the period of gestation when it is allowed. However, based on their own experience of pregnancy and childbirth, most of them could guess the correct gestation period. People need to be made aware that abortions should not be used as a method of family planning or spacing between children. Given the unmet need for contraception, dissemination of knowledge about different contraceptive methods needs to be stepped up. The supply of contraceptives also needs to be regularised, so that couples are motivated to use them rather than abortion to space their children. Women also need to be made more aware of the potential risks of abortion and of post-abortion problems. They should be educated about the health hazards, particularly those that impact their reproductive health, posed by repeated abortions. They should also be made to understand that abortions conducted after 20 weeks of pregnancy are risky and unsafe, and should be avoided.

Most women disapprove of abortion and sex detection on moral grounds. However, sex detection is acceptable when a family has only daughters and no son. Our FGDs revealed that, in the study area, sonography is seen as being synonymous with sex selection. Information, education and communication activities in this context need to be increased to enhance women's awareness of relevant laws. In addition, as a first step towards eliminating son preference, gender inequalities need to be reduced. Enhancing the status of women will bring down the number of sex-selective abortions.

That the decision on abortion is taken carefully after much thought is reflected in the feelings women experienced after abortion. While some felt guilty, many just felt relieved. Some women also said that they had no feelings one way or the other. Thus, while they might not approve of abortion in theory, most women are practical and accept it when they feel they have no other alternative. However, they did say that did not wish to go through any more abortions 'ever again'.

Recent years have seen the introduction of a new, non-surgical method of abortion—also called medical abortion—that uses oral abortifacients (mifepristone and misoprostol) and has to be conducted within 56 days of the last menstrual period. Research by Winikoff et al. (1997) reveals that medical-abortion techniques are safe and effective and therefore accessed by many women in developing countries. According to private doctors, many women in India, too, have already started accepting medical abortion and its use is expected to increase significantly, especially in urban areas. The question is: will this help or add to our difficulties in the estimation and understanding of abortions in urban or urban-fringe areas?

Notes

A number of people have contributed towards making this project a successful one. I thank HealthWatch Trust and MacArthur Foundation for their unstinting support. Also Dr Leela Visaria, Ms Shveta Kalyanwala and Dr Bela Ganatra for their guidance throughout this endeavour. I am particularly grateful to Professor Tara Kanitkar, who was our project consultant. Her constant encouragement and support have been immensely valuable. My thanks also to Dr Sanjeeanee Mulay who helped us clarify the ethical issues involved, as well as to Dr Shireen Jejeebhoy, whose valuable comments on the study report helped us to finalise this document.

Last but not least, I would like to thank all my respondents who, without any expectations, shared their experiences of a very sensitive and personal issue.

REFERENCES

Bandewar, Sunita. 2002. 'Quality of Abortion Care: A Reality from Medical, Legal and Women's Perspective'. Report. Mumbai: CEHAT.

Bankole, Akinrinola, Susheeela Singh and Taylor Hass. 1998. 'Reasons Why Women have Induced Abortions: Evidence from 27 Countries'. *International Family Planning Perspectives* 24 (3), September.

———. 1999. 'Characteristics of Women who Obtain Induced Abortions: A Worldwide Review'. *International Family Planning Perspectives* 25 (2), June.

Bart, Johnston Heidi and Kenneth H. Hill. 1996. 'Induced Abortion in Developing World: Indirect Estimates'. *International Family Planning Perspectives* 22 (3).

Chhabra, R. 1996. 'Abortion in India: An Overview'. *Demography India* 25 (1).

Chhabra, R. and S. Nuna. 1994. *Abortion in India: An Overview*. New Delhi: Ford Foundation.

Chhabra, S., N. Gupte, Anita Mehta and Arti Shende. 1988. 'Medical Termination of Pregnancy and Concurrent Contraceptive Adoption in Rural India'. *Studies in Family Planning* 19 (4), July–August.

Ellertson, C., J. Koenig and J. Bull. 1997. 'How Many US Women Need Emergency Contraception?' *Contemporary Obstetrics/Gynaecology*, October.

Ganatra, Bela. 2000. 'Abortion Research in India', in Radhika Ramasubban and Shireen J. Jejeebhoy (eds), *Women's Reproductive Health in India*. Jaipur and New Delhi: Rawat Publications.

Ganatra, Bela and Siddhi Hirve. 2002. 'Induced Abortions among Adolescent Women in Rural Maharashtra, India'. *Reproductive Health Matters* 10 (19), May.

Ganatra, B. R., S. S. Hirve, S. Walawalkar, L. Garda and V. N. Rao. 1999. 'Induced Abortions in Rural Community in Western Maharashtra: Prevalence and Patterns'. Ford Foundation working paper, New Delhi.

George, S. and R. Dahiya. 1998. 'Female Foeticide in Rural Haryana'. *Economic and Political Weekly* 23 (32).

Gupte, Manisha, Sunita Bandewar and Hemalata Pisal. 1997. 'Abortion Needs of Women in India: A Case Study of Rural Maharashtra'. *Reproductive Health Matters* 9, May.

ICMR (Indian Council of Medical Research). 1989. 'Illegal Abortion in Rural Areas: A Task Force Study'. Report. New Delhi: Indian Council for Medical Research.

Jesani, Amar and Aditi Iyer. 1993. 'Women and Abortion'. *Economic and Political Weekly* 28 (48).

Khan, M. E., Sandhya Barge and R. Chandrasekar. 1990. 'Study of MTP Acceptors and Their Subsequent Contraceptive Use'. *Journal of Family Welfare* 26 (3).

Khan, M. E., Sandhya Barge and George Philip. 1996. 'Abortion in India: An Overview'. *Social Change* 26 (3 and 4).

Mundigo, Axel I. and Cynthia Indriso (eds). 1999. *Abortion in the Developing World.* World Health Organization, New Delhi: Vistaar Publications.

Oomman, Nandini and Bela R. Ganatra. 2002. 'Sex Selection: The Systematic Elimination of Girls'. *Reproductive Health Matters* 10 (19).

Pachauri, Saroj. 1995. 'Defining a Reproductive Health Package for India: A Proposed Framework'. South and East Asia regional working paper No. 4, New Delhi: Population Council.

Shah, A. and S. Taneja. 1991. 'What do Males and Females of Delhi Think about Female Foeticide'. *Journal of Family Welfare* 37 (2).

Shrotri, A. N., J. V. Panvalkar and U. D. Sutaria. 1980. 'Reasons for Delay in Seeking Abortions'. *Journal of Obstetrics and Gynaecology of India* 30 (4).

Solapurkar, M. L. and R. N. Sangam. 1985. 'Has the MTP Act in India Proved Beneficial?' *Journal of Family Welfare* 31 (3).

Sinha R., M. E. Khan, B. C. Patel, S. Lakhanpal and P. Khanna. 1998. 'Decision Making in Acceptance and Seeking Abortion of Unwanted Pregnancies'. Paper presented at the International Workshop on Abortion Facilities and Post-abortion Care in the Context of the RCH Programme, New Delhi.

Srinivasa, D. K., K. A. Narayan, A. Oumachgui and G. Roy. 1997. 'Prevalence of Maternal Morbidity in a South Indian Community: Final Report. Pondicherry: Jawaharlal Institute of Postgraduate Medical Education and Research.

Tiwari, Sudha. 1994. 'Report of Thematic Meeting on Reproductive Health: The Need for Comprehensive Policy and Programme, May 4–5'. Ahmedabad: Organised by CHETNA.

Tsui, Amy, J. N. Wasserheit and J. G. Haaga (eds). 1997. *Reproductive Health in Developing Countries: Expanding Dimensions, Building Solutions.* Washington D. C.: National Academy Press.

United Nations. 1993. *Abortion Policies: A Global Review*, Vol. II.

Visaria, Leela. 1999. 'Proximate Determinants of Fertility in India: An Exploration of NFHS Data'. *Economic and Political Weekly*, Oct 16–23.

VHAI (Voluntary Health Association of India). 1999. 'The Independent Commission on Health of India'. New Delhi.

Winikoff, B., I. Sivin, K. J. Coyaji, E. Cabezes, X. Bilian, G. Sujunan, D. Ming-kun, U. R. Krishna, A. Eschen and C. Ellertson. 1997. 'Safety, Efficacy and Acceptability of Medical Abortion in China, Cuba and India: A Comparative Trial of Mifepristone–Misoprostol versus Surgical Abortion'. *American Journal of Obstetrics and Gynaecology* 176 (2).

V

Sex-Selective Abortion in Gujarat and Haryana: Some Empirical Evidence

Leela Visaria

With the passage of the Medical Termination of Pregnancy (MTP) Act, 1971, India became the first country in the developing world to legalise induced abortions, albeit under certain conditions. The Act clearly specifies not only the reasons for which abortion can be legally performed, but also who can perform it in what sorts of facilities.[1] Abortion can be legally procured in the following circumstances: if a pregnancy carries the risk of grave physical injury to a woman; if it endangers her mental health; when it results from contraceptive failure; if it is the result of rape; or if it is likely to result in the birth of a child with physical or mental abnormalities. Methods to detect deformities in the foetus, such as amniocentesis and sonography, which use ultrasound technology to provide valuable and early information on a range of physical problems, have become widely available in the country, thanks largely to the private medical practitioners who are eager to use newer technologies for diagnosis. However, the technologies that help detect physical or mental abnormalities in the unborn child can also identify the sex of the foetus at no extra cost or effort.

There is increasing indirect evidence from some parts of India that termination of pregnancy is sought not for the reasons stated under the Act but because there is a strong son preference among our people. Modern technology is thus being used to abort foetuses of the unwanted sex. Nor surprisingly, female-selective abortions are on the rise.[2] The trends in the juvenile sex ratio, evident from the 1991 and 2001 Censuses of India and the two *National Family Health Surveys* (NFHS) conducted in 1992–93 and in 1998–99, point to a significant deficit of girl children in the age group 0–6 years (measured as the number of female children per 1,000 male children), a deficit that has almost steadily increased over time (Miller 1989: 1229–36; IIPS 1995; IIPS and ORC Macro 2000).[3] Between 1991 and 2001, the decline of females in the juvenile sex ratio was sharpest in some districts in Haryana, Punjab, Gujarat and Maharashtra. This has led to the belief that sex-selective abortions are becoming widely prevalent and are increasing in these areas (Malik 2002).[4]

An analysis of NFHS–2 data on children ever born five years preceding the survey conducted by Arnold, Kishor and Roy (2002: 759–85) indicated that at the all-India level, the male to female sex ratio of the last births was 1,434 (for every 1,000 girls), which was much higher than the sex ratio of 1,069 of all the earlier births. However, there were significant inter-state variations, with states like Haryana, Punjab and Gujarat manifesting strong son preference in the sex ratio of last births, which ranged between 1,752 and 2,173. This meant that for every 1,000 girls who were last births, there were more than 1,750 boys who were last births. As the authors point out, this is a powerful indicator of the effect of gender preference on reproductive behaviour. The distortion may be due to the use of sex-selective abortions, which would help parents rid of the birth of unwanted daughters, or because parents may have decided to stop having children once the minimum desired number of sons were born. In either case, the preference for sons is evident in the behaviour of couples.

However, what has attracted the attention of many women's groups and others is that this gender bias is flagrantly aided, on the one hand, by medical technology that helps detect the sex of the foetus, and on the other, by the liberal nature of the abortion law which leaves it vulnerable to abuse. The government responded to a petition made by non-governmental organisations (NGOs) and women's groups by passing an Act that prohibits the practice of prenatal diagnosis to determine the sex of the foetus (the Prenatal Diagnostic Techniques [PNDT] Act of 1994). Under the Act, individual practitioners, clinics or centres cannot conduct tests to determine the sex of the foetus or inform the couples about it. However, despite the existence of monitoring systems, both at the state and central levels, and even with the Act having been in place for six to eight years at the time of the 2001 Census, it is fairly evident that in many places the Act has been violated with impunity. The 2001 Census-based juvenile sex ratios show a larger increase in the deficit of girls compared to the ratio in 1991, particularly in those regions of the country where son preference is historically known to be strong. Since it is easy to hide the link between the two activities—sex detection of the foetus and abortion—particularly if carried out in discrete locations, it is perfectly possible to evade the law in connivance with the clinics that have ultrasound facilities and offer sonography. According to the 2001 Census there were 49 districts in India where, for every 1,000 male children, there were less than 850 female children in the 0–6 age group. The majority (38) of these districts were located in just three northern and western states: Punjab, Haryana, and Gujarat (Census 2001).

However, we have an extremely limited understanding of many issues surrounding the practice of female selective abortion, at the level of the household or from the perspective of women who undergo such abortions. For instance, we do not know, enough about what actually compels couples or their families to resort to this practice, who the real decision-makers in the family are, and what impact aborting the female foetus has on the physical or mental health of the woman who undergoes such abortion. Also, we have only a sketchy understanding of how the interlinkages of sex-selective abortion and decline in fertility or in the desired number of children are perceived and articulated by women, couples or their extended families. The question often raised is: does the desire for fewer children compel parents to regulate their fertility behaviour in order to produce children of the sex that they want (or that societal norms dictate they should want)?

Research Objectives and Methodology

We undertook this research study to explore these issues and attempt to answer at least some of these questions by collecting primary data—both qualitative and quantitative—from women in Haryana and Gujarat, as well as from a few providers of abortion services in Gujarat.[5] As shown above, based on the juveline sex ratio estimated from the Census data, the deficit of girls has increased in these states, especially since 1981.

Objectives

The main objectives and concerns that guided our research were:

- **To determine the woman's role in the decision-making process:** A woman's fertility is not just a function of her body. It is a complex interplay of gender relations that determines her freedom of choice in all issues relating to sexuality and sexual relations. The patrilocal structure and formation of households makes a new bride's status in the conjugal family very subordinate in the initial years of marriage. This also happens to be the period when childbearing occurs. We felt it would be interesting to explore whether, even in a situation where choice is limited, the woman has some space to articulate her point of view. We also wanted to understand if increase in the level of education makes a difference in terms of decision-making, i. e., do educated women enjoy a greater degree of freedom than illiterate women? Regarding sex-selective abortion, the fundamental question before us was: does the woman have any say in the decision to have a sex determination test and/or a subsequent abortion if the foetus is that of a girl child? We decided to explore this issue by talking to women in groups.
- **To determine the husband's role and that of other members of the woman's affinal and natal families:** It was relevant to explore whether, and the extent to which, a woman accepts and is influenced by the views of her husband and/or other senior members of the family. A related issue was to see whether the woman's natal family has any influence on the decision-making process.
- **To examine the issue of son preference:** While the preference for sons is well documented not only in India but also in many Asian countries, what needs to be explored is the extent to which the decline in the desired or ideal family size affects the desire for sons and how it influences and impacts the practice of sex selective abortions (see, for example, Das Gupta and Visaria 1996). Has the desire for fewer children eroded son preference or is it still as strong? If the desire for a given number of sons has remained unaffected, then the

implication is that fewer girls are wanted. This issue needs to be understood because it has major policy implications.

- **To study the availability of abortion services and the role of service providers:** We need to look at the various sources that women use for sex-selective abortions, as well as the perspective of service providers from whom women obtain these services. Do providers feel that women are justified in aborting a female foetus if they desire a male child? Do they view the PNDT Act as an imposition that restricts their practice? For the act to become effective, and for its violation to stop, providers' views are important to gauge.
- **To make an inter-state comparison:** Haryana and Gujarat were selected in order to understand why and how similar practices with regard to the elimination of girls have evolved in these regions. Exploration of this issue will require very detailed historical research in the two states; however if some light is thrown on the socio-cultural and economic similarities between them, our understanding of the issue will be deeper.

Choice of Location

We decided to locate our research on the determinants of sex-selective abortion in Gujarat and Haryana,[6] where the sex ratio of children over time, especially between 1991 and 2001, became distinctly biased against girls. Between 1991 and 2001, the number of girls per 1,000 boys aged 0–6 years declined in almost all the districts of Gujarat and Haryana, though the extent of decline varied; in 13 out of 19 districts in Haryana and 7 out of 24 districts in Gujarat the decline was over 5 per cent or 50 or more per 1,000 children. Census data further revealed that the deficit of girls had assumed alarming proportions in certain districts of these two states.

Both Gujarat and Haryana have witnessed relatively rapid economic development. However, except for a notable increase in female literacy, the fruits of development have not been equally shared between women and men. Historically, the social and health status of women in both these states has been poor. Violence against women is quite widespread; in fact, among all states in the country, Gujarat also enjoys the dubious distinction of recording the highest number of deaths due to burning, among women in the prime of their life.

Haryana (which was a part of Punjab before bifurcation of the state in 1966) is historically known to have a masculine sex ratio, which is usually attributed to the higher mortality that women in this region have experienced from infancy to well into their reproductive years (UNFPA 2001; Yadav 2001). Two significant longitudinal studies undertaken in the Punjab region in the 1950s and 1970s demonstrated that the cultural practice of neglecting female children and delays in provision of health care during illness led to significantly higher mortality among girls compared to boys (Kielmann et al. 1983: 172–214; Wyon and Gordon 1971). A revisit in the 1980s to the Khanna *tehsil*, studied by Wyon and Gordon, suggested that discriminatory attitudes towards girls and women had hardly changed in the intervening period (Das Gupta 1987: 77–100). The expression of such attitudes, however, has aquired another dimension with the development of new technologies that help not only to detect congenital abnormalities in the foetus but also its sex.

Judging by the hoardings even in small towns, and the regular advertisements in local newspapers and magazines before the passing of the PNDT Act in 1994, it is evident that clinics conducting sex-determination tests had already mushroomed in Haryana. While no longer openly advertised, this lucrative practice continues to flourish unabated after the passing of the Act: it has simply gone underground. The decline in the sex ratio of girl children in the 0–6 age group in Haryana, from 879 girls per 1,000 boys in 1991 to 820 according to the 2001 Census, suggests that the neglect of female children, including the practice of the abortion of the female foetus, continues to be a cultural norm in the region. (The deficit of girls in the child population is even greater in the case of Punjab; from 875 girls per 1,000 boys in 1991, the ratio declined to 793 in 2001.[7])

The drop in the girl child ratio by 60–83 points in the span of just one decade cannot be solely related to the discrimination against girls that has been practised in this region for several decades, because at no other time in the region's history of census-taking has the sex ratio of children declined so drastically. The use of female-selective abortions is almost certainly an added factor. Because of their simplicity and easy availability, such abortions have become very popular.

Apart from the contiguous belt comprising Punjab, Himachal Pradesh, Chandigarh, Haryana and Delhi in North-West India, where the girl count in the juvenile sex ratio reached a level lower than 900 in 2001, Gujarat in western India is another state where, between

1991 and 2001, the girl count declined by 50 points, from 928 to 878. In this relatively economically developed state, prenatal diagnostic techniques like sonography as well as chorionic biopsy[8] have been available for quite some time through private clinics and nursing homes, even in small towns. Anecdotal evidence suggests that strong competition has led to a reduction in the charges for these services. Easy access is, to a certain extent, a response to increasing demand. Female foeticide thus can be seen as a new form of discrimination, in addition to the old culture of neglect of the girl child, the practice of infanticide among certain communities, and sex differentials in the provision of medical care in the region.

Both Gujarat and Haryana have fairly good road networks, with frequent and efficient bus services and well-connected villages and towns. This has increased the mobility of women, who often travel (alone in Gujarat and accompanied by male relatives in Haryana) to nearby towns for various chores, including visits to health providers. There are several private health or medical facilities, even in small towns with a population that is often not more than 30,000. Clearly these facilities survive and prosper because of the clientele from the surrounding hinterland.

Study Design

To understand the extent of awareness and use of abortion services by rural women, we purposively selected in each state, one district that had the lowest juvenile female to male sex ratio according to the 2001 Census of India. In Haryana, Kurukshetra district had the lowest sex ratio among children aged 0–6 years. In fact, with 770 girls per 1,000 boys, Kurukshetra had the lowest sex ratio among all the 591 districts of the country for which 2001 Census data are available. Within Gujarat, between 1991 and 2001, there was a higher decline in the juvenile sex ratio in the districts of Kheda, Mahesana and Gandhinagar, the latter having been carved out of the adjacent Mahesana and Ahmedabad districts, where historically the practice of female infanticide has been well documented. We selected Mahesana district for the study, which, according to the 2001 Census, reported the lowest juvenile sex ratio of 798 girls to 1,000 boys within the state.

Having done that, we turned our attention to the rural areas of the two districts (Mahesana and Kurukshetra). Although clinics providing abortion services are generally located in urban areas, the use of these services is also quite high among women living in nearby villages, indicating the efficacy of the demonstration effect. Therefore, from each district we first selected two *taluka*s or blocks with the lowest juvenile female to male sex ratio according to the 2001 Census. The talukas selected from Mahesana district were Unja (sex ratio: 744 girls per 1,000 boys) and Vijapur (sex ratio: 778 girls). In Kurukshetra the selected talukas were Thanesar (sex ratio: 868) and Pehowa (sex ratio: 865). For all villages in these talukas, information was compiled on the percentage of literate women and scheduled castes and tribes in the population, the number of households, the total population, the juvenile sex ratio and the distance from the nearest town. This information was generally based on the 1991 Census because village-level information from the 2001 Census was not available when the villages were selected. As shown in Table 5.1, the number of villages in each of the selected talukas varied a great deal. The variation in the juvenile sex ratio was also quite wide, even if outliers at both ends are not taken into account. Generally, the juvenile sex ratio does not vary as much as the sex ratio of the total population. The latter can usually be explained in terms of sex-specific migration

Table 5.1: Juvenile sex ratio: selected talukas in Gujarat and Haryana (1991 Census)

	Total number of villages	Sex ratio of rural population (girls per 1,000 boys)	Range in sex ratio of 0–6 population (boys–girls)	Range in 0–6 sex ratio of bottom third (Mahesana) or half (Kurukshetra) of villages (boys–girls)
Gujarat:	1,093	957		
Mahesana district				
Unja taluka	31	987	1,178–687	865–687
Vijapur taluka	56	954	1,416–691	829–691
Haryana:	389	883		
Kurukshetra district*				
Thanesar taluka	281	884	1,563–578	856–578
Pehowa taluka	88	880	1,529–564	828–564

Note: *Some of the listed but uninhabited villages have been excluded from consideration in the case of the Kurukshetra district.

(usually by adult men in search of work, boys for education or training, etc.), but it is difficult to explain why the sex ratio of children in the 0–6 years age group should vary so much. Such young children would normally be with their parents or move with them. However, it is possible that data error could be responsible for some of the observed anomaly.

After listing all the villages in each taluka in descending order of juvenile sex ratio, we randomly selected three villages from each taluka. In Gujarat, the selection was made from the bottom third of the villages, since they were closer to the taluka average on most of the selected indicators, including the distance from the nearest town. In Haryana, however, the selection of three villages from each taluka was made from the bottom half of the villages arranged in descending order of juvenile sex ratio.[9] Thus, a total of six villages from Gujarat and six villages from Haryana formed the universe of our study.

Research Tools

Although our focus was essentially on understanding the perspective of women—whether and why they resort to sex determination tests and abort female foetuses—we felt that in order to understand their motivation more clearly, it was also necessary to get a handle on the extent of sex-selective abortions that take place. We therefore decided to combine the qualitative approach with some quantitative information. We obtained the latter by listing all the households in the selected villages and collecting information on the pregnancy history of all currently married women between 15 and 49 years of age in those households. The schedule designed to collect this information was quite short and, apart from some socio-economic background information, no additional questions were asked. While collecting information on the outcome of each pregnancy that a woman had gone through, provision was made to record all possible outcomes, including spontaneous or induced abortions. However, despite our attempts to record all events, analysis of data indicates an under-reporting of abortions.

As mentioned earlier, in all six villages selected from each state, efforts were made to collect some basic household-level information and the pregnancy history of all currently married women in all households as part of the house-listing exercise.[10] Only a few questions were asked, pertaining to current age, age at marriage, education, activity, caste and ownership of land. The answers were taken, at face value and used mainly to identify women for FGDs (focus group discussions) in each village. The primary focus of the research was, by using the qualitative approach, to gain an in-depth understanding of such issues as the decision-making process relating to abortion and son preference; it was also felt that a detailed pregnancy history of the women would give us an opportunity to indirectly estimate the extent of sex-selective abortions in the two areas and get a quantitative handle on the characteristics of women who had used this practice.

Focus group discussions (FGDs) conducted with women belonging to different socio-economic strata within each village constituted the qualitative component of our research. The number of FGDs varied from village to village. In multi-caste villages FGDs were conducted with most of the numerically significant groups. As shown in Table 5.2, 28 FGDs were conducted in the six villages of the Mahesana district in Gujarat and 16 in the six villages of the Kurukshetra district in Haryana. The total number of women who participated in the discussions was 298 in Gujarat and 135 in Haryana. On an average, three to four FGDs were conducted in each village, keeping in mind the caste composition of the population. Since the two sets of data complement each other, we decided to integrate them for our analysis.

Two independent teams were constituted to do the fieldwork—one for Gujarat and the other for Haryana. Knowledge of the local language and its nuances is very important if one is to probe a sensitive issue like abortion. All research tools were therefore prepared in both Gujarati and Hindi, the languages of the field areas. The principal

Table 5.2: Focus group discussions in Gujarat and Haryana: profile of woman participants

	Mahesana	Kurukshetra
Number of focus group discussions	28	16
Total number of women participants	298	135
Average age of women	29.5	31.4
% of high castes	32	49
% of other backward castes	53	25*
% of scheduled castes	15	26
% of literate women	59	41

Note: * Includes one Muslim and nine women whose caste names as recorded by the investigators made it difficult to identify the category in which they would fall.

investigator provided orientation and training, including a discussion on ethical issues, to both teams,[11] each of which consisted of three field investigators and a supervisor.

Ethical Issues

Given the sensitive nature of our inquiry, ethical concerns were addressed right in the beginning. First, a project-specific ethics committee was constituted with the principal investigator as a member. Other members included people from the NGO (non-government organisation) community, a lawyer and a gynaecologist. The director of a well-established NGO was appointed as the convener. An initial meeting apprised the committee members of the purpose, objectives and methodology of the research being undertaken, and the suggestions they gave were incorporated into the design of the research tools. It was agreed that, initially, community leaders would be contacted and informed about the purpose of our research.. When the draft of the consent letter for FGDs was shared with the committee members, the overwhelming response was that it should be written in an easy-to understand language. The issue of obtaining the signature of the respondent on the consent letter was discussed and it was finally decided that in instances where respondents were unwilling to sign the letter, we would have to go ahead with their oral consent. Similarly, it was emphasised that any question that required identification of individuals should be deleted from the house-listing schedule as well as from the interview guide.

The orientation given to the field investigators emphasised the importance of privacy, confidentiality and respect for women's right to withdraw at any stage of the interview or discussion. It was also emphasised that while it was all right to obtain information on household characteristics from any adult member of the household, pregnancy history should be obtained only from the women themselves. Further, care should be taken to ensure that this information was not collected in the presence of other family members without express permission from the woman respondent. In addition, investigators would need to reassure all respondents that the information provided by them would be used for research purposes only and not be shared with anyone else. Nor would their identity, under any circumstances, be revealed to anyone within the family or to any member of the community or village.

As we had anticipated, written consent was difficult to obtain.[12] Putting their signature on a piece of paper was unacceptable to most respondents, even though we offered to give them a copy of the letter along with the name, address and telephone number of the member–convener of the ethics committee. They also found it difficult to keep their attention from wandering when reading the page-long consent letter. We therefore had to make two compromises. One, we had to convey the content of the letter to the respondents orally. And two, we had to accept their oral consent for participating in the research.

A major issue that came up in Gujarat was the awareness among women that some abortions (the sex-selective variety) were illegal; they feared that if they spoke about them, it would place the doctor who had performed the abortion in a difficult situation. Even though we did not insist on knowing the sex of the aborted foetus, the respondent women tended to hold back on the number of abortions they had undergone. We did not succeed in convincing all of them that no information provided by them would be shared with anyone else, or that we were not in a position to take any action against anyone.

Profile of Women in the Two States

Some of the salient characteristics of the surveyed women are presented in Table 5.3. There were clearly certain differences between the two regions, especially in terms of their educational attainment and activity status, caste composition, household type and ownership of land. However, we did not place too much emphasis on these elements, because of the distinct possibility that, had some of the questions during the house-listing been posed differently, we might have elicited different responses. It was also possible that some of the responses were interpreted or coded differently in the two regions. Be that as it may, close to half the women in both Gujarat and Haryana reported themselves as being illiterate, although during discussions with field investigators it emerged that when young, some of them had been enrolled in school for two or three or more years. However, their reading and writing skills were either minimal or had rusted from being rarely used after leaving school, such that they had virtually relapsed into illiteracy. Some of the women therefore felt that it was not worth reporting their level of formal education, since they had not acquired any literacy skills, and were therefore, for all practical

Table 5.3: Profile of women interviewed in Gujarat and Haryana

Characteristics	Gujarat		Haryana	
	Distribution	Av. no. of live births	Distribution	Av. no. of live births
No. of currently married women	1,388	2.9	1,121	3.0
Age of women (%)				
< 20	9.1	}	10.8	
21–24	17.1	} 1.9	15.3	1.8
25–29	22.7	}	21.4	
30–34	20.3	} 2.9	18.5	2.8
35–39	18.3	{	16.8	
40 +	12.5	} 3.6	17.2	3.9
All ages	100.0		100.0	
Education				
Illiterate	47.6	3.5	44.2	3.5
Primary level (Class IV)	10.9	2.8	3.3	2.6
Upper primary level (Class VIII)	22.5	2.5	39.5	2.5
Above upper primary level	19.0	2.0	13.0	1.8
All	100.0		100.0	
Occupation				
Cultivation-cum-animal husbandry	30.4	2.8	0.3	4.3
Agriculture/manual labour	33.7	3.4	29.7	3.7
Other misc. economic activity	3.1	3.0	1.5	2.8
Housework	32.8	2.5	68.5	2.7
All	100.0		100.0	
Caste composition				
Upper castes	38.8	2.3	42.1	2.6
Other backward castes	53.2	3.3	28.1	3.2
Scheduled castes	7.1	}	29.6	
Scheduled tribes	0.8	} 3.3	0.2	3.6
All	100.0		100.0	
Household type				
Joint	33.8	2.5	44.4	2.6
Nuclear	66.2	3.2	55.6	3.4
% households owning land	57.0	2.7	38.7	2.5

(*Table 5.3 continued*)

(*Table 5.3 continued*)

Characteristics	Gujarat		Haryana	
	Distribution	Av. no. of live births	Distribution	Av. no. of live births
% households not owning land	43.0	3.2	61.3	3.4
Average number of children born per woman		2.9		3.0
Sex ratio of live births (no. of females per 1,000 males among all parity children)	843		855	

purposes, illiterate. All the same, the percentage of women with education beyond the lower primary level in the Haryana villages (52.5) was higher than that in Gujarat (41.5).

The two regions also differed substantially on the question of the type of work women were engaged in. In our field area in Haryana, more than two-thirds of the women reported household work as their primary activity. Clearly, some of the work that women did as unpaid family workers, including taking care of cattle or milch animals, was not perceived as having any economic value but viewed as part of their domestic duties.[13] In Gujarat, on the other hand, only a third of women said they were not engaged in any economic activity. Animal husbandry was reported as the major occupation in which a third of the women were engaged.

Another important difference between the two states was in the caste composition. In the Gujarat villages, the economically and socially backward communities (known as 'other backward castes' or OBCs) constituted more than half of the population, while scheduled castes constituted only 7 per cent of the total population; in the Haryana villages, on the other hand, scheduled castes accounted for 30 per cent of the population, while OBCs accounted for 28 per cent. The upper castes were a residual category and accounted for about two-fifths of the population in both survey areas.

The average number of live births to women in both the states followed a pattern observed in many surveys. The average number in both the states was estimated to be 2.9–3.0 children per woman. Illiterate women had, on an average, 50 per cent more children compared to women who were educated beyond the upper primary level.[14]

This differential was also observed with regard to other variables such as caste, landownership and the activity status of women. Women belonging to upper castes or landed households had, on an average, one child less than those who belonged to the lower castes or landless households. The pattern observed among the better-off in society had linkages with the sex composition of the few children that they had or desired.

For us, the most interesting finding was that not only was the average number of children born to women almost the same in both states, but that the sex ratio of all live births was also very similar: the number of girls per 1,000 boys was 843 in the case of Gujarat and 855 in the case of Haryana.[15]

Deficit of Female Children

As has been mentioned earlier, we instructed the investigators to record all pregnancies and their outcomes, including the sex of the live births. However, the pregnancy histories collected by them show that a very small percentage of pregnancies resulted in abortion. (In both Gujarat and Haryana, induced and spontaneous abortions together accounted for just about 7 per cent of all pregnancies.) As observed in most other studies, including NFHS surveys, women's reluctance to report abortions is evident in our study as well. We therefore had to ascertain the practice indirectly by calculating the sex ratio of all live births by birth order as well as the sex ratio of the last birth occurring to all women. The results for Gujarat are presented in Table 5.4 and for Haryana in Table 5.5. The sex ratios have been calculated based on the background characteristics of women, such as age, level of education, work status, caste and landownership. (The information on husbands' education and work status is not shown in the tables.)

A noteworthy finding for Gujarat (Table 5.4) is that overall, the preponderance of male children or deficit of girls increased as the birth order increased. Although the sex ratio of the first birth was greater than the normally acceptable range of 104–107 boys per 100 girls, by the time women had their fourth or higher parity child, the chances of it being female diminished greatly. Assuming that the sex ratio at birth (without any interventions) was around 950 girls per 1,000 boys, the deficit of girls increased to almost 25 per cent.

Table 5.4: Sex ratio of births and background of women in Gujarat

Characteristics	Sex ratio of all live births	Sex ratio of 1st live birth	Sex ratio of 2nd live birth	Sex ratio of 3rd live birth	Sex ratio of 4th and higher order births	Sex ratio of the last birth	Total no. of live births
All	844	867	853	849	780	479	3,708
Age of women							
15–24	927	882	916	1,098*	1,072	732	527
25–34	860	983	841	722	824	460	1,704
35 +	799	716	839	973	730	353	1,477
Women's education							
Illiterate	900	892	993	947	783	557	2,128
Primary level	824	698	838	1,143*	788	611	405
Upper primary level	767	887	707	562	944	366	721
Above upper primary level	742	893	659	618	286	360	454
Women's activity							
Cultivation-cum-animal husbandry	747	769	822	769	539	421	1,101
Agriculture/manual labour	931	891	926	949	972	598	1,481
Other misc. economic activity*	967	1,053	1,000	1,100	714	360	118
Housework	820	928	787	772	667	431	1,008

Caste composition							
Upper castes	727	838	654	978	588	358	1,065
Other backward castes	886	883	952	935	773	565	2,306
SCs + STs	971	889	1,143	769	1,138	524	337
Landownership							
Yes	800	874	778	824	642	409	1,898
No	893	857	956	881	887	578	1,890
No. of births	3,708	1,274	1,074	696	664		

Note: * The number of women with these characteristics was very few in the total universe and therefore the estimated sex ratios based on a few cases cannot be accepted as stable.

Table 5.5: Sex ratio of births and background of women in Haryana

Characteristics	Sex ratio of all live births	Sex ratio of 1st live birth	Sex ratio of 2nd live birth	Sex ratio of 3rd live birth	Sex ratio of 4th and higher order live births	Sex ratio of the last birth	Total no. of live births
All	853	951	824	829	774	553	3,030
Age of women							
15–24	863	1,020	742	560	800	755	382
25–34	836	962	833	716	716	434	1,228
35 +	868	935	848	859	824	385	1,420
Women's education							
Illiterate	870	903	883	906	782	483	2,006
Primary level*	852	–	–	–	–	500	52
Upper primary level	815	1,168	649	482	947	404	787
Above upper primary level	854	887	934	583	–	614	185
Women's activity**							
Agriculture/manual labour	889	904	907	990	775	576	971
Housework	839	978	813	700	761	420	1,591

Caste composition							
Upper castes	801	973	792	571	686	414	1,200
Other backward castes	853	867	778	918	873	612	889
SCs + STs	926	1,067	935	903	789	443	966
Landownership							
Yes	815	980	786	573	782	415	1,089
No	876	970	858	882	773	503	1,942
No. of births	3,030						

Note: *In Haryana there was a total of only 50 births to women whose education was up to the primary level. As shown in Table 5.3, women in Haryana who enter the school system continue to pursue education beyond the primary level. As a result, no stable estimates are possible of sex ratio by birth order for women with primary level education.

**The number of women in the categories of cultivation-cum-animal husbandry and other miscellaneous activities was very small and hence the sex ratios of the children of these few women have not been estimated.

However, this overall picture masks some of the significant and larger differences by certain characteristics of women. For example, the deficit of girls among second and third children was much greater for women who were educated beyond the primary level, women who were not engaged in any economic activity or who reported themselves as housewives, women who belonged to upper castes and those whose families owned land. The high correlation between these variables suggests that in Mahesana district women who belong to upper castes, such as Chaudhury Patel, tend to be more educated than women from other communities. In addition, their families own land and they do not participate in any economic activity outside their home. Until almost the 1970s, there was no tradition of sending girls to school among the Patels of Mahesana, but this has changed in the past two or three decades. Partly in response to the demand among educated boys for educated brides, Mahesana Patels have started educating their girls. The overall assertion made by many that the sex ratio is much more adverse to females among the economically better-off population groups in relation to others does indeed hold true for our research area.

The number of fourth and higher order births were fewer, but by then the socio-economic differentials in the sex ratio of these births are of considerably less significance, implying that many women, regardless of their level of education, caste or economic status, ensured that they produced sons.

The situation in Haryana was very similar to that in Gujarat. Sex-selective abortion for first pregnancies did not appear to be the norm and was not practised, but by the time women had their second or the third child, almost 50 per cent more boys were born compared to girls. This preponderance of males or deficit of girls was observed more among women who were better educated, who belonged to higher castes and whose families were landed. As in Gujarat, these women belonged to the dominant Chaudhury caste. Interestingly, the Chaudhury Patels of Mahesana district informed us that, about 200 years ago, they had migrated into this region from Haryana, bringing with them some of their social practices and customs, which are current even today. The similarity between the two groups where treatment of women is concerned is also striking. Female infanticide has been known to exist in both groups and, with the advent of new technology, this practice has apparently been replaced by sex-selective abortion.

The FGDs that were conducted with women belonging to diverse socio-economic and educational groups corroborated these findings. Women's reasoning about the sex composition of the children was as follows: the majority of women accept the outcome of the first pregnancy regardless of whether it is a boy or a girl. However, if the first child is a daughter, upper-caste women are overtly or covertly pressured to take appropriate measures to ensure that the second or the third child is male. Although this pressure is much less among the lower castes, many have started either emulating women from the upper castes or have begun thinking the same way.

Sex Ratio of Last Births

Tables 5.4 and 5.5 also show the estimated sex ratios of the last live births of women in both states. These estimates relate to all women and not just women who have finished with childbearing. It is quite likely that some of these women will go on to have more children. Our estimates clearly show that the sex ratio of last births had a greater deficit of girls than the sex ratio of all other births. There were less than half as many girls as boys among the last births for most groups of women. The ratio was most skewed among women who belonged to upper castes, whose families were landed, who had some education and who were older in age. Among these women, for every 100 boys that were last births, there were only around 40 girls. This suggests that if the last birth was that of a boy, couples who had attained the desired number of sons refrained from having another child. But if the last conception or birth was a girl (who would either be allowed to be born or aborted), they continued to bear children until they had a son. This is a rather powerful indicator of the effect of gender preference on reproductive behaviour. The analysis of the NFHS–2 data for women who had completed their childbearing also showed a similar trend. At the all-India level, the sex ratio of last births (100 girls 143.4 boys or 70 girls per 100 boys) was highly in favour of boys compared to the sex ratio of all other births (106.9 per 100 girls). The same pattern was observed in every state, but more pronounced in the western Indian states of Haryana and Punjab, where the sex ratio of last births was 188 boys per 100 girls compared to 103 for all other births (Arnold, Kishor and Roy 2002).

Son Preference

Son preference was very evident among all social groups in both Gujarat and Haryana, even though the desired number of children had come down to two or three. During the FGDs, none of the women said that they wanted more than two or three children. They had fairly rational explanations for why many children were not desirable in the current socio-economic context—a clear indication that the small-family norm has spread across all groups and is widely accepted. Women also indicated that they had seen television advertisements on the advantages of having a small family and had also heard similar views from health providers who visited their areas. As one upper-caste woman in Gujarat said:

> Things have become so expensive. It is necessary to take proper care of the children. If we have two children, we can take care of them properly. We can't if we have more children. Therefore, we should have less children so as to manage things properly. We can provide good clothes to them, good food and good education.

Similarly, a woman in Haryana said:

> There is hardly anybody today who wants a family of ten! Everybody wants a *chhota parivar, sukhi parivar* [small family, happy family]. If we have a small family, we can manage with our limited resources in terms of agricultural land.

However, in spite of wanting fewer children, the women were quite clear about their choice of sex for these children. Their responses revealed a widespread and open son preference. In order to filter out the influence that other family members might exert on their decision, we asked the women to imagine a hypothetical situation where they had complete freedom to choose the number and sex composition of their children. Among those who indicated a preference for three children, the overwhelming response was for two sons and one daughter. Some women who wanted to limit their family size to two children indicated that they would want at least one of them to be a son. If, however, both turned out to be girls, they would almost certainly opt for a third child in the hope that it would be a boy. Though women did admit that not all sons support parents in their old age, the desire for sons was nevertheless very strong among women of all social groups. As a woman from a backward community in Gujarat put it:

> Yes, we wait for the son. We must have a son, howsoever he may turn out to be. We will always hope for a son. After all, a daughter will go away after she gets married. A son will stay with us and take care of us.

Women from the upper castes (Chaudhury in Haryana and Chaudhury Patel in Gujarat) which practise dowry even said that if their first child were a boy, they would be satisfied with just one child. The menace of the dowry system is a strong deterrent to having girls, along with the fear that the daughter may be sent back to the parental home if her in-laws are not satisfied with her dowry, or for some other reason. According to these upper-caste women (in both states), giving gifts, money, etc., to daughters is a lifelong activity, in addition to the large cash payment as dowry to the groom's family at the time of marriage. On almost every important occasion (the birth of a child, the birth of a son, marriage, the death of close members of the affinitive family) the daughter is given something appropriate by her parents to mark the occasion. The dowry payment to the groom's family varies depending on many factors, such as the economic status of the dowry givers as well as receivers, and the educational attainment and employment status of the groom. Factors such as the age and appearance of the girl are also taken into account in determining the dowry amount. In spite of all this, the fear that the girl may be sent back by the in-laws or her husband on some pretext or the other looms large in the minds of many mothers.

> There is trouble for daughters. They may find a good family or a bad one after their marriage. The times are not good. They [the daughters] may come back home. If they have trouble with their in-laws, they may be sent back by their in-laws. In earlier times, women used to do backbreaking labour, look after the cattle after their marriage. These days they don't do things like that. If there is an economic problem, the in-laws just send the bride back to her parental home. So a girl is always a reason for tension for her parents. (Patel woman from Gujarat)

> A girl requires a dowry if she is to be married. This is a cause for anxiety. Finding a suitable groom and hoping that she will settle down happily in her new home is a source of worry. (Woman from Haryana)

On the other hand, although women from backward communities and scheduled castes also indicated a preference for small family size, their willingness to modify their behaviour in the light of the sex of the children born to them appeared greater than among the higher-caste women. For example:

> Although three children are enough, if two of them are daughters then we must have another [one more] son. It is like that in our Thakore community. Because if something untoward happens to one son, then at least we should be left with another one who would continue the family line. If you have only one son and he dies, what do you do? Upper-caste people can afford that. We can't. Upper-caste people go for only two children—one son and a daughter.
>
> People prefer more sons because the daughter goes off to another family after marriage. We hope that a son will get married, bring a bride and look after us when we are old. A daughter will go to her in-laws after marriage. Some may get a good family; others may not be as lucky.

Sex Determination

As is evident from the sex ratio of live births presented earlier, the almost universal desire for more sons than daughters does find expression in actual behaviour. In the FGDs, women from all communities categorically indicated that if the first-born child is a daughter, then couples do want to know and take steps to discover the sex of the next child. All women who participated in the discussions knew exactly where to go for sex-determination tests, how much they cost, and so on. They were aware that such tests are not done in public hospitals but in private facilities, the majority of which also provide abortion services. The women could also describe the sex-determination procedure quite accurately and in great detail.

The women participating in the FGDs also indicated that when they became pregnant again after the birth of a daughter, there was some pressure from the elders in the family to ensure that the next child would be a boy. At the same time, the desire for producing a son came across as very strong among the women themselves. There was clearly a deep internalisation of patriarchal values, which appeared to be linked to their sense of security. By and large, both husband and wife took the decision for a sex-determination test. The higher-caste women also reported that they didn't even have to inform family elders about the test.

We asked the women whether, if they had the freedom to choose, they would still decide to undergo a sex-determination test. Son preference appear to have been internalised to such an extent that women had no hesitation in saying that they would want to know the sex of the foetus if they already had one daughter and saw nothing wrong with this. Almost all of them had to consult their husbands and/or get their permission for the test (partly because of the cost involved).

> We have to go for the test if the first child is a girl. If we don't, we may end up giving birth to three daughters in the false hope of getting a son. (Kshatriya woman in Gujarat)

> Women definitely get the test done.... If it is a girl they abort the foetus and if it is a boy they keep the baby. Everybody knows about the test.... The women themselves want to know whether they are carrying a male or a female child. (Chaudhury woman in Haryana)

Women from backward communities had an additional reason for obtaining the husband's consent before going in for a sex-determination test. When asked whether they would get it done without their husband's permission, the general response was:

> No, we can't go alone. We can't go without asking our husbands. Our husbands might say that we want to keep the child, or that the child may be from someone else and therefore we are going. So we can't even step out of the house without asking them.

Although a woman's parents or in-laws might have produced several children, it appears that they do not wish a similar fate for their sons and daughters-in-law. As the women explained, since the facilities (for sex determination and abortion) did not exist in earlier times, their parents had no choice but to have several children. Now they, especially the mothers-in-law, themselves suggest that their daughters-in-law get the test done, especially if they have already produced one or more daughters.

> Mothers-in-law also have changed with the times. They are also aware of the price rise. They might have managed to raise their children, but it is difficult to raise more children today. (Backward-caste woman)

> If we already have one son and one daughter, the in-laws ask us to go for a test and if the test reveals the foetus to be a daughter, they ask us to abort. (Chaudhury Patel woman)

However, some women living in nuclear families indicated that they did not always have to consult other family members for the test. It also emerged from the discussions that the decision about and visit to the clinic for sex detection were usually kept secret by the husband and wife. They would go to a nearby town on the pretext of shopping or visiting relatives and get the test done, with no one in the family any the wiser.

> No one in the family would know, not even the elders. We would tell them that we were visiting our parental house, board a bus, get the test done and return. The husband reaches the hospital on his own. We get the test done, and if need be, even have an abortion performed and return home as if nothing has happened. (Patel woman in Gujarat)

During the FGDs, we also asked women whether they informed or consulted their own parents or other members of the natal family about the test. Usually, given India's patriarchal society, once a girl is married, her parents have practically no influence in their daughter's life. In every single group discussion, women indicated that their parents had no say whatsoever in the matter. However, some women did say that, knowing how much their daughters' well-being and status in the in-law's family depended on their ability to bear sons, parents do want them to produce at least one son and therefore pray to God to bestow a son on them.

> Our parents do not say anything. Only our in-laws express their preference for sons. But our parents would want that their daughter should have a son. If she has one son, then she should have another too. For this, they would also offer prayers. (Backward-caste woman in Gujarat)

The Decision-making Process about Female-selective Abortion

We also asked the women about the decision-making process involved if the foetus was found to be female. According to them, if a woman had already given birth to one or two girls but had no son and was pregnant again, then everyone in the extended affined family would ask her directly or indirectly to get the sex of the foetus detected. The Chaudhury Patel and other high-caste women almost uniformly reported this practice. However, according to women from some of the lower castes, since aborting any foetus was considered a sinful act, the question of sex detection and subsequent abortion did not arise.

Since the test is done in the second trimester, the act of abortion if the foetus is female was usually known to the family. The elders generally approved of the couple's decision or gave it their tacit consent. If, however, the couple wanted an abortion in the first trimester regardless of the sex of the foetus, then the abortion was often performed without the knowledge of others. Women also indicated that the decision to abort the female foetus was almost entirely that of their husbands and/or mothers-in-law. Women could not take this decision on their own. At the same time, they did not express or convey any remorse about aborting female foetuses. Since these women had virtually no decision-making power, they accepted whatever their conjugal families, including husbands, wanted. They simply went along with the decision made for them by others. But we could see some differences between women belonging to higher social groups and those who belonged to scheduled castes and other backward communities, with regard to the influence of in-laws in these matters. While high-caste women had to inform and consult their in-laws, women from the lower castes had to obtain only their husbands' consent for abortion. Since a large proportion of the latter tend to live in nuclear settings, this could be one reason for the low involvement of their extended families in decisions pertaining to their lives.

> A woman cannot take a decision on abortion on her own. If her husband does not want a daughter then he asks her to have an abortion. And if he wants a daughter, then she keeps the daughter. If our husbands are ready to support us and stand by us, we can be firm and go for abortion or not go for abortion. In any case we need to consult our husbands. (Patel woman)

> There is no such pressure from the family to abort a female child. Only the wish of the husband prevails, no one else's. Even if other members of the family say that they do not want a girl but the husband wants to have a daughter, then he has his way. Similarly, if other family members want the child but the husband does not, then we have to have an abortion. (Woman from a potter community)

Women also reported that sometimes they themselves wanted to abort a female foetus because they already had one or two daughters. This feeling was stronger among women belonging to social groups like the Patels and Kshatriyas, who value sons much more than daughters. They unhesitatingly said that they would opt for abortion. But even in such cases, they would have to obtain the permission or consent of family elders to exercise their wish.

> If the first two children are girls and the third one is also a girl, then we need to take the permission of the elders to have an abortion. We have to follow the advice of the elders. (Thakore woman from Gujarat)

> We decide to go in for abortion if we find out that it is a girl child. What can the husband say? He would also advise us have an abortion. If we already have a girl, then why should we go for another girl or collect many girls? The family members exert pressure only when we have girls. But mostly women themselves realise that they already have daughters, so they should go for abortion on their own. (Woman from Haryana)

Service Providers

The majority of women in both states knew which towns had private doctors with nursing or maternity homes that provided sex-determination and abortion services. They were also familiar with the prevailing rates for sex-determination tests and abortions. Surprisingly, there was very little variation in the information provided by the women, both between the two states and, within the states, between the different social groups. However, awareness about the legal status of sex-determination tests was higher in Haryana than in Gujarat. The Haryanvi women, therefore, got the sex-determination test done at one place and the abortion at another, without disclosing the fact that they had had the test and that they knew the sex of the foetus. They also said that although the doctors were not supposed to tell them whether the foetus was that of a boy or a girl, 'it is still going on'—meaning that they did inform the women.

Based on information provided by the women in Gujarat, we decided to contact a few private practitioners in towns around the surveyed villages. Since we had already given them the consent letters which clearly indicated that they were under no obligation to participate in our research, we were pleasantly surprised to find that all eight doctors whom we contacted in one town and one village of Mahesana district were willing to talk to our research team. We were also very surprised to learn that in Mahesana town, which has a population of 31,000 according to the 2001 Census, there were nine maternity homes with an average of ten beds each, and all of them had ultrasound facilities and did sonographic tests.[16] Understandably, women from nearby villages used these facilities not only for delivering children but also for the other services offered. All the nursing homes had very prominently displayed notice-boards—one indicating that abortion services were available at the facility, and another proclaiming that information on the sex of the foetus would not be provided, nor would requests for such information be entertained.

The majority of doctors belonged to the upper castes and were from the same area. They therefore had a good understanding of the social customs, norms and economic profile of the area. All except one doctor owned an ultrasound machine, but indicated that they no longer carried out sex-determination tests and used the machines to detect abnormalities in the foetus. Nevertheless, they indirectly indicated that while they themselves were not doing these tests, other doctors in the area could well be doing them since the demand for such tests was very high, especially among the higher castes and among those from the lower castes who already had two or three daughters.

The doctors confirmed our impression based on the FGDs and the indirect estimations of the use of female foeticide, and said that son preference continues to be very strong in the region. At least one son is a must and almost all couples, regardless of caste, do not desire more than one daughter. They also indicated that the pressure on women of the Patel community to determine the sex of all pregnancies, including the first one, is quite high. However, women from other caste groups do not experience such pressure for the first child.

All the doctors were aware of the PNDT Act and its ramifications, as well as of the consequences of aborting female foetuses. Some of them indicated that the PNDT Act should be implemented very strictly and that violators should be punished. However, one doctor, who was more candid than the others, said that, while all of them may not admit to it, most doctors (including himself) in the region continued to perform sex-determination tests. When there is a high demand for a service, and if it would fetch good returns, not many people would be able to resist the temptation. He also said, 'If I do not do the test, the patient will go to someone else. Patients who come to me for other services will also stop coming. That will have an adverse effect on my work and income.'

Conclusions

The in-depth FGDs with women from all social groups in both Gujarat and Haryana brought home some hard-hitting truths. One, there is an all-pervasive collusion between cultural or social norms and technology. Son preference is so strongly entrenched, and the well-being and status of girls so precarious once they are married, that couples tend to avoid having girls. Facilities for conducting sex-detection tests with ultrasound machines began proliferating in both states some 15–18 years ago and are now even found in some of the relatively large villages.

Two, in both states, despite the spread of schooling among girls in recent decades, the patriarchal social structure still survives. Women derive value and position only as mothers of sons. Their happiness and social status in their conjugal homes is thus dependent on producing sons. Women themselves have internalised these values to such an extent that even when they say that daughters take better care of old parents or are more emotionally attached to their mothers, their statements sound hollow because in spite of such feelings, they desire more sons than daughters. In the pursuit of sons, they have become, with some pressure from their families, consumers of the new ultrasound technology that allows them to bear only sons.

Three, the shift to a small family size, evident in India in recent decades, has not been accompanied by a simultaneous shift in the economic and social pressures to have sons and avoid daughters. As was stated by women in both states, they want fewer children, but only if at least one, if not two, of them is a son. This has led to an increased acceptance and use of sex-selection tests to achieve the parental preference to have sons while not exceeding the desired number of children.

However, awareness about the illegality of sex-determination tests was fairly widespread among the women in our study area. In another study conducted in a town in Maharashtra, 14 per cent of women, 18 per cent of their husbands and 28 per cent of married men felt that women should be able to have an abortion if the foetus was female (Clark et al. 2001). Many of our own respondents also felt that the ban should be removed and couples should have the freedom to decide the sex composition of their children. At the same time, they were also aware that the requisite services are easily accessible from private providers. Government legislation against the use of ultrasound technology for sex detection has only driven it underground and raised its cost, but it is extensively available and used. However, the fees charged are still within affordable limits and in any case, as many respondents pointed out, the cost of the test and related abortion is much lower than the cost of providing a dowry and the other monetary obligations that are due to a daughter after marriage. As one of our researchers pointed out: 'The alarm bells ringing in the corridors of power about the missing girls in the demographic picture do not find an echo in the dusty by-lanes of the villages of these districts.'

The practice of getting rid of daughters, which is known to have existed in these regions for centuries, is such that certain social groups in both states have started facing a deficit of brides for their sons. According to a number of women we spoke to, some men are forced to remain bachelors, while for others brides are being imported or bought from scheduled tribes and other groups by paying bride price. We have no hard evidence on the extent of this practice, but it might well turn out to be a lesson in social integration. However, despite the deficit of women, a fact that is becoming increasingly evident, societal norms do not yet seem to be responding to this emerging phenomenon.

The prevalent social norms and practices raise a number of questions. In this context, is the passing of a national legislation to regulate prenatal diagnostic technologies any kind of effective answer? If its blatant misuse is anything to go by, the law has proven to be largely ineffective. The issue now is: will regulatory mechanisms, even if clamped at all levels or with better implementation, prevent the misuse of these technologies? Will the impounding of ultrasound machines in unregistered clinics and maintaining of detailed registers on their use in registered clinics help to reduce their use for the detection of the sex of the foetus? We believe that what is needed is a concerted effort to address the bias against girls at the source, and every action and every group that can address this issue would contribute to improving the status of women in our society.

Notes

This study would not have been possible without the help of several people. Gratefully acknowledged are the two research teams consisting of Shakuntala, Meena and Kusum in Gujarat, and Vandana, Bhanu and Vimal in Haryana. Ila Mehata in Gujarat and Manisha Chaudhary in Haryana supervised the two teams. Without Manisha's insightful inputs, both during the focus group discussions and later, while we were analysing and writing them up, the report would have become pedantic and academic. Shveta Kalyanwala's enthusiasm knows no bounds and she has contributed, with gentle persuasion and active participation, at all stages of this research. Jignasu Yagnik and Bharat Adhyaru at the Gujarat Institute of Development Research very ably shouldered the responsibility of data management. Continuous support from Sudarshan Iyengar has been very valuable in completing the task. The comments of the two reviewers have been very helpful and are acknowledged with thanks.

1. The stipulated conditions are such that abortions performed by trained doctors who are not registered in facilities specifically approved for abortion services are termed illegal. In India the number of illegal abortions may be 8 to 11 times higher than legal abortions (Chhabra and Nuna 1993). The intention is to provide women with safe, legal and timely

abortion services; however, given the stringent nature of the Medical Termination of Pregnancy Act, many safe abortions may be classified as not legal. At the same time, the availability of and access to legal abortion services is so limited for a large proportion of women living in remote rural areas that, despite the fact that it is now three decades since the Act was passed, many abortions not only take place outside the ambit of the Act but are often performed in unsafe conditions, leading to post-abortion complications and sometimes even death (Clark et al. 2002).

2. There is enough empirical evidence of son preference in India and its relation to the sex ratio of births (see, for example, Booth et al. 1994: 1259; George and Dahiya 1998: 2191–98).
3. The international practice is to estimate the sex ratio in terms of number of males per 1,000 females. However, in India, the convention has been (following the British practice, which has recently changed in accordance with international practice) to estimate sex ratio in terms of number of females per 1,000 males. We have, in this report, followed the Indian convention, since the issue is debated within the country in terms of deficit of girls or women rather than in terms of increase in men or boys.
4. The Indian Census does not collect data on pregnancies aborted, use of sex-determination tests, or sex ratio at birth. It therefore cannot provide any direct evidence that sex-selective abortions are increasing in the country and that they are responsible for the current imbalance in the sex ratio of young children.
5. We could not interview any providers in the state of Haryana for several reasons. They were very sensitive about the fact that they were violating the law and conducting sex-selective abortions clandestinely. The investigators feared that, if approached, the providers would not respond to their calls or cooperate; on the contrary, they might also influence the community to not cooperate with them.
6. The principal investigator's knowledge of the local languages and familiarity with the two regions were major considerations in the selection of the two states. Also, unlike Maharashtra, there have been no major studies on sex-selective abortions in Haryana and Gujarat, although both states historically are known to have practised female infanticide.
7. Data on sex ratio at birth are limited since a significant proportion of births occurring at home are not registered. A detailed analysis of hospital births is warranted in view of the gravity of the situation.
8. Unlike ultrasound sonography, which is generally accurate in the second trimester only, chorionic biopsy is a relatively simple technique involving a cervical smear that can be done during the first trimester of pregnancy.
9. Proximity to the nearest town and the easy availability of transport services to the villages were important considerations in the selection of villages in Haryana.

10. However, it is possible that at the time of fieldwork, some households may have been locked due to the temporary migration of the people concerned. We have omitted such households from our estimations.
11. Since all the field investigators in Gujarat were recent postgraduate students and unmarried, a trained medical person provided them with orientation on reproductive health issues. The Haryana team, it was felt, did not need such a structured orientation. However, the supervisor discussed the issues with them in the field as and when the need arose.
12. In Gujarat, a *sarpanch* of one of the villages insisted on reading the consent letter himself. However, without discussing the letter with the field supervisor, he surmised that all the doctors who conduct abortion in the region would be taken to task. He therefore instructed the villagers not to provide any information on abortion to the investigators. It took a lot of effort to clear this misunderstanding.
13. The responses to the activity question probably reflect both the societal norms relating to women's work and duties within the household, and the differentials in the field experience of the two teams. In Gujarat, the question was likely to be probed because the field investigators had been trained to probe this question in a number of other studies undertaken, on women's economic activity, by the employing organisation.
14. While the inverse relationship between education and fertility is well accepted and demonstrated in the literature, it is quite likely that illiterate women were somewhat older than literate women, affecting the differential in fertility schedules to a certain extent.
15. In Haryana, the sex composition of children who were not alive at the time of the survey was not available. The investigators failed to collect or ask that question. It is difficult to assess the effect of this lack of information on the overall sex ratio of children born to the women.
16. The other place that we visited was a rural area which had two maternity homes, both equipped with sonography facilities and owned by doctors belonging to the upper castes. However, the maternity wards of both facilities had no patients at the time of our visit. It appears that the bulk of their practice was comprised of outpatients.

References

Arnold, F., S. Kishor and T. K. Roy. 2002. 'Sex-selective Abortions in India'. *Population and Development Review* 28 (4), December.

Booth, B. E., M. M. Verma and R. S. Beri. 1994. 'Foetal Sex Determination in Infants in Punjab, India: Correlations and Implications', *British Medical Journal* 209.

Census. 2001. Series-1, India, Provisional Population Totals, Paper 1 of 2001, Supplement, District Totals. New Delhi: Office of the Registrar General of India.

Chhabra, R. and S. C. Nuna. 1993. *Abortion in India: An Overview*. New Delhi: Veerendra Printers.

Clark, Shelly, Batya Etul, Shubha Ambardekar, Ann Leonard and Kurus Coyaji. 2001. *Husbands, Wives and Legal Abortion in India*. University of Chicago: Harris School of Public Policy.

Das Gupta, M. 1987. 'Selective Discrimination Against Female Children in Rural Punjab, India'. *Population and Development Review* 13 (1).

Das Gupta, M. and L. Visaria. 1996. 'Son Preference and Excess Female Mortality in India's Demographic Transition', in Korea Institute for Health and Social Affairs (KIHASA), *Sex Preference for Children and Gender Discrimination in Asia*. Research Monograph 96–02. Seoul: KIHASA.

George, S. and R. S. Dahiya. 1998. 'Female Foeticide in Rural Haryana'. *Economic and Political Weekly* 33 (8 August).

IIPS (International Institute for Population Sciences). 1995. *National Family Health Survey, India 1992–93*. Bombay.

IIPS (International Institute for Population Sciences) and ORC Macro. 2000. *National Family Health Survey, India 1998–99*. Mumbai.

Kielmann, A. A., et al. 1983. 'Analysis of Morbidity and Mortality', in A. A. Kielmann, C. E. Taylor, C. DeSweemer, R. L. Parker, D. Chenichovsky, W. A. Reinke, I. S. Uberoi, D. N. Kakar, N. Masih and R. S. S. Sarma (eds), *Child and Maternal Health Services in Rural India: The Narangwal Experiment, Vol. 1: Integrated Nutrition and Health Care*. Baltimore: The Johns Hopkins University Press.

Malik, R. 2002. *A Less Valued Life: Population Policy and Sex Selection in India*. Maryland: Centre for Health and Gender Equity.

Miller, B. D. 1989. 'Changing Patterns of Juvenile Sex Ratios in Rural India, 1961–1971'. *Economic and Political Weekly* 22 (2 June).

UNFPA (United Nations Population Fund). 2001. *Sex Selective Abortions and Fertility Decline: The Case of Haryana and Punjab*. New Delhi: UNFPA.

Wyon J. and J. Gordon. 1971. *Khanna Study: Population Problems in the Rural Punjab*. Cambridge, Mass.: Harvard University Press.

Yadav, B. 2001. 'Haryana's Setting Daughters'. *Economic and Political Weekly* 36 (24 November).

VI

Community Perspectives on Abortion: An Ethnographic Exploration of Rural Pune

Sudhakar Morankar, Bhupali Mhaskar, Vidula Purohit, Mrudul Patil and Abhay Kudale

In the history of public health in India, there were two landmark events that impacted directly on women's health. The first was in 1952, when India became the first country to adopt a national family-planning programme; the second was in 1971, when, with the adoption of the Medical Termination of Pregnancy (MTP) Act, India became one of the first countries to legalise abortion on moderately liberal grounds.

But it is because of this Act that Indian women are fortunate enough to have access to legal abortion services. Many people consider the Act to be revolutionary, for it allows women to both avail abortion care due to failure of contraception and have access to abortion without the husband's consent (Bandewar 2001: 35). Yet today, a quarter of a century later, it is estimated that the number of illegal abortions is two to five times more than the legal ones (Ganatra 1999). Amongst the various reasons postulated for the failure of the MTP Act, poor implementation is considered to be the chief one (Gopalan and Shiva: 2000).

Situation in India

With only about 1,000 of the 15,000 doctors trained to perform abortions practising in rural areas, safe abortion facilities are not yet within the reach of rural populations. According to 1992 statistics,

India had 11 million abortion cases, of which induced abortions accounted for 6.5 million and spontaneous abortions for 4.5 million (Gopalan and Shiva 2000: 256–59). Women often resort to abortion when they have an unwanted pregnancy, either due to contraceptive failure or due to non-utilisation of contraceptive methods. Lack of access to good-quality contraceptives is cited as one of the main causes of abortion (*ibid.*). The other major cause is its use to limit family size or as a method birth spacing. In several cases, abortion represents an act of desperation on the part of women, as the physical, economic and psychological stress of having an unwanted child overrides any feelings of guilt and/or fear of complications they might experience. The husbands are often unwilling to use contraception, leaving women to suffer or cope alone (Bandewar 2001: 35).

Until the 1980s, most abortion research was hospital-based and focused on such aspects as the socio-demographic characteristics of women, the reasons for abortion, morbidity and the cost of abortion care, and was mainly governed by a perspective that viewed MTP as a means that the state used to achieve its goal of population control. The unit of analysis was pregnancy and not women who experienced pregnancy or abortion. It was only in the 1990s that research on abortion began to be conducted with a focus on women, their reproductive health needs and the decision-making process. Also, the quality of abortion care, and the socio-cultural, legal and political context of abortion became the new thrust areas. The purpose, the underlying philosophy, as well as the methodologies employed, changed. Instead of hospital-based studies, research became community-based. A new professional rigour and researchers' attempt to understand the ground realities from the women's perspective often combined to challenge the findings of earlier research.

The available data demonstrates that induced abortion is very common in the developing world, despite the fact that contraceptive prevalence rates have increased dramatically in the last 30 years. Although the frequency and distribution of abortion vary, there is no country where abortions do not occur (Axel and Indriso 1999). Many researchers have estimated that the incidence of induced abortion is increasing worldwide. The reason for this is attributed to a variety of changing trends, including a desire for smaller families, shifts from rural to urban residences and an increase in non-marital sexual activity (*ibid.*)

Research Objectives and Methodology

Abortion is an extremely personal matter that frequently requires maintaining secrecy and discretion, particularly when the pregnancy occurs through an extra-marital relationship or where the woman is unmarried, separated or widowed. This need is especially acute in rural areas. Since privacy is the critical factor, women tend to seek practitioners who offer speedy, one-time services without the need for follow-up. In such cases, access to abortion services away from home and the scrutiny of curious neighbours becomes more important than the expenditure to be incurred (Ganatra 1999; Gopalan and Shiva 2000; Gupte et al. 1997: 77–87).

In keeping with the rights-based approach recommended by the International Conference on Population and Development (ICPD) in 1994, the Government of India launched a target-free Reproductive and Child Health-I (RCH-I) programme in 1997. Since community-needs assessment is an integral part of the RCH programme, and safe abortion one of the services it offers, it becomes imperative to assess the community's needs with regard to abortion services. Yet, existing research on abortion has failed to take into account the social, cultural, economic and political context of communities in which abortion-seeking behaviour takes place. In a patriarchal setup, this behaviour is varied, intricate and sometimes hidden, but it is also simultaneously influenced by gender, social structure and culture. An understanding of the larger community's perspective is thus necessary to obtain a holistic picture of this complex issue. We therefore decided to focus our research on understanding the community's views on abortion and abortion-related needs. Our main objectives were:

- to understand the cultural meanings of abortion in the community;
- to understand the perceptions and the socio-cultural factors influencing decision-making related to abortion and abortion-related care among women; and
- to determine the perceptions, practices and experience of village-level health providers such as traditional *dai*s and community health volunteers (CHVs) with regard to abortion and abortion-related care.

Locating the Research

The study was carried out in 14 villages (covering a total population of about 10,000) of the Velhe *taluka* (sub-district) in the Pune district of Maharashtra. Though one of the better-developed districts of western Maharashtra, the Velhe taluka comprises a hilly and drought-prone area and is relatively underdeveloped, even though it is located just 65 km. from Pune city. The Maharashtra state government has listed it as the most backward taluka of the Pune district. Despite its proneness to drought, agriculture is the people's primary occupation, with rice and *ragi* comprising the main crops. Due to the hilly nature of the terrain, the agricultural yield is low. Since there are no irrigation facilities, people can only practise rain-fed agriculture. A subsidiary occupation is the production of milk. There are no industries in the area and youth and men migrate to the nearest cities, such as Pune and Mumbai, to earn their livelihood.

Velhe enjoys good public and private transport facilities and the taluka is well connected to Pune, Mumbai and Saswad. Almost all villages have telephones, although often they are non-functional. The taluka also enjoys good educational facilities—in fact, there is even a college. Almost every village has a primary school up to Class VII, but children have to travel a distance of about 5 km. if they want to study further. In general, however, the literacy rate in the area is low. Apart from some grocery stores, there are no other shops in the villages.

The population in the area comprises mainly Marathas and Kunbis—higher castes—along with some artisan castes like potters, cobblers and carpenters. In terms of health infrastructure, Velhe has one rural hospital (RH), one primary health centre (PHC) and six sub-centres, nine private practitioners and at least one traditional dai in almost every village. However, there is no medical facility or chemist available at the village level. Once a month, auxilliary nurse midwives (ANMs) visit the villages to conduct the immunisation programme.

Tools of Data Collection

The study used vignettes as a tool to collect data from the women in the community, in focus group discussion settings or individual in-depth interviews. Focus group discussions (FGDs) and in-depth interviews were conducted with 50 key informants (25 males and 25 females). Interviews with them were used to identify the community's views and perceptions relating to abortion. These informants were chosen from among opinion leaders, *gram panchayat* (village assembly) members and presidents of *mahila mandals* (women's groups).

Eight FGDs (focus group discussions, four each with women and men of the 14 villages) spread over different age groups were conducted at Velhe, the central village in the study area. Each FGD comprised about 8–10 participants. There was also one FGD each with adolescent (16–19 years) boys and girls. The boys, who were studying in Class IX through Class XII, were more vocal than the girls, who were a bit shy. In the girls' group, three were studying in school while four were dropouts. In the young adult (20–35 years) male group, all but one participant (who was a shop-owner) were farmers. In the young adult female group, one was a widow while the rest were married with at least two children. In the middle-aged (36–50 years) male group, all participants were farmers. Women in the middle-aged group were all housewives who also did agricultural work in their own fields. The two groups for the elderly (51+ years) had seven male and 13 female participants respectively.

Informal, in-depth interviews were conducted with 40 community members (20 males and 20 females) purposively selected from six villages. The sample was chosen on the basis of caste in order to understand the caste dynamics of the issue. All respondents were over 25 years old and engaged in farming. These interviews were carried out to help us flesh out the identified concepts.

Presenting Vignettes

Vignettes are imaginary situations/scenarios narrated to respondents to stimulate thought and to elicit their views on particular social problems. We used this method to help our respondents think objectively about the issue of abortion and give us their views. A total of five vignettes were presented to the respondents. These were:

Vignettes for Ever-Married Women

- A married woman who currently has one son and two daughters becomes pregnant for the fourth time and does not want to bear a child.

- A married woman who has four daughters becomes pregnant for the fifth time.
- A young widow of 23 years becomes pregnant in a village similar to that of the respondents.
- A young woman of 25, who has been separated from her husband (i.e., not living with her husband) for the last 2 years, becomes pregnant in a village similar that of the respondents.

Vignette for Pregnancy Outside Marriage

- A 16-year-old unmarried adolescent girl becomes pregnant in a village similar to that of the respondents.

After presenting each vignette, respondents were asked questions about the physical, social, financial and psychological problems that they thought the woman was likely to undergo. They were also asked to explain what, according to them, were the reasons/causes for her condition and what sort of help-seeking behaviour would she adopt given her circumstances.

Comprising two females and one male, our research team was multidisciplinary with a background in health sciences, social work and anthropology. While the female researchers spoke to our women respondents, the male investigator focused on the men.

Data Collection

For the interview of key informants and community members, schedules were prepared, pre-tested and finalised in consultation with experts. Interviews with key informants were conducted in all 14 villages with the help of the Village Health Guide (VHG). Interviews with the community members were conducted by the research investigators. The respondents' availability and choice of venue for the interview were given prime consideration.

Visiting the villages in the evenings when people had some free time, consulting them about the data collection process, and seeking their consent to undertake the study also helped us establish rapport with them. During the phase of data collection, researchers stayed in the villages and participated in the villagers' day-to-day chores—both on and off the farm. They even took part in the festivals that fell during this period. In turn, the community shared their problems and views with the researchers.

Since the study was conducted in the month of April, marriages sometimes made it difficult for us to access the respondents. Also, although agricultural work was at a standstill, people were busy completing their house repairs, making some of those people unavailable for the study. Sometimes, interviews had to be fixed very late in the evening when people were relatively free.

Initially, the women were hesitant to speak about abortion. But after the researchers had become familiar with the villagers through frequent visits to the villages, they became more open and frank in their discussions. During FGDs, adolescent girls were initially too shy to discuss topics like menstruation, pregnancy and abortion in the presence of researchers. After some effort, we somewhat succeeded in making a few of them participate in the discussion. Overall, girls were more hesitant than boys to speak in the presence of others.

Ethical Concerns

Given the sensitive nature of the issue, it was not possible for researchers to approach the topic head-on. It was therefore decided to begin the interviews with a discussion on general health problems and then gradually steer the respondents into talking about abortion. Since our study is based on the community's perspectives, we did not include the actual experiences of abortion seekers in our data.

For each interview, we sought the oral consent of respondents after explaining what our project was about and assuring them of confidentiality and anonymity. When the interviews/discussions/vignette presentations were being transcribed, care was taken to replace original names with dummy ones. Explaining the project and its purpose was especially necessary to obtain the consent of the village elders, who were initially hesitant to talk about abortion. Similarly with adolescents: only those who were willing to speak were considered for participation in FGDs.

Profile of Respondents

As mentioned earlier, more than two-thirds (85 per cent) of the population in Velhe comprises the Marathas. Their dominance in size and upper-caste status enables them to wield a lot of influence on the other castes who live there. Tables 6.1a and 6.1b and 6.2 present a profile of all those who participated in in-depth interviews and FGDs.

Table 6.1a: Profile of female respondents

Female respondents	Key informants (N = 25)	In-depth interviews (N = 20)
Mean age	Mean: 42.00	Mean: 43.15
	Min.: 25; Max.: 70	Min.: 23; Max.: 65
Marital status	Married: 76.0% (19)	Married: 90% (18)
	Widowed: 24.0% (6)	Widowed: 10% (2)
Caste	Maratha: 72% (18)	Maratha: 25.0% (5)
	Brahmin: 8% (2)	Brahmin: 20.0% (4)
	Others: 20% (5)	Others: 55.0% (11)
Occupation	Housewife and farming	Housewife and farming
Average years of schooling	4.44	1.75
	Min.: 0; Max.: 11	Min.: 0; Max.: 10

Table 6.1b: Profile of male respondents

Male respondents	Key informants (N = 25)	In-depth interviews (N = 19)
Mean age	Mean: 54.79	Mean: 49.63
	Min.: 40; Max.: 79	Min.: 29; Max.: 72
Marital status	Married: 100%	Married: 89.5% (17)
		Widowed: 10.5% (2)
Caste	Maratha: 78% (21)	Maratha: 42.1% (8)
	Brahmin: 12% (4)	Brahmin: 36.8 % (7)
		Others: 21.1% (4)
Occupation	Farming	Farming: 78.9% (15)
		Service: 5.3% (1)
		Other: 15.8% (3)
Average years of schooling	7.04	4.85
	Min.: 3; Max.: 15	Min.: 0; Max.: 12

Table 6.2: Profile of FGD participants

Male respondents				
Age group	16–20	21–35	36–50	51+
Mean age	16.62	28.75	46.44	65.08
Marital status	Unmarried	Married	Married	Married (4)*
				Widowed (4)

(*Table 6.2 continued*)

(*Table 6.2 continued*)

Male respondents				
Occupation	Schooling	Farming	Farming	Farming or unemployed
Caste	Maratha	Maratha	Maratha	Maratha
Average years of schooling	11	11	7.5	2.8
Female respondents				
Age group	16–20	21–35	36–50	51+
Mean age	16.12	27.37	39.71	60
Marital status	Unmarried	Married: 87.5 Widowed: 12.5	Married	Married (5)* Widowed (6)
Caste	Maratha	Maratha	Maratha 71.42	Maratha
Average years of schooling	8.6	5.8	2.2	Illiterate

Note: * Parenthetical figures denote number of participants.

Cultural Meaning of Abortion

Although, with the passage of the Medical Termination of Pregnancy (MTP) Act in 1972, abortion was legalised in India, morbidity and mortality due to unsafe abortions continue to pose a major public health challenge. All communities have their own ways of dealing with the processes of birth, growth, development, maturity, decline and death, with due regard for differences in age and sex (Herskovits 1956: 52). A 'deviant' occurrence like abortion, particularly if it is outside marriage, can threaten the structured relationships between individuals, family and community. To address the challenge of unsafe abortions, it is therefore necessary to understand the cultural context of the community in which the abortion-seeking behaviour takes place.

Fertility

Getting pregnant is regarded as a very important event for a woman in the respondent community. Since her main function is to provide the family with an heir, pregnancy not only elevates her own status in society, but also, if she successfully delivers a son, that of her family.

According to our respondents, Indian women are expected to become pregnant within one or two years of marriage.

There was some variation in the community's perceptions about which days are considered to be the most fertile for conception. About half the respondents said that the fourth and fifth days after menstruation are the most conducive for pregnancy. In this two-day period, not only is the uterus totally clean, its opening also becomes wider, making it easier for the sperm to enter. In addition, there are some months, like *Aashad* (July) and *Shravan* (August), and the days immediately preceding and following festivals like *Holi* (the 'festival of colours' in March) that are more fertile than others. For generations the community has believed that these holy months and days come with God's blessings, and are therefore auspicious periods in which to conceive a child.

Conception

The community did not differentiate between embryo and foetus but referred to both as the 'child in the womb'. On further probing we discovered that up to the third month of pregnancy the conception is usually referred as the 'ball of flesh'; thereafter, until the time of delivery, it known as the 'child in the womb' because it is only in or after the fourth month of pregnancy that life starts. However, instead of differentiating between the two stages of pregnancy, sometimes the pregnant woman is referred as someone with child.

It is also believed that life in the female foetus starts earlier (in the third month of pregnancy) than in the male foetus, which only begins in the fifth month. The belief that females become active earlier was based on women reportedly experiencing female foetus movement at approximately two and a half months of pregnancy, whereas it begins at the fifth month when the child is male. The foetus is considered to be alive only when it begins to move.

Miscarriage or Spontaneous Abortion

When asked about spontaneous abortion, most respondents described it as an 'unfortunate incident'. For a woman, miscarriage is synonymous with bad luck and family members are quick to accuse her of having caused it by eating forbidden food. Almost all the respondents said that the main reasons for miscarriage are a small uterus or one with a wide mouth, the age of the mother (if she is very young), eating 'hot' (heat producing) or not enough food, and lifting heavy loads.

When 'hot' foods like papaya, jackfruit, the first milk of the cow or buffalo, bananas and groundnuts are consumed in large quantities by a pregnant woman, she is likely to miscarry within the first three months of pregnancy. No woman who wants a child would ever risk consuming such foods: 'Why to test poison?'

Almost all respondents stated that in earlier times miscarriages were not very common. Older women recalled that when they were pregnant, they did all the work that normal women did. Now pregnant women are asked to rest from the second month of pregnancy and, despite that, the general perception is that they face many complications. However, in spite of such perceptions, miscarriages are not very common.

Women who have miscarriages or abortions are considered to be ritually polluted and are therefore expected to observe certain rites. This is particularly the case with some castes or in families wherein 'God' resides (i. e., some member(s) of the family are said to be possessed by a god/goddess and regarded as godmen or godwomen). These rites can extend from twelve to fifteen days, during which period the woman is not allowed to enter the kitchen or the room that has been set aside for worship. However, the period for observing ritual pollution can vary, depending on the caste. And in families where there are no other women to do the day-to-day chores, this period has been conveniently shortened to four or five days. Of course, the main advantage of this ritual is that it offers women some respite from housework.

Bleeding after miscarriage is considered normal. Usually, no medical help is sought unless the bleeding is heavy or excessive, i. e., if the woman needs to change her menstrual cloth/pads more than five times in a day. Normally, women change their menstrual cloth only twice a day. Respondents said that the incidence of medical intervention after miscarriage is rare. Medical aid is available at the taluka headquarters but, due to lack of good transport and other infrastructure, it is difficult to access medical help at night or during the monsoons.

Induced Abortion

Many communities in India place high value on women's ability to produce live children, and have their own rituals and precautionary measures to help women conceive and carry them through to a safe delivery. In the community covered by our study, children are viewed as 'God's gift': God gives a couple children because they have done something good in their past life. All respondents said that it is all right if a couple does not want another child. But to 'drop' (abort) a child or foetus is equal to 'child murder' and therefore a sin. If couples do not wish to have children, they have several contraceptive options available to them, such as tubectomy, oral pills or abstinence. There is thus no need for abortions.

Unsafe/Safe Abortion

According to our respondents, abortion is *always* unsafe because it makes a woman weak and undermines her physical health. However, under certain conditions, abortion is acceptable if performed before the pregnancy reaches a certain stage—i. e., up to the fourth or fifth month.

Although abortion is not socially acceptable, given the immense pressure that families are under to provide daughters with a dowry, the community does make allowances if a woman has only girls, or more girls than boys. Son preference is evident, and sons are sought not only because they continue the lineage but also because they are considered to be the ones who will take care of the parents in their old age.

All respondents said that women with '*izzat*' (honour) do not opt for abortion, but of course there are always a few exceptions. It is important to follow community norms and keep within the prescribed socio-cultural limits. Married and unmarried women who become pregnant despite using contraception do often seek abortion.

Most women in the study villages were observed as wanting to get pregnant within a year of marriage. Postponing pregnancy might lead to not being able to bear a child later, which is a shameful prospect. They could also be accused of infertility. We also, noted that, despite being aware of temporary contraceptive methods, women are unwilling to use them due to the misconception that the Copper-T affects the heart and pills lead to infertility. They prefer more permanent methods, among which tubectomy is the most widely used. After having the desired number of children, women usually get their tubes tied.

Izzat/*Aabru*

Culture provides the basis for the social, political and economic organisation of any society. It comprises a set of guidelines—both explicit and implicit—which tell the individual how to think, feel, and act as a male/female member of that society (Helman 1990: 131, 153). Any deviation from these guidelines is considered a threat to the well-being of that society.

We found that izzat (honour) is given prime importance in the study villages. The role of men is to protect family honour, whereas women have to exercise considerable self-control to ensure that their behaviour, both in private and in public, does not transgress prevailing social norms. Women are respected in the community if they show strict adherence to these norms, since their 'honour' is closely linked with that of their family and community. Family honour and social worth are constantly under scrutiny and male members should use their authority within the family to ensure this. For instance, if a woman or any other person in the family deviates from these norms the man, as head of the household, should correct the transgression, either by punishing or banishing the person concerned from the family.

Earlier, all transgressions were considered a threat to the family's as well as the village izzat (individual izzat was given comparatively little importance). Older men would get together and decide on the severity of the transgression and punish the transgressor accordingly. But with exposure to the outside world, the individual is gaining more importance and the community no longer openly questions errant behaviour, because there is always the lurking fear that the next culprit might well be a daughter or a son of those who sit on judgement.

Paradoxically, while abortions are generally frowned upon, abortions among married women are viewed with sympathy. All respondents stated that no married woman would opt for an abortion without compelling reasons, such as if she has only female children or if the pregnancy poses a threat to her life. Since sex is permitted only after marriage and within wedlock, pregnancies out of wedlock are not acceptable. All respondents held family izzat to be of utmost importance. Pregnancies that occur outside marriage threaten the family honour and have to be dealt with differently.

Decision-Making Dynamics

The dynamics of decision-making at the family level play a critical role in arriving at an understanding of abortion at the community level. In order to comprehend the community's viewpoint on abortion, and to understand the possibilities suggested by the community in case of undesired pregnancies, we have done a vignette-wise analysis, providing a separate abortion-seeking-process flow-chart for each vignette (see Figures in Appendix). After interviewing key informants to identify the concepts to be used, five vignettes were presented to every respondent. Some respondents did not respond to all vignettes, while others came up with various scenarios of what might happen in each case. Therefore, the denominator varies in each flow-chart (Figure). Since we discovered that the community supports abortion only in the case of women who have more or only female children, or if there is a threat to her health or life, the vignette about the woman with four daughters was also presented to the respondents of in-depth interviews (40), to obtain a more rounded picture of the identified concepts.

Since abortion is viewed as the killing of a foetus, some members of the community felt that a married woman should not undergo abortion. At the same time, abortion by a woman who has several female children is socially acceptable. It does not condone pregnancies outside wedlock; only women who are married and living with their husbands may become pregnant. The following vignettes present profiles of five women who become pregnant.

Vignette 1: A Married Woman with One Son and Two Daughters

A married woman who already has one son and two daughters becomes pregnant for the fourth time and does not want to bear the child.

In a case like this, the respondents felt that there are less chances of a woman undergoing abortion (74 out of 86 respondents). Though the woman may want the abortion, the family may refuse her the necessary permission. Since she can only have an abortion with the family's approval, if she were to end up having an abortion, she would first obtain permission from her husband and other family members.

According to several respondents (50), there are many valid reasons for a woman to have an abortion: poor economic circumstances, bad health and female children. However, in the sort of situation just described, the majority of married women would wait in the hope that the child might turn out to be another son. Of 86 respondents, 77 were of the opinion that family members, especially the in-laws, would not allow women in such a situation to undergo abortion. If the woman is living in a joint family, she would not be able to ignore what the in-laws say. Seventy respondents said that abortion is child murder and the onus for it lies more with the woman than with the husband.

Vignette 2: A Married Woman with More or Only Girl Children

A married woman with four daughters gets pregnant for the fifth time. This vignette was presented only to the respondents of our in-depth interviews. Out of 40, only 32 responded. All 32 said that a woman with four daughters would want only a male child as a result of the fifth pregnancy. Her family members would also have the same expectation. A woman is always blamed if she is not able to deliver an heir for the family; in fact, the blame is also extended to her parents.

It was clear that there is no objection to abortion in such a case because several female children are an economic drain on the family. Dowry, marriage and paying constant 'respect' to the daughters' in-laws places an immense cultural and social burden on parents. Several respondents (29) said that abortion is not a sin in these circumstances; 11 said that if the woman continues with the pregnancy and the outcome is again a female child, there will be further blame heaped on her. All 32 respondents claimed that the family and community would be supportive of such women if they decided to have a sex-determination test and undergo abortion if necessary.

Vignette 3: A Young Widow

A young 23-year-old widow becomes pregnant in a village similar to the study village.

In general, the community has some sympathy for a widow who has lost her husband at a young age. Young widows need to be supported, economically, socially and psychologically, and sometimes these needs can put her in a situation where she can be sexually exploited. But if such a situation occurs with her active consent—she may, for instance, form a relationship with a man due to economic pressures—then she is likely to incur the community's displeasure.

All 74 respondents said that the widow would be blamed if she became pregnant. Her partner would not be held responsible at all (64 respondents). However, 33 also said that such a woman could have a negative influence on other women in the village. The villagers would therefore boycott her or minimise their social dealings with her. In such cases, the honour of the village (*gavachi* izzat) was more important than that of the woman's; 64 respondents felt that such a woman would have no other alternative but to have a secret abortion. Very few (5) respondents suggested remarriage as a solution.

In addition, the entire family would be upset if a widow's pregnancy became public knowledge. The natal family might offer some moral and emotional support, but her in-laws would definitely reject her, even if the person who had sexually exploited her belonged to the husband's family. In fact, twenty-five respondents said that it was likely that family members would ask her to leave the house, while the rest felt that her inability to control her sexuality after her husband's death should be condemned.

Vignette 4: A Young, Separated Woman

A young 25-year-old woman, who separated from her husband two years ago, becomes pregnant in a village similar to this one.

It appears that the community does not condone pregnancy in the case of a woman who is separated from her husband; 57 out of 84 respondents blamed the woman since she chose to have a relationship with another man despite having a husband. They said that such a woman is totally shameless and needs to be reprimanded for her behaviour. Separated women find it difficult to get support from either their natal or husband's family. According to 15 respondents, the immediate reaction of the family and community would be that she should commit suicide. Therefore, the woman would have no option but to abort the child. As many as 17 respondents said that they would not want her to stay on in the village. Even family members would not accept her. However, some did admit that while such women are accused, the man who is responsible for her pregnancy does not face any criticism from the community.

Vignette 5: An Unmarried Girl

A 16-year-old unmarried, adolescent girl becomes pregnant in a village similar to this one.

There was some difference of opinion about whether a girl in such a case should be regarded as guilty or innocent. Some respondents felt that she must have been exploited and has become pregnant as a result. Others were convinced that she must have consented to have sex with the man; if she hadn't, why had she not screamed for help when he was forcing her to have sex? However, most (64 out of 77) respondents conceded that now that she had made the mistake which led to pregnancy, she had no other alternative but to abort unless, as 15 respondents pointed out, the man who was responsible for her pregnancy was of the same or a higher caste and accepted her as his wife.

These responses have several implications for the issue of pregnancy and abortion among unmarried girls. As 26 respondents pointed out, even when the boy is ready to accept the girl as his wife, the caste dynamics of the village might not allow it. If the boy is of a lower caste, it would not be acceptable to the girl's family and other people of her caste if news about her pregnancy were to leak out. The girl's parents or family members would prefer to keep the pregnancy under wraps and send the girl to a distant place for an abortion. If the girl's pregnancy becomes public knowledge, the fear is that they will not be able to arrange a suitable marriage for her because the prospective groom's relatives will be sure to make enquiries about her character and the family's status in the village. The family will definitely think about the loss of their izzat which, once damaged, cannot be recovered. Some respondents (34) pointed out that the community is very severe in its condemnation of a family whose daughter's 'misdeed' threatens the village izzat.

Thus we can see that while, in general, the village community condemns abortion, the severity of condemnation depends on the marital status of the woman. For instance, such condemnation is much reduced in the case of a married woman who already has four daughters and decides to abort the fifth.

Post-Abortion Complications

Several women die after abortion due to complications or lack of proper care. In Velhe district, there are no post-abortion care facilities available at the village level. Women who undergo abortion might therefore have to face a plethora of problems—physical, psychological, social and economic.

For instance, some women may experience physical problems like heavy bleeding, severe body pain, lower abdominal pain and, sometimes, infertility. If they are not properly treated, they may become very weak due to heavy blood loss. However, none of the 14 villages included in our research reported any incidence of severe morbidity due to abortion. Psychological problems, on the other hand, are more common. After abortion, women constantly think about the 'killing' of a foetus that they have committed. This guilt is far more acute among women who conceive out of wedlock, as they cannot even talk about their feelings with anyone. They are thus unable to express their emotions or mental anguish.

Knowledge of the MTP Act

Our data reveals that the respondents are neither aware about the MTP Act and its provisions, nor about the facilities available for abortion. This is true even of the village-level health functionaries. As a consequence, government facilities are very poorly utilised.

Not surprisingly, respondents' familiarity with the tools and techniques used in performing abortions was also poor. About half the respondents said that they knew of some surgery called curettage that is used in abortion, but their knowledge did not extend beyond this.

Abortion and Post-Abortion Care

The general view was that there is no real need for abortion services at the village level. Even if they were available, women conceiving out of wedlock would not use them. Regarding post-abortion care, respondents felt that, instead of just abortion facilities, integrated health services should be provided in villages. This would be more useful because in emergencies it is very difficult to transfer the case to some facility outside the village. The need for easy access to basic health services was strongly emphasised.

The Decision-making Process

The following indicators were used to analyse decision-making relating to abortion:

- Disclosure of pregnancy
- Decision to abort
- Seeking information about abortion facility
- Choice of provider
- Expenses for abortion
- Accompanying person

Disclosure of Pregnancy

About two-thirds of the respondents said that if a married woman with one son and two or more daughters became pregnant, she would inform her husband of the fact. It is customary in the villages for menstruating women to observe 'menstrual pollution'. Family members, particularly the mother-in-law, keep a close watch on the daughter-in-law's menstrual cycle and, if she has failed to observe this custom, the mother-in-law automatically knows that she has missed her period. However, as the respondents pointed out, in cases where pregnancy occurs outside wedlock, a woman will try to hide her pregnancy by pretending that she is still having her periods and may therefore continue with the ritual. According to nine out of 77 respondents, an unwed girl will also do this (see Appendix, Figure 6.5; all Figures referred to subsequently are in this Appendix), but only for two or three months. Subsequently, as 18 respondents said, she will either tell her mother about the pregnancy herself, or her mother will know about it through her changed behaviour (Figure 6.5).

Almost all respondents said that experienced women can tell if a woman is pregnant through certain signs women in this condition display, such as dry vomiting, glowing skin, increase in breast size and a distended stomach.

Of 74 respondents, 64 said that a pregnant widow will try and have an abortion as early as possible; 38 out of 84 (Figure 6.4) said the same about a separated woman. This is something such women decide on independently and may not inform even their parents. By and large, they keep their pregnancy and abortion a secret. They may, however, disclose their pregnancy to the man who is responsible for it. Or, if they do not have the courage to take the decision to abort on their own, they might confide in their mothers, sisters or some other persons close to them.

Decision to Abort

If a married woman with two or more daughters and just one son becomes pregnant, her family members usually ask her to continue with the pregnancy and get a tubectomy done after delivery (70 out of 86 respondents, Figure 6.1). Such a woman carries on the pregnancy unless there is some other major problem like lack of money or risk to her health. Even if she is poor, she will beg and feed her children but will not abort her child. She will consider abortion only if her family does not want the child. Since the majority of families in the villages are still joint families, the daughter-in-law's first duty is to obey the family elders. In these families, the decision for abortion is usually taken by the mother-in-law in consultation with her son. In nuclear families, the final decision-maker is the husband. Respondents mentioned that although all male members of the family are involved in the decision-making process, the final say lies with the mother-in-law and/or husband.

When a married woman with only daughters becomes pregnant, the family usually advises her to have a sonography. She obliges because, according to the Hindu religion, every man should have at least one son (Dawis 1981: 419, 421). If the foetus is determined to be female, she is advised to have an abortion. All respondents (32, Figure 6.2), said that, in the present inflationary times, it is not possible to raise so many daughters and get them married. The amount likely to be spent on a daughter's marriage ranges from Rs 100,000 to Rs 150,000, according to some of the respondents.

Very few respondents said that there is no difference between sons and daughters. However, they did say that, instead of waiting for a son, it is better to get a tubectomy done after two or three children. According to them, a family needs both daughters and sons. When parents die, a son is needed to perform the death ceremonies that will assure their salvation, and a daughter is needed to mourn them. Without a daughter's wailing and weeping, heaven does not 'open' its doors for the dead. Thus, people take a practical view of abortion in instances where the woman has only daughters: 'If a son is not in her fate, then there is no need to give birth to more girls.'

The respondents listed certain steps that a woman who conceives out of wedlock (including separated women) follows when she decides to abort. She first tries to hide her pregnancy by pretending that she is having regular periods. In the meanwhile, she also tries various options like eating papayas and other 'hot' foods. When she fails in her efforts, she informs her sexual partner who, if he is supportive, takes her to the clinic. However, most respondents felt that in such cases, the partner very rarely supports the woman. Men just use women for fun.

Some years ago, if a widow living with her in-laws got pregnant, she would have been packed off to her natal home and the in-laws would have broken off all relations with her. If she was living in her natal home, her parents too might have treated her in a similar fashion. However, adapting to the times, villagers have become a bit liberal these days. Instead of throwing her out, the widow's family may well take her secretly for an abortion. If the widow belongs to a dominant caste, people may not talk about the abortion openly; but if she is from a lower caste, the villagers will discuss the incident avidly and publicly.

Separated women usually take the decision to abort on their own. This is rarely the case with widows and unmarried women, unless they have money over which others do not have control. Relatives are generally not consulted for decisions relating to abortion. Kinship involvement is necessary only for arranging marriages; no one involves relatives in their personal decisions.

Seeking Information about Abortion Facility

When asked how people know where to go for abortion, the spontaneous response was that now everybody has become very clever, no one is ignorant. The main source of information about abortion facilities is advertisements in newspapers and magazines and on state transport buses. The villagers are also in close contact with Pune city, which they visit frequently. It is therefore not difficult for them to find out about the facilities available there. Also, in every village there are a few people—an ANM, a literate woman, an Anganwadi worker, the village health guide, a dai, a multipurpose health worker (MPW), or even the village gossiper—who know of several facilities. They become a major source of information for the villagers.

However, most people do not ask for such information directly. It is usually sought under the pretext that someone else needs it. Women gather this information from other women when walking to the river to wash clothes, while working in the fields, or while fetching water; men get it during gossip sessions with friends.

All respondents stated that information about abortion facilities includes the name of the clinic and the time and money required for the procedure.

Choice of Provider

The choice of provider is an important indicator of the decision-making process for abortion. Apparently, about 20–25 years ago, abortions were carried out in the village itself which was risky, both for the abortion seeker and the abortion provider. Now that modern medical facilities are within easy reach, there is no traditional method used for abortion in the district. Most were of the opinion that a married woman wanting an abortion will probably go to the government hospital. Since the abortion is her family's decision, she can do this openly. The lengthy procedures followed in government hospitals also do not pose a problem; she does not have anything to hide and the abortion does not need to be done hurriedly. But if the woman comes from a rich family or if her family is concerned about her health, she will choose a private clinic.

On the other hand, widows, and separated or unwed women prefer to use private clinics. Since their pregnancy is socially unacceptable, secrecy is of paramount importance. Women who conceive out of wedlock also use private facilities, and the farther away they are the better. Such clinics offer very quick services with minimum or no paperwork. They also do not require follow-up visits. Using some plausible excuse to explain her absence from the village, a woman can thus visit the clinic in the morning and be back home by the evening.

Expenses for Abortion

Cost is an important consideration while taking a decision about abortion. Married women use a nearby place, such as the government hospital, where the charges are not very high. Abortion is often delayed if the family is economically constrained or if the money cannot be raised in time. However, if the woman already has several daughters, or if the pregnancy is an unsanctioned one, no thought is given to expenses. Particularly in the latter case, the women (or their families) take loans or pawn jewellery and vessels to manage the expenses, because, while getting rid of the unwanted pregnancy is important, of even more importance is that this be done secretly. To maintain secrecy, they are willing to spend any amount of money.

Accompanying Person

Because there is no secrecy involved, it is the mother-in-law who usually accompanies a married woman seeking abortion. However, our question about who accompanies women aborting an out-of-wedlock pregnancy elicited varied responses. According to the majority of respondents, it is the parents who accompany the woman in cases of socially unsanctioned pregnancies, although they may do so under the pretext of visiting relatives. According to other respondents, a woman in such circumstances would have to go either alone or with some close female relative like an elder sister or aunt. Another option mentioned was the male partner responsible for the pregnancy.

Cultures are never static; influenced by other groups and cultures, they are in a state of constant flux (Jha 1994: 69). This is certainly true of our study area. Earlier, abortion and pregnancy outside marriage were strongly stigmatised and the transgressor was usually rejected by the family and the community. With the passage of time, and especially with the proliferation of nuclear families, the strong sense of communal belonging has become diluted and has been replaced by a more individualistic outlook. So long as it is not done openly, even an abortion outside marriage is accepted, albeit reluctantly. The attitude now is: 'These days, everything is permitted. It has happened to someone else today. What if tomorrow it happens in our family?'

Table 6.3 Community's understanding of abortion

Variables	Vignettes: Married woman with 1 son and 2 daughters	Married woman with 4 daughters	Widow	Separated woman	Unwed woman
Blame for pregnancy	No	Female foetus	Yes	Yes	Yes
'Izzat'	—	*	****	*****	****
Community approval for abortion	Apathy	Yes Sympathy	Yes Strong stigma	Yes Strong stigma	Yes Strong stigma Little sympathy
Final decision-maker for abortion	Mother-in-law/Husband	Mother-in-law/Husband	Self/ Parents	Self	Self/ Parents
Providers	Govt or private	Private and/or govt	Private	Private	Private
Consideration of economic affordability for abortion	Yes	?	No	No	No
Secrecy maintained	No	No	Yes	Yes	Yes
Accompanying person	Mother-in-law	Mother-in-law	Parents/Sister/ Aunt/Partner	Alone/Partner/ Friend	Parents/ Aunt/Partner

Notes: ***** Indicates maximum threat to Izzat and '—'indicates no threat; '?' means that there is no economic consideration for sex determination, but for abortion government facilities may be used.

Village-level Providers' Perceptions of Abortion and Abortion Care

The MTP Act permits abortion under a broad range of social and medical conditions: if the woman's life is at risk; when her mental and physical health need to be preserved; when the pregnancy is the result of rape or incest; when the foetus is impaired; and when there is contraceptive failure. Except in the case of medical emergency, abortions are legally allowed only within the first 20 weeks of pregnancy and must be performed by a registered physician in a government facility or in a facility approved by the government. In contravention of these conditions, it has been shown that about 90 per cent of induced abortions take place at other than registered institutions. According to a community-based study in rural Maharashtra, abortions take place mostly in the private sector (Ganatra 1999). To explore the community's perceptions about abortion and abortion-related care, it is therefore necessary to take into account perceptions of health functionaries.

The providers covered by our research are village-level health care providers. Six dais, one male community health volunteer (CHV), one private practitioner (an ayurveda doctor) and two ANMs were interviewed as key informants.

Need for Abortion

All six dais said that married women, barring those who have only daughters, should not have abortions. All of them believe that abortion is '*bal hatya*' (child murder) or '*bhruna* [foetus] hatya'. They were also very clear about the fact that they are *facilitators for childbirth*, not for abortion. They admitted that although, until about 15 or 20 years ago, they did perform abortions, this was very rare. But now that medical facilities are available, there is no need for them to do so. According to them, in the first two months of pregnancy the embryo is just a ball of flesh. It is only by the end of fourth or fifth month that life starts in an embryo. So, if abortion is the only alternative, it is better to have it by the fourth month.

The private practitioner and government health functionaries were more concerned with the reasons for abortion than with its socio-cultural aspects. Government providers mentioned that if a married woman wants to undergo an abortion due to contraceptive failure, then she must immediately adopt some contraceptive measure after the procedure. They pointed out that, in villages, daughters-in-law do not have any say in the family. It is therefore very difficult for them to adopt any family-planning method. Sometimes, due to the heavy load of household work, women do not get the time to visit the hospital and find out what family-planning methods are available, and they are too shy to ask others about contraceptives. Both the private and government health care providers corroborated that there *are* a few cases of abortion outside wedlock in the villages and they all go to a nearby town for abortion. Because of the need for secrecy, such cases rarely come to them. They too felt that abortion must be carried out within the third or fourth month of pregnancy because after that there are chances of complications.

According to all the functionaries we interviewed, the major reasons for abortion are poverty, female children, a threat to the health of the expectant mother and pregnancies outside wedlock.

Methods of Abortion

In the days when abortions were conducted in the village, the dais said they would tie a *neem* stick to a length of string and insert it into the uterus. Although they have heard about curettage, they have no knowledge of the modern methods used by doctors.

The private practitioner and government health care providers also stated that Dilation and Curettage (D&C) is the most widely used method. Some of them are aware of other methods, but cannot use them due to the non-availability of the requisite facilities in the area.

Safety of Abortion

Dais stated that abortion is never safe because it is a forced procedure, like squeezing pulp from a raw mango. The private practitioner and government health care providers were more realistic. They said that abortions carried out after the fourth month could be risky. They also cautioned that abortion seekers need to take proper care in order to avoid post-abortion complications like heavy and continuous bleeding, low backache and problems of the uterus.

Knowledge of MTP Act

Knowledge about the MTP Act among the providers appears to be very poor. Dais knew nothing about the Act, but they were aware that sex-selective abortions are legally prohibited. Their source of this knowledge was television. None of the providers had any accurate information about the legal aspects of abortion, though the ANMs did know a bit more than the others. The private practitioner could not even say which methods are available for abortion.

It is clear from our data that, more than those of the other health providers; the views of traditional dais on abortion seem to coincide with those of the members of the community. This is not surprising, considering that dais belong to the same milieu and share the same cultural beliefs.

Summing Up

In most parts of India, and certainly in the Velhe district, sexual relations are permitted only after marriage and only with the spouse. There is also a strong belief that a woman should become pregnant within a year or two of marriage and provide the family with an heir. Since knowledge about the father's identity is essential for social approval, the social stigma associated with out-of-wedlock pregnancies is very strong. Blame is usually attached to the woman, who is castigated for breaking community norms and seeking sexual relations outside of marriage. Given the high premium placed on 'izzat', even her family is unwilling to support her. She is therefore left with only two alternatives: leave the village or secretly terminate the pregnancy. Secret abortions are therefore a mode of social survival.

One reason for the low use of contraceptive measures is the excessive pressure the community puts on women to prove their fertility soon after marriage. This is compounded by the fact that there seem to be several misguided notions about contraceptives. For instance, people believe that the Copper-T causes heart problems and oral pills lead to infertility. The refusal to use temporary contraceptives means that there is less spacing between children.

When a married woman gets pregnant she occupies a special place in the community, which celebrates her pregnancy with several rituals that have a special significance in recognising woman's transition from a wife to a mother. Well-wishers in the community also help the woman avail the nutritional and emotional support she requires during this transition. Family members have begun to pay more attention to women's health, particularly during pregnancy. This may due to the advent of various national programmes such as RCH and the Integrated Child Development Scheme (ICDS), which have made women more conscious of their health needs.

The community also advocates certain precautions that help carry a woman through to a safe delivery. The main one is to restrict the pregnant woman's consumption of 'hot' food. For generations, 'hot' foods have been considered harmful during pregnancy. It is believed that consuming food like papaya, banana, and millet during pregnancy leads to miscarriage. Caught as they are in the transition from traditional to modern, younger women, though not quite subscribing to this belief, are nevertheless hesitant to risk flouting it.

While not condoning abortion, the community does make some concessions in certain circumstances, particularly if a woman has a large number of daughters or only daughters. Since girls are viewed as a drain on the family's financial resources, such women are permitted to have an abortion, provided the foetus is determined to be a female. A community-based study done in Punjab (Nayar 2002: 39) also points out that the practice of female foeticide has the approval of the general public, the leaders, health workers and doctors. It seems that there is not much variation in how sex-selective abortions are viewed at the all-India level.

Out-of-wedlock pregnancies are viewed with disfavour. However, there is some sympathy for widows, since they are seen as having been cheated of their husbands by a trick of fate. Premarital sex is also frowned upon. However, considering their youth and innocence, and the likelihood that they may have been duped by some man, unmarried girls are viewed somewhat sympathetically by the community. But women who have separated from their husbands and have sexual relations with other men are a different kettle of fish. The community has a very negative attitude towards them, particularly if they get pregnant. To avoid suffering public humiliation, such women opt to have their pregnancy terminated in secret.

Still, there is some indication that our study community has begun to recognise that as human beings, everyone needs some measure of emotional and sexual support. It is perhaps this recognition that prompted respondents to suggest that a widow should be allowed to remarry, that a separated woman should return to her husband or divorce him and get married to the man of her choice, and that unmarried girls should get married. A study conducted by CEHAT (Gupte et al. 1994–96) reports that women had secret abortions to avoid the stigma attached to pregnancies due to sex outside marriage.

There is a high degree of correlation between the community's attitude to abortion and the decisions relating to it. As has been pointed out, the community supports abortion in the case of a married woman who has many or only female children. Since such a woman would have an abortion not for her own but her family's sake, her behaviour is considered to be well within societal norms. Since abortion among married women does not have to be hidden, expense is an important consideration in the choice of provider. A nearby facility—government or private—that is affordable is generally preferred. In such cases, the decision-making process for abortion is less complicated and therefore not likely to cause much mental stress to the woman or her family.

Where pregnancies out of wedlock are concerned, both the decision-making process and the abortion are kept secret. In such cases, women tend to choose a facility that is far away and offers quick service and confidentiality. Given the immense pressure to maintain secrecy, cost considerations are not important. However, since pregnancy and abortion outside wedlock threaten the family and village izzat, socio-cultural factors like village honour, personal and family humiliation, and social survival play a major role in the decision-making process.

At the village level, health care is provided by CHVs, ANMs and traditional dais. ANMs and CHVs are more programme-oriented and view abortion as merely a medical procedure. However, the providers covered by us did not play any specific role in providing abortion services. While the ANMs and CHVs are at least aware of the existence of the MTP Act, the dais are clearly influenced by the prevailing social and cultural norms. All providers we interviewed are against having abortion services in the villages. They feel that such services might increase the incidence of unwanted pregnancies, including pregnancies outside marriage.

Appendix

Figure 6.1: Abortion-seeking process of a married woman with one son, two daughters

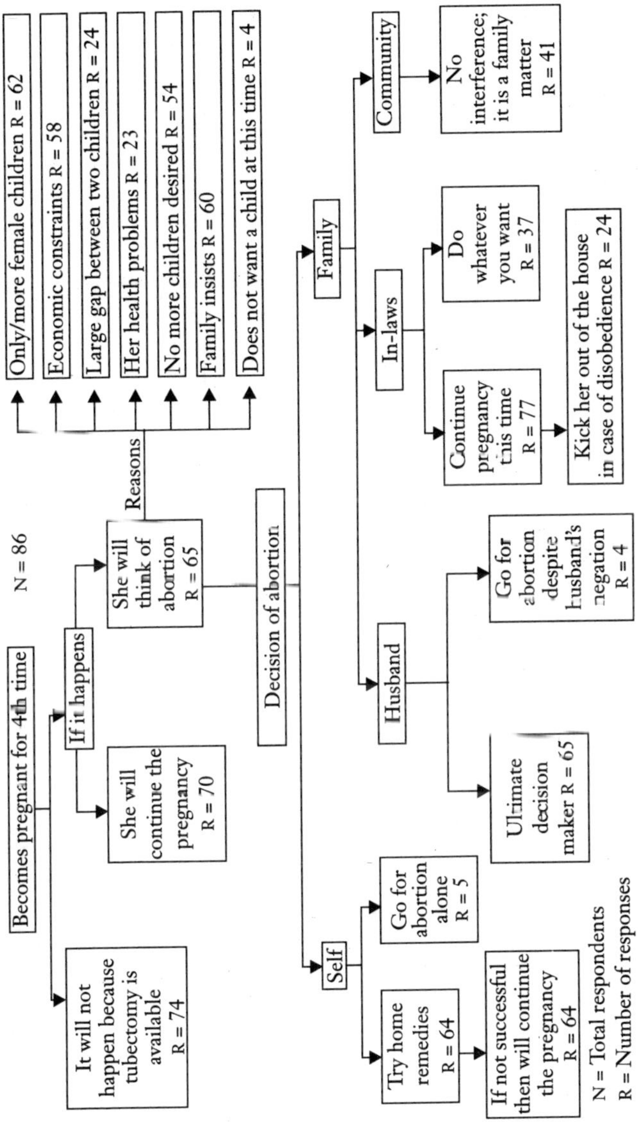

Figure 6.2: Abortion-seeking process of a woman with four daughters

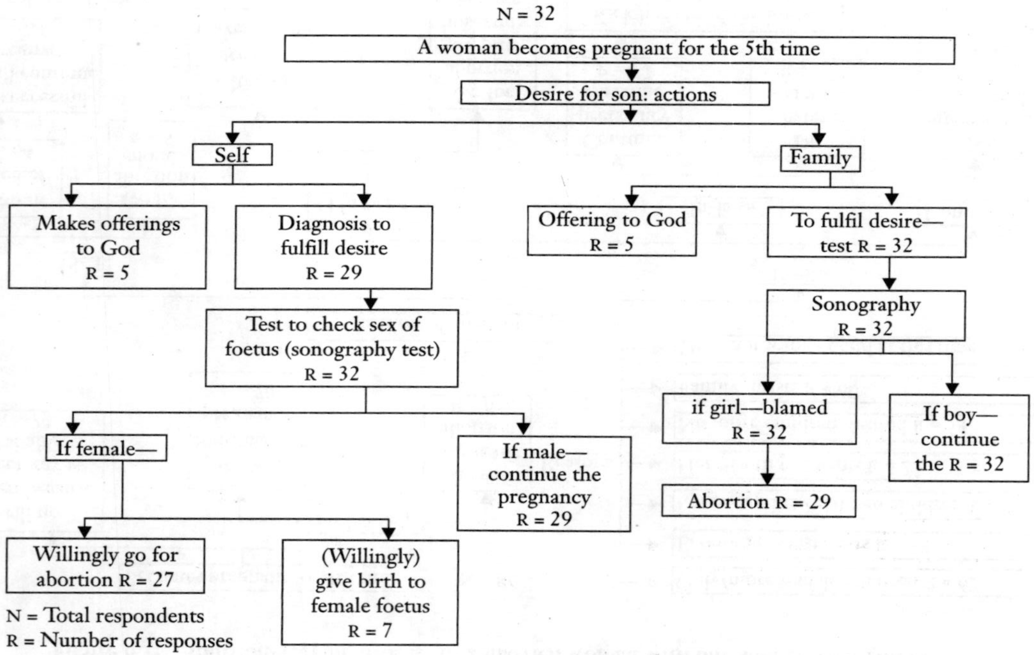

Figure 6.3: Abortion-seeking process: a widow

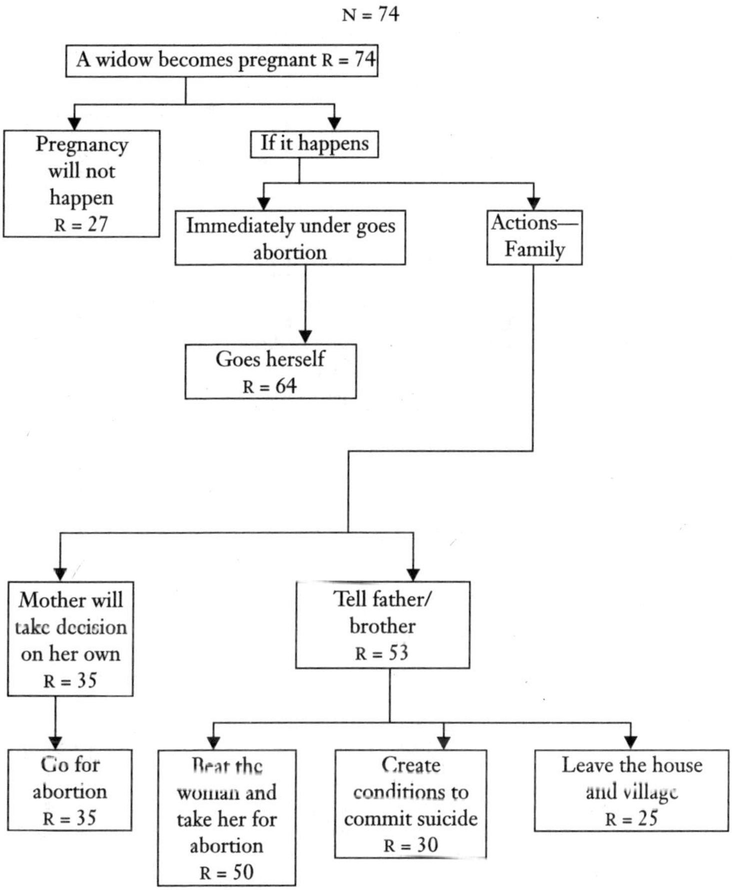

N = Total respondents
R = Number of responses

Figure 6.4: Abortion-seeking process of a separated woman

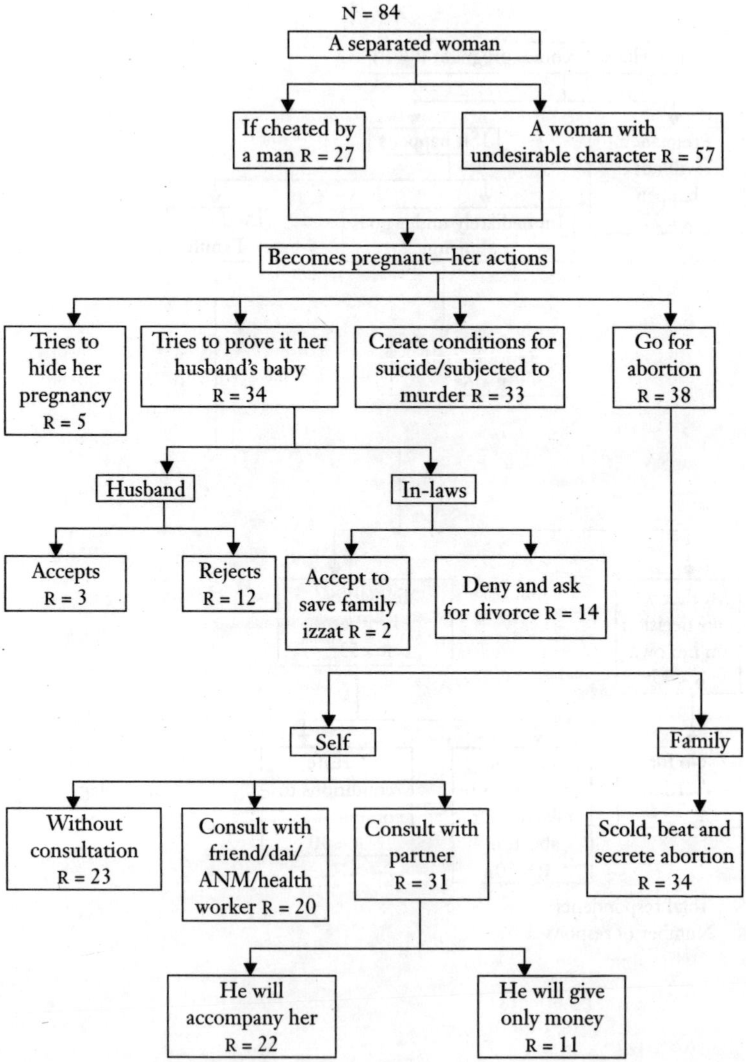

N = Total respondents
R = Number of responses

Figure 6.5: Abortion-seeking process of an unmarried girl

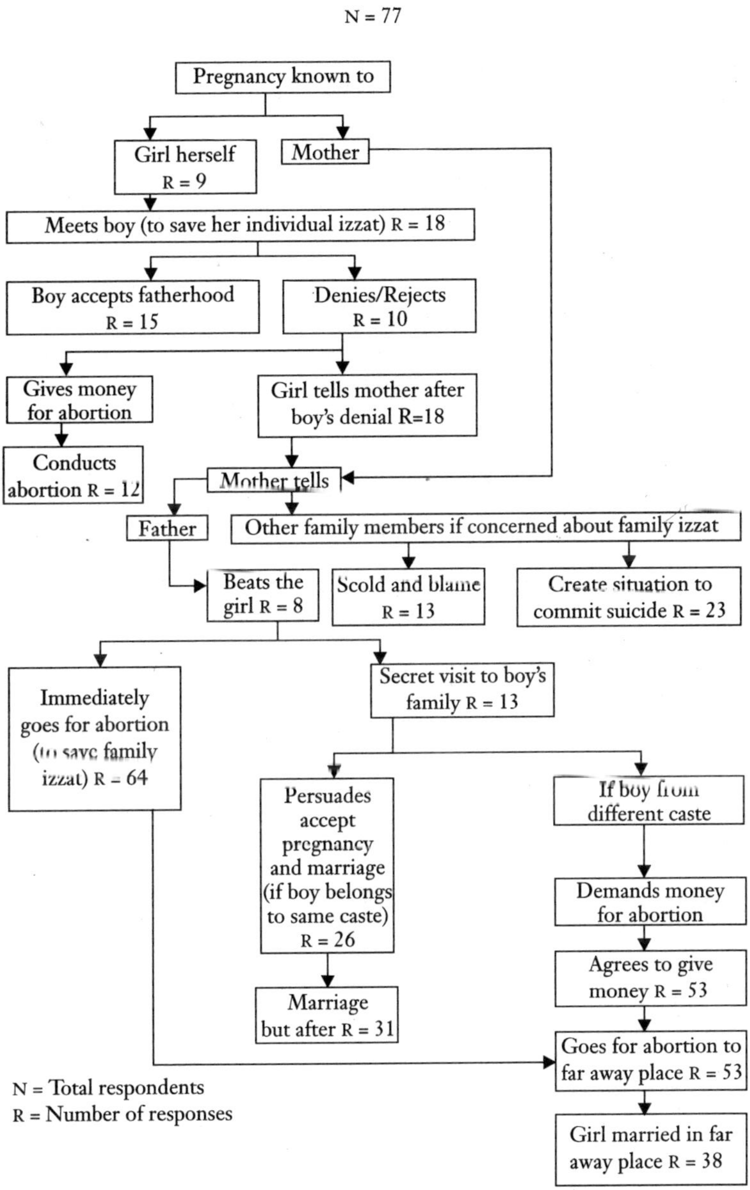

Notes

This project would not have been possible without the active support of several people. We gratefully acknowledge their invaluable contribution and apologise for not being able include all the names here.

Our heartfelt thanks to Professor R. K. Mutatkar and Dr B. V. Bhanu for their constant support and guidance during the course of this study; Dr Bela Ganatra, Siddhivinayak Hirve, Hemant Apte, Sunita Bandewar and Professor Pelto for their expert advice; and Dr Sudha Tewari and Dr Mala Ramanathan for reviewing the draft report.

Shri Kaka Vaidya, Sau. Nirmala Hande, Sau. Parvati Jadhav, Sau. Malan Jadhav and Uma Dhavale, who introduced the researchers to the community and supported us during data collection. We could not have managed without you!

To Neelam Joshi and Reshma Shende, who helped in transcribing and translating taped data, and to Ujwala Tapadia and Vinayak Amle for their efficient administrative support, our deepest appreciation and thanks.

We are also grateful to Dr Leela Visaria and Ms Shveta Kalyanwala of HealthWatch India for all their administrative and technical support. We are especially grateful to HealthWatch India, New Delhi, for giving us the financial support to carry out the study. We would also like to place on record our thanks to Aalochana and CEHAT for providing us with library support and our colleagues at MAAS–CHRD, who supported us constantly and in other ways.

And last but not least, a big 'thank-you' to all the people from 14 villages who participated in the research: without you there would be no study!

References

Bandewar, Sunita. 2001. 'Unsafe Abortions'. *Health Panorama* 2.

Datta, B. 2002. *What About Us? Bringing Infertility into Reproductive Health Care*. New York: Population Council.

Dawis, K. 1981. *Human Society*. Delhi: Surgit Publications.

Ganatra, B. R., S. S. Hirve, S. Walawalkar, L. Garda and V. N. Rao. 1996. 'Induced Abortions in Rural Community in Western Maharashtra: Prevalence and Patterns'. Abstract included in D. Vasundhara, R. Shah and G. Misra (eds). 2000. *Abortion in India: An Annotated Bibliography of Selected Studies, 1990–2000*. New Delhi: Creating Resources for Empowerment Action (CREA).

Ganatra, B. R. 1999. 'Induced Abortions Among Adolescents Girls in Rural Maharashtra'. Ford Foundation working paper.

Gopalan, S. and M. Shiva (eds). 2000. *National Profile on Women, Health and Development: Country Profile—India*. New Delhi: Voluntary Health Association of India and the World Health Organisation.

Gupte, Manisha, Sunita Bandewar and Hemlata Pisal. 1994–96. 'Women's Perspective on the Quality of Health and Reproductive Health Care: Evidence from Rural Maharashtra'. Abstract included in D. Vasundhara, R. Shah and G. Misra (eds). 2000. *Abortion in India: An Annotated Bibliography of Selected Studies, 1990–2000*. New Delhi: CREA.

Gupte, M., S. Bandewar and H. Pisal. 1997. 'Abortion Needs of Women in India: A Case Study of Rural Maharashtra'. *Reproductive Health Matters* 9.

Helman, C. 1990. *Culture, Health and Illness: An Introduction for Health Professionals*. Oxford: Butterworth Heinemann.

Herskovits, M. 1956. *Man and His Works: The Science of Cultural Anthropology*. New York: Alfred A. Knopf.

Jha, Makhan. 1994. *An Introduction to Social Anthropology*. New Delhi: Vikas.

Mundigo, Axel and Cynthia Indriso. 1999. *Abortions in the Developing World*. New Delhi: Vistaar Publications.

Nayar, U. 2002. 'Doomed Before Birth: Study of Declining Sex Ratio in the Age Group 0–6 Years in Selected Districts of Punjab and Haryana'. Abstract included in D. Vasundhara, R. Shah and G. Misra (eds). 2002. *Abortion in India: An Annotated Bibliography of Selected Studies, 1990–2000*. New Delhi: CREA.

VII

Post-Abortion Care in the Public Health System

M. Prakasamma

Roughly 15 per cent of annual maternal deaths that occur in India are due to unsafe abortions (Johnson 1999). Most of these take place because of low-quality abortion services and poor post-abortion care leading to bleeding, infection and sepsis. Almost all these deaths are preventable.

Despite a reasonably flexible Medical Termination of Pregnancy (MTP) Act, most abortions in India are performed outside the legal and public health system, resulting in a high number of unrecorded and unsafe abortions (ICMR 1989; Mathai 1998; United Nations 1993). It is estimated that 13 per cent of all illegal abortions worldwide occur in India (WHO 1991). Although the country saw a five-fold increase in the number of institutions offering MTP services between 1972 and 1997, the number of MTPs (1.4 per cent) performed in these facilities did not witness a proportionate rise. In addition, most of these facilities lacked the functional equipment and the trained manpower—or both—to provide MTP services (Chhabra and Nuna 1994: 244–47).

The principal reason for induced abortion in a marital situation is unwanted pregnancy. The other reasons are health problems, financial constraints and marital status (Barge et al. 1997; Jejeebhoy 1998: 1275–90; Sinha et al. 1998). Most abortions that married women under-go are due to poor awareness and inadequate contraception-related services (Gupte et al. 1997: 77–86). The decision to undergo abortion or continue pregnancy is often made not by the woman herself but by other family members—husband, mother, mother-in-law or others. The socio-cultural and gender factors associated with abortions out of wedlock further complicate access to services, due to the need for confidentiality.

The most recognised, frequently occurring complications arising from unsafe abortions in India are: pelvic infection followed by sepsis, incomplete abortion, haemorrhage, and uterine and cervical injuries (Barge et al. 1997; Greenslade et al. 1994: 1–4; Kerrigan et al. 1995; Maitra 1998). These can be tackled with the help of carefully planned post-abortion services delivered through an efficient outreach and referral system. Peripheral health services (village, sub-centre and primary health centre [PHC]) are unable to deliver post-abortion follow-up care to women who undergo abortion in their area. The poor coordination between primary and secondary health systems and the poor linkages between public and private services do not facilitate such service. In fact, abortions are frequently unrecorded.

The role of peripheral health workers such as the auxiliary nurse midwife (ANM) in the provision of abortion services is generally limited to referral and follow-up of abortion cases. They are not trained to perform abortions even in early pregnancy. In addition, because ANMs do not usually live in the villages they serve, women are hesitant to seek their services for abortion. They prefer to approach illegal providers who are easily accessible or, if they can afford it, go to private clinics and hospitals. The potential of mid-level and peripheral service providers in abortion care thus needs to be re-examined and expanded, and the access to and the quality of abortion services in both the public and private sectors improved. In addition, safe and easy-to-use abortion technology needs to be piloted and promoted in outreach areas, to improve access and to reduce the hazards of unsafe abortion.

This is easier said than done. Before initiating any interventions, it is critical to first identify and examine both the perspectives of and the problems faced by women who have undergone abortion in government hospitals and assess the coverage and quality of post-abortion services that they received. It is equally essential to look at the practices of and problems encountered by service providers in delivering abortion-related services, as well as to understand their perception of clients and the issue of abortion in general.

Research Objectives, Questions and Methodology

Aims and Objectives

We undertook a study of abortion-related issues in Medak district of Andhra Pradesh. Our main objectives were:

- To assess post-abortion follow-up services provided to women who have undergone abortion in a government hospital
- To assess the profile, perceptions and problems of women undergoing abortions in government hospitals
- To identify women in a selected community who had abortions within a year prior to commencement of research and assess the services they received from the public health system
- To assess the perceptions, practices and problems of service providers: doctors, nurses, ANMs and others

While interacting with the women, we sought to determine the following:

- Do they receive post-abortion care and counselling from public health providers?
- How many of them access the services of ANMs or other service providers, and what is the content and quality of these services?
- What are the factors that hinder them from actively seeking the help of public health service providers during and after abortion?
- What do they expect from service providers in relation to abortion and post-abortion care?
- What are the economic and health consequences when they cannot access services from the public health system?

From the providers of abortion services, we tried to elicit views on the following issues:

- How sensitive is the health system in general and service providers in particular to gender concerns such as confidentiality, decision to seek abortion, and privacy?
- What factors hinder the provision of post-abortion service by ANMs and other service providers and what needs to be done to improve the provision of post-abortion care and counselling?

- In their perception, how is postnatal care different from post-abortion care? Are women treated differently depending on what kind of care they require?
- What, according to the providers, is the relationship between abortion, MTP and family-planning acceptance?

For the purposes of our study we defined *post-abortion care* to include assessment and management of complications following abortion, post-abortion family planning counselling, and provision of support to the women and their families. The *post-abortion follow-up period* was defined to cover a period of six months after abortion. *Service providers* denoted all those who had a role in providing services either in the selected hospital or in the villages covered by the selected PHC. They included doctors, nurses, ANMs, female health supervisors and public health nurses.

Location

Our research was conducted in Medak, a backward and predominantly rural district of Andhra Pradesh. With a population of 2.65 million, the literacy rate in the district is lower than the national- or state-level rate and stands at 34.8 per cent for females. Besides the district hospital that has 300 beds, Medak has nine more small hospitals which together have a total of 278 beds. There are also 57 PHCs, 382 sub-centres and 68 private nursing homes and hospitals spread around the district.

Research Design

Our research consisted of three components—the follow-up or prospective component, the community or retrospective component, and service provider and facility assessment. Since the sample, site and instruments varied for all three components, each was conducted as an independent study, though the findings were pooled together for presentation and analysis. A community hospital (ZH) located on a major highway was selected for the follow-up component, and three villages covered by a nearby PHC were selected for the community study. The final sample consisted of 40 women who had experienced abortions, 13 of whom were chosen through community-based identification and 27 through hospital-based recruitment. Our research also included 17 service providers and two health facilities—a hospital and a PHC.

Follow-up of Women after Abortion: Prospective Component

The cases of 27 women who underwent abortion in a small government hospital were followed up for six months to assess the post-abortion services provided to them by government service providers. The women were recruited between March and August 2002 and followed up until March 2003. Each woman was interviewed four times:

First interaction	:	immediately after abortion, at the hospital
Second interaction	:	two weeks after abortion, at home
Third interaction	:	two months after abortion, at home
Fourth interaction	:	six months after abortion, at home

Women in the Community: Retrospective Component

For this we chose three villages covered by a PHC located closest to the selected hospital. The three villages together had a population of 6,636. A house-to-house survey was conducted to identify women aged between 15 and 49 years, the childbirths they had had and the abortions that they had undergone during the previous 12 months. Among the 1,494 married women that were identified, 143 had been pregnant during the previous 12 months. Of these, 16 claimed that they had an abortion during the 12 months preceding our study. Since we could interview only 13 of these 16 women, our findings in this context pertain only to them. It is important to point out here that while this sample is too small to arrive at any definite conclusions, it does provide useful insights into women's experiences and the quality of services in the periphery.

Service Providers and Facilities

Two categories of service providers were interviewed: those working in the hospital, and those in PHC (which therefore have field-based duties). In all, four doctors, three staff nurses (from hospital), nine ANMs and one health visitor (from the PHCs) were interviewed. Facility assessment was done in the selected community hospital and PHC.

Post-Abortion Care

The standard of care that should be provided to women at two weeks, two months and six months after abortion was formulated during workshops with the help of an expert group comprising gynaecologists, nurse–midwives and public health specialists. This group also reviewed the research tools and examined the ethical issues related to the study.

Based on the framework that emerged during the workshops (see Table 7.1), interview guides were developed for interacting with women during each follow-up visit, and for interviewing service providers. A facility checklist was prepared and used for assessing facilities in the hospital and the PHC. Field investigators were trained in different topics related to pregnancy, its problems, and the different types of abortion, methods of abortion, and post-abortion complications and care. They also received practical training in interviewing, counselling, and maintaining privacy and confidentiality.

Ethical Issues

In order to ensure confidentiality and continuity, only one person—qualified, senior ANM—was used to recruit women throughout the six months. Each woman was apprised of the purpose of our research and her consent for participation was sought before she underwent abortion. If she agreed to participate, she was observed and interviewed after the procedure. Her address was noted down and the time and place for follow-up visits were fixed. Privacy and confidentiality while visiting her home were ensured.

It was recognized that, while confidentiality was a concern in all cases, some cases required extra vigilance; keeping this in mind, women were divided into three groups: married women whose abortion was known to family members and neighbours; women (including those who were married) who had undergone or were planning to undergo induced abortion but did not want certain family members

Table 7.1: Framework for post-abortion care and follow-up

Immediately after abortion	Two weeks after abortion	Two months after abortion	Six months after abortion
Observe for bleeding from vagina: amount, consistency, colour, odour. Check vital signs—TPR, BP, pain. Check retraction of uterus. Observe abdominal distension. Observe signs of perforation such as increased pulse rate, pain and breathlessness. Give perineal care Administer analgesics and other medications as prescribed. Reassure the client. Check if urine is passed. Observe if there is any discharge from nipples. Arrange baby care, if needed. Reassure relatives by giving post-abortion advice on perineal care, rest, sexual activity, family planning, diet, cleanliness. Also, talk about review visit.	Take history of bleeding, fever, white discharge, foul smell, burning micturition, haematuria, and pain or distension of abdomen. Observe perineum. Give reassurance. Ask about doubts and give information. Reinforce messages on perineal care, rest, sexual activity, diet, cleanliness. Counsel on family planning. Refer for problems.	Find out about abnormal bleeding, white discharge and smell. Find out about abdominal pain and distension. Ask whether menstruation has started. Find out history of using any family-planning methods and the type used. If not used, ask when and what type she is planning to use. Counsel on use of family planning methods. Ask when she wants next child. Ask about doubts and give information. Give reassurance. Refer for problems.	Find out about regularity of menstruation. Take history of amenorhea. Ask history of abortion or abnormal bleeding with discharge of products. Take history of chronic fever, burning micturition, abdominal pain and white discharge. Ask history of using any family planning methods and the type. Counsel on use of family planning. Counsel on risks of repeated MTPs. Ask when she is planning for next child. Refer for problems.

(the mother-in-law, for example) to know about it; and high confidentiality cases where utmost care had to be exercised. These comprised unmarried girls, widows and women separated from their husbands. In such cases, only one staff member—the one who recruited the women—made all subsequent visits, often meeting the women in public places. The follow-up visits were kept strictly confidential, with the field investigator being debriefed after each visit.

Follow-up became a problem in some cases when women gave incorrect or incomplete addresses during their first interaction with our staff (immediately after abortion). We took this to indicate that they did not want to be visited and so no further effort was made to contact them again. Two women went to their maternal homes for abortion. When they returned to their marital homes, it was difficult to meet them without breaking confidentiality. Hence, follow-up was done only for 27 women, although 33 had initially consented to participate.

The Women's Perspective

As mentioned earlier, our findings relate to the 27 women who were followed up for six months and the 13 women from three villages who had undergone abortion during the year prior to the study. Of the 27 women 15 had undergone induced abortion (MTP) and 12 had suffered either bleeding or abdominal pain at home before they approached the hospital for treatment and complete abortion. On the other hand, all 13 women who were identified in the community insisted that they had spontaneous abortions. Because the three groups differed on several variables, such as age, order of pregnancy and period of gestation, they were dealt with separately. However, wherever possible, our findings on them have been integrated.

Profile of Women Who Underwent Abortion

Within easy access of nearly 100 villages, the government hospital we selected is a referral hospital located on a national highway. The majority of women (19 out of 27) were from villages that fell within a 25 km radius of the town in which the hospital is located. However, one woman lived about 100 km away but chose to use this particular hospital because her mother lived near it; eight women came from other *mandal*s.

We discovered that most of the women were poor, illiterate, landless labourers from socio-economically underprivileged communities. About half of them (14 out of 27) were illiterate and only two had studied beyond the high school level. The majority were housewives or daily-wage labourers; only three worked in their own farms or had their own (petty) trade. Over 50 per cent (16 out of 27) belonged to the Scheduled Caste or Tribe communities and nine were Muslims (see Table 7.2).

Table 7.2: Socio-economic, demographic and health profile of the women

Socio-economic profile	Freq.	Demographic and health profile	Freq.
Literacy and education		Present marital status	
Illiterate	19	Married	35
Primary school or able to read/write	12	Widowed/separated	1
		Unmarried	4
Studied up to high school	7		
Studied above high school	2		
Occupation of women		Age at marriage in years	16
Housewives	17	Less than 15	7
Daily wage labourers	18	15–17	8
Owning trade/farm	3	18–20	4
Others	2	Above 20	5
Occupation of husbands		Age at abortion in completed years	
Daily wage labourers	17	Less than 20	5
Owning trade/farm	9	20–24	11
Service/employed	8	25–29	7
Not mentioned/not applicable	6	30 and above	4
Caste		Duration of pregnancy at the time of abortion in weeks	
Scheduled castes	19	Upto 12	5
Scheduled tribes	4	13–16	11
Other backward castes	7	17–20	7
Others	8	More than 20	4
Religion		Order of pregnancy	
Hindu	19	First	8
Muslim	9	Second	6
Christian	10	Third or more	13
Others	2		
Type of house		Number of abortions	
Kachcha	9	One	24
Pucca	8	Two	2
Semi-pucca	23	More than two	1
Number of rooms		Number of childbirths	
1	18	None	11
2	15	1	4
3	7	2 or 3	6
		4 or more	6
Household size		Number of living children	
Between 2 and 5	22	None	11
Between 6 and 8	14	1	4
9 or more	4	2 or 3	6
		4 or more	6

Most women lived in one-room houses in joint families (17 out of 27), with the household size being more than six in the case of half the women. Very few families had assets such as land. Only 12 owned bicycles or other two-wheelers. Some families owned a few goats and a few had cattle for farming. Two families had sewing machines and were engaged in tailoring. A few families had a television set and a radio. Only five said they did not have day-to-day financial problems.

A similar picture obtained for the 13 women identified in the three villages. The majority belonged to the lower socio-economic strata and had low education and income levels. Four women had completed primary education, while seven were illiterate. Most of the women and their husbands were daily-wage labourers. Only four of the 13 women lived in concrete houses, while five lived in kachcha homes. Box 7.1 indicates the socio-economic status of the majority of women who underwent abortion in the government hospital. In this box, as also throughout this chapter, the names of respondents have been replaced with initials to protect their identities.

Box 7.1: Socio-economic status of women

An illiterate, scheduled caste woman (SG) was living with her mother; her husband had left her because she was not good looking. Her mother had to leave the comfort of living with her son to care for her abandoned daughter because SG's brother did not want them living in his house. They rented a small room without electricity or water for Rs 100 per month. Taking up whatever work was available, each managed to earn about Rs 20 per day whenever they were fortunate enough to get work. But because SG was not able to work for many days after the abortion, they did not earn enough even to buy food. At the time of our research, SG and her mother were worried that they might have to move out of the rented room since it was becoming difficult to pay the rent. All they owned were a few clothes and vessels.

SF was a 30-year-old Muslim woman with seven children. Both she and her husband worked as daily-wage labourers. Besides vessels and clothes, they also owned two goats. If they managed to get work, their combined income amounted to about Rs 70 per day. After she had the abortion, SF could not work for some days and the family did not have enough to eat.

Age and Type of Abortion

Over 50 per cent (16 out of 27) of the women were below 25 years (Table 7.3). Women who underwent an induced abortion were slightly older than those who had a spontaneous abortion. The mean age of women who had induced abortions was 24.8 years compared to 21.5 years for those who had spontaneous abortions.

Table 7.3: Age and type of abortion

Age in years	Spontaneous abortion	Induced abortion	Total
18 or younger	1	3 (unmarried)	4
19–24	8	4	12
25 and above	3	8	11
Total	12	15	27

Period of Gestation and Type of Abortion

Two-thirds of the women (18 out of the 27) had their abortion in the first trimester. Among the nine women who had it in the second trimester, five aborted between 13 and 16 weeks, three between 17 and 20 weeks and one woman at 22 weeks. Of the nine women who had their abortions in the second trimester, three had induced abortions whereas six had spontaneous abortions. Only three of the 15 women who had induced abortions delayed till the second trimester. There were more women who had induced abortions in the first trimester compared to those who had spontaneous abortions.

All the women who had abortions stated that their pregnancy was unwanted. Each had different reasons. The three who delayed abortions until the second trimester gave the following reasons: One had not expected to get pregnant, because she had had a tubectomy; the second said she was afraid of the social repercussions of her pregnancy; and the third said she could not take oral pills early because she had high blood pressure, and had to wait until it became normal. These narratives are presented in Box 7.2.

Box 7.2: Why did women delay seeking abortion services?

CR did not expect to become pregnant since she had undergone tubectomy the previous year. She already had four children and did not want any more. When she observed her increasing abdominal size and other signs of pregnancy, she thought she had a tumour. She went around clinics and hospitals saying she had undergone tubectomy and now had a growth in her abdomen. The growth was confirmed as pregnancy when she was 14 weeks pregnant. The news was a shock to her. She did not know what to do. She was ashamed since she felt that pregnancy after sterilisation would perhaps be taken by others to mean that she was a promiscuous woman. Hence, she did not approach the ANM. Finally she spoke to her mother-in-law and went to the government hospital for an abortion at 16 weeks.

(*Box 7.2 continued*)

(Box 7.2 continued)

NM was an 18-year-old, unmarried, scheduled-caste girl. She engaged in sexual relations with a boy next door. She was afraid of the changes in her body and confided her fears to her sexual partner, who refused to accept responsibility. When things became worse, she was compelled to inform her mother, who approached the boy and requested him to marry her daughter. The boy refused since he belonged to an upper caste. These negotiations took some time. NM and her mother finally went to the hospital when she was 16 weeks pregnant.

SF, a Muslim woman with seven children, worked as a daily-wage labourer and had a history of hypertension. She did not want any more children. She went to the PHC for oral pills but the ANM did not give them to her because her blood pressure was high. She went to the government hospital for tubectomy, but here too the doctor advised her to wait until her blood pressure was normal. He gave her some tablets and asked her to come back again. In the meantime she conceived. She could not take time off for abortion since work was available at that time and she could not afford to forego the wages. She did not tell the ANM because she would not be of much help. She finally approached the government hospital for help when she was almost 20 weeks pregnant.

Order of Pregnancy, Order of Childbirth and Number of Abortions

For nearly one-third of the women (8 out of 27), the abortion was of the first pregnancy (Table 7.4). But for about half of them (13 out of 27) it was the third or subsequent pregnancy. Five of them had experienced five pregnancies. One woman was pregnant for the ninth time: she had seven living children and had had two induced abortions. Another woman was pregnant for the eleventh time, with four living children and seven induced abortions. Among the 12 women who had spontaneous abortions, it was the first pregnancy for one-third (4) of them, whereas amongst those who had induced abortions it was the third or subsequent pregnancy for nine out of 15 women.

Table 7.4: Order of pregnancy and type of abortion

Order of pregnancy	Spontaneous abortion	Induced abortion	Total
First	4	4 (unmarried)	8
Second	4	2	6
Third or more	4	9	13
Total	12	15	27

Number of Abortions per Woman

Though the majority of women (24) had only one abortion, two women had two abortions each. In both cases, one was induced while the other was a spontaneous abortion. One woman had seven induced abortions. Among the 13 women in the community-based sample, ten women had one abortion each and three had two or more abortions. One woman in the community had three pregnancies, all of which had ended in abortion.

Number of Childbirths/Living Children and Type of Abortion

Of the 27 women who were followed up, 11 had not had a single childbirth (Table 7.5). Four women had one child each, six had two or three children each and another six had four or more children. In the case of women who had spontaneous abortions, only five of the 12 women had at least one living child. Among the seven women who had no living children, it was the first pregnancy for four women and second pregnancy for the remaining three. One of them (one each had a stillbirth, a neonatal death and one had two spontaneous abortions. On the other hand, all 11 married women who had induced abortions had at least one living child. Women who had induced abortions appear to have had more children compared to those who had spontaneous abortions.

Table 7.5: Number of childbirths and type of abortion

No. of children	Spontaneous abortion	Induced abortion	Total
None	7	4 unmarried	11
1	2	2	4
2 or 3	2	4	6
4 or more	1	5	6
Total	12	15	27

Reasons for Abortions

The most common reason for induced abortion appears to be inadequate contraceptive information and services. Of ten women living in a marital relationship, seven had an induced abortion for spacing childbirths. All seven said that they had to abort their pregnancy because their last child was too young. Only three of these ten women underwent abortion for other reasons, such as health problems, tubectomy failure or reservations about the use of modern spacing methods. Another fairly common reason (five out of 15) was 'socially unacceptable pregnancy'. Four had abortions because their pregnancy was the result of an illicit sexual relationship, and one young woman was the victim of rape. Box 7.3 and Box 7.4 describe what some of the women reported as social and other reasons for opting for induced abortion.

Box 7.3: Induced abortion of socially unacceptable pregnancy

Five of the 27 women underwent abortion because their pregnancy was not socially approved. Among these, four were unmarried one was a widow.

PD (18 years) developed a relationship with a married neighbour who was related to her. When she became pregnant, he told her not to reveal this to anyone. He approached a staff nurse living in their neighbourhood, who advised them to go to the government hospital for abortion.

NM (18 years), educated up to Class X, was staying at home while her parents worked in the fields because they could not afford to send her for higher education. She developed a relationship with a boy next door, who denied the relationship and refused to marry her. So her mother took her to the government hospital for an abortion.

BK (20 years) had a boyfriend who belonged to a different caste. Both sets of parents refused to accept their relationship; hence marriage was not possible. When she became pregnant, her mother took her to hospital for an abortion.

BM was 15 years old and studying in Class VIII in the next village. One day, on her way back from school, four young men kidnapped her, took her to a field and gang-raped her. She was too shocked and afraid to tell anyone. Her mother took her to a private doctor for irregular periods. When the doctor confirmed BM's pregnancy, her mother was afraid to tell her husband, who was BM's stepfather. The doctor advised them to go to a government hospital for abortion because they could not afford her fee.

SV (28 years) was a widow with three children. After her husband's death six years earlier, she had been living in her husband's joint family. She developed a relationship with her husband's married cousin who was their neighbour. When she became pregnant, the man did not want the relationship to be revealed. He accompanied her to the hospital for an abortion. When she went to the government hospital, she did not reveal that she was a widow.

Box 7.4: Other reasons for induced abortion

Not ready for the next child: A graduate, SR, was a housewife with a two-year-old daughter. She wanted to do her B.Ed and become a teacher. When she became pregnant for the second time, she felt that having another child would hinder her from a teaching career. She convinced her husband and underwent abortion without informing the other family members.

Sterilised but pregnant: AA had undergone tubectomy after four children. As a labourer, she could barely feed her children on her earnings. The ANM of her village had taken her for tubectomy at a DPL camp. When her pregnancy was confirmed, she spoke to her mother-in-law and they went to the government hospital for abortion.

Desperate to get rid of unwanted pregnancy: A 35-year-old Muslim woman with four children (two boys and two girls), GB did not want any more children but she was not using any contraception. When she was 12 weeks pregnant, she went to the government hospital and had a Dilation and Curettage (D&C) done. When the bleeding continued for over a week, she thought that the abortion was not complete; went to a private clinic and had another D&C done. When she did not get her period for more than a month, she became anxious and went to a doctor in the city and had a third D&C done. At the end of six months, GB started using oral pills. She no longer believed in sterilisation.

Seven induced abortions in 10 years: An illiterate, 35-year-old woman from a poor family, AS worked as a labourer. She had four children and did not want any more. The ANM visited her several times and advised a family-planning operation. But she could not undergo tubectomy because, as she claimed, 'the spirit of the goddess enters me frequently'. On such days, AS falls into a trance (this type of hysterical behaviour called *Banamati* is common in Medak). She thought, 'What if the goddess were to enter my body during the operation? What would happen to me?' She refused the operation and would have an abortion, every time she missed her period for two consecutive months. Her husband did not want to undergo vasectomy. However, other family members felt that she should undergo tubectomy.

The Sex of the Child and Abortion

Our sample was too small to permit inferences to be drawn about gender preference. However, we did find that in the case of four of the six women who underwent abortion for spacing, the last child was a daughter who was less than a year old.

Conception after Abortion

Eight of the 27 women became pregnant within six months after abortion. Six had had spontaneous abortions and wanted to conceive again. The remaining two had had induced abortions. One was afraid she might become infertile if she waited too long and the second was a widow who could not use contraception because of her marital status.

Post-Abortion Problems and Complications

Most women faced complications after abortion; 17 of the 27 women said that they had developed complications within two weeks of the abortion. This number rose to 21 in the case of complications that occurred between two weeks and two months. And at the end of six months, three women still had problems related to abortion. Most women who faced complications said that they took action to deal with them (18 out of 21). Twelve went to a hospital or doctor for medicine and advice. In the case of the remaining six, a family member obtained medicines from a doctor, health worker or healer. Some examples of kinds of post-abortion complications reported by women are shown in Box 7.5.

Box 7.5: Post-abortion complications

JD had three children (two daughters and one son). She wanted one more son. During the twelfth week, she had slight bleeding and went to the government hospital where she had a D&C. She had continuous bleeding for 15 days after the procedure, so she went back to the hospital where the doctor prescribed some medicines. When the bleeding did not subside, she was referred to the district hospital. But JD went to a private hospital instead because she did not trust the government hospital to deal with her problem. Six months later, JD was again 12 weeks pregnant and hoped to get a son.

SR had bleeding, white discharge and swelling of the face and feet for two months after abortion. She went to a private doctor who suggested scanning and D&C. SR was afraid and went to her mother's place in the city for treatment. After the complications subsided, she became apprehensive about becoming infertile and was therefore anxious to conceive again. She did not use contraception. At the end of six months she was 14 weeks pregnant.

SP was married at the age of 15 years. She gave birth to a girl child three years after marriage. But the child died six days after birth. After this, she had two abortions within a span of two years. She changed three doctors in the hope of receiving treatment that would help her to conceive. But after eight years of marriage she had still not managed to have any children. Her sisters-in-law and other relatives accused her of infertility and threatened to get her husband remarried. But the husband was supportive of her.

When RK did not conceive again for five years after her first delivery, the neighbours began saying that she might never conceive again. She approached the village *dai* (it is believed that dais can treat infertility). The dai gave RK

(*Box 7.5 continued*)

(*Box 7.5 continued*)

some tablets and she became pregnant. Unfortunately, the doctor told her that it was a molar pregnancy and she had to abort the pregnancy. Family members and friends were angry with her for approaching the dai as they felt this was the cause of the abortion.

Post-Abortion Contraception

For both groups of women, menstrual regularity, contraceptive utilisation and pregnancy status were assessed at two and six months after abortion. Data revealed that only one woman was using contraception at the end of two months. Though she did not want any more children, she did not believe in permanent sterilisation. At the end of six months, only five women were using contraception. Two had started using oral pills, two had an intra-uterine device (IUD) inserted and one underwent tubectomy. Eight had become pregnant again within six months. The rest did not use any contraception.

Abortion Used as Contraception

Six of the 15 women who had induced abortion used it as a spacing method. Four of them said that they had undergone abortion because their last child was too young when they got pregnant again. Two had abortions because the timing of the pregnancy was not convenient or because there was no one to take care of a child at the time. Some cases of women who used abortion as contraception are presented in Box 7.6.

Box 7.6: Post-abortion contraception

Sterilisation for social reasons: SG underwent tubectomy two months after abortion though she did not have any living children. She was separated from her husband and, according to her neighbours, was too poor to feed herself. Her mother and neighbours pressed her to undergo sterilisation since she did not have a husband. The operation was performed in the government hospital.
Oral pills after abortion: GB had four children—two boys and two girls. She did not want any more children. She started taking oral pills. RD, on the other hand, had only two children—one son and one daughter. The two-and-a half-year-old son had not started talking yet and the daughter was less than a year old. RD did not want to undergo sterilisation till the boy could speak and hence started using oral pills.

(*Box 7.6 continued*)

(Box 7.6 continued)

IUD after abortion: JK and MT have studied above high school and are from a middle-class background. Both had an IUD inserted at the government hospital because they were familiar with it. In the case of JK, her mother worked there. In the case of MT, her mother's house was next to the hospital and she knew the staff. JK did not want to have a tubectomy because she felt that it would make her weak. She was trying to convince her husband to have a vasectomy. MT wanted to delay the birth of her second child.

Reasons for Not Using Contraception

Among the 14 women who were not using contraception at the end of six months, four were unmarried girls. Of the remaining 10, four wanted to get pregnant or wanted to have a male child. One was scared of operations and the other, who had completed the desired family size, did not undergo sterilisation or use any other form of contraception because it was against her beliefs. ZB, a Muslim woman with four children, did not approve of modern contraception methods and preferred to use herbal medicines instead.

Cost of Abortion

Many women chose the government hospital because they could not afford private hospitals and because they thought government services would be free. But doctors in the government hospital also charge a fee, though it is lower than that in private hospitals (Table 7.6). Women found it difficult to find the money to pay for abortion and had to struggle to repay loans taken for the purpose. The doctor's fee constituted 90 per cent of the abortion cost. Only two out of 27 women did not pay the doctor for abortion.

Table 7.6: Cost and type of abortion

Fee paid to doctor	Spontaneous abortion	Induced abortion	Total
Below Rs 500	5	9	14
Above Rs 500	6	5	11
Total	11	14	25

The average fee for abortion in the government hospital was Rs 612 (Table 7.7). The average fee for spontaneous abortion was slightly higher (Rs 633) compared to induced abortion (Rs 590). The maximum amount charged was Rs 1,500. The doctor's fee would vary depending on the women's economic status and the intensity of their need for abortion. Bed charges were extra. Besides the doctor, the women also had to pay the dai, who generally charged Rs 30. The maximum amount paid to a dai was Rs 50. As a rule, the hospital nurse did not expect any direct payment. However, in two cases the women said they paid her Rs 30, but then they did not pay anything to the dai.

Table 7.7: Hospital fee

Cost of abortion	Amount in Rs
Average fee to doctor	612.0
Maximum fee to doctor	1,500.0
Average fee to dai	30.0
Maximum fee to dai	50.0
Average hospital charges	11.5
Maximum hospital charges	50.0
Average cost of medicines	145.7
Maximum cost of medicines	600.0

The hospital also levied a nominal charge of Rs 5 if the woman had to stay on for a short while, but this charge went up to Rs 50 if she had to remain there for a whole day. Four of the 27 women said they paid Rs 50 as hospital charges. On the whole, however, the average hospital charge paid by the women was Rs 11.5. The average travelling cost per woman was Rs 50 and the average amount spent on medicines was Rs 145.74. Barring one woman, who did not spend on medicines at all, the maximum amount spent on medicines was Rs 600 and the minimum was Rs 50. Box 7.7 overviews some such abortion costs.

Box 7.7: Economic burden of abortion

For AA, the total cost of abortion, including doctor's fee and treatment charges, was about Rs 1,250. Her husband, who is a daily-wage labourer, did not have the money. Her mother-in-law had to borrow it from the village headman. AA had to sell two goats to repay the money that her mother-in-law borrowed. The cost was high because they did not believe that she was pregnant, and had to use the services of a private hospital for scanning to confirm pregnancy.

BM's mother, a labourer, was charged Rs 1,000 because her daughter was unmarried and therefore needed the abortion. Her pregnancy was the result of rape. BM's mother had to arrange for the money secretly. She borrowed Rs 300 from the village *patel,* for which she had to pay 5 per cent interest. In addition, she had to sell her gold beads and BM's silver anklets. BM's mother earned only Rs 20 per day and was struggling to repay the loan. BM had to discontinue her studies.

(*Box* 7.7 *continued*)

(Box 7.7 continued)

JB had to sell personal belongings like her watch and jewellery. She borrowed money from her brother-in-law at 10 per cent interest. It took her three months to arrange for the money. Due to repeated visits to the hospital for complications and treatment, JB's husband lost two months of work.

PR took two days to arrange for the Rs 1,300 required for her treatment. She had to take a loan on interest. PR complained she was not able to work after the abortion.

MG said she borrowed money at 5 per cent interest and was planning to work hard to save money to repay the loan.

RK was a DWCRA (Development of Women and Children in Rural Areas) group member. She borrowed Rs 10,000 from DWCRA women's group at 3 per cent interest. She had to return the money within six months. She was planning to repay the money by cutting down on family expenses. RK had to spend more since she also had an operation.

The cost of abortion services varied for all 13 cases in our community sample. The doctor's fee ranged from Rs 150 to Rs 2,760. The minimum cost was Rs 150 (this was the amount spent by a poor woman who used the services of a government hospital). One woman said that after paying the high fee for abortion, she could not afford a post-abortion check-up. Another woman said she could not have a complete check-up due to financial constraints; and because she could not afford private services, she was forced to put up with the rude behaviour of one of the hospital staff.

Most women had to borrow money at 5 per cent interest. Some had to sell their assets like jewellery and cattle. Apart from financial costs, abortion also affected the work, education and livelihood of women and their families. Sometimes they lost their jobs because of their absence from work. Women who were daily wage workers suffered the most, because they could not work and earn to feed themselves and their families. Those who were engaged in petty trade lost their businesses after abortion.

Family Support

We found that women considering abortion generally turned to their husbands, mothers and mothers-in-law for support; 12 women said they first approached their husbands or sexual partners to discuss the problem before deciding on abortion. However, even if the husband agreed to help pay the bills, he did not in all cases accompany the wife to the hospital; for that, the women sometimes approached their mothers (8) or mothers-in-law (6).

We found that husbands in nuclear families were more supportive, particularly when the women chose to have induced abortions. Of the three women who were involved in premarital relationships, two received some support from their partners.

In two cases, while the husbands were initially supportive, they turned against the women when there were complications. One woman did not inform the husband at all: 'I already had four children. I took the help of the ANM and went to the hospital. I told him afterwards.' Husbands got upset if the abortion was of a wanted child, particularly when it happened spontaneously.

Mothers provided pycho-social and economic support even if they were not the first ones to be informed about the abortion. They even kept the daughter's pregnancy or abortion a secret from their own husbands if the pregnancy was a result of a premarital relationship. In some cases, mothers-in-law were also supportive and played a key role in decision-making about abortion.

Responsiveness of the Public Health System

Two government health facilities were assessed for the presence of service providers, equipment and facilities for carrying out the abortion procedure. One of these was a block hospital and the other a primary health centre. The PHC had only one doctor and nurse, with no facilities to conduct MTPs. Our observations therefore pertain only to the block hospital.

Abortion Facilities and Services

The hospital had three doctors—two female and one male. There were also three nurses who assisted during abortion and provided immediate post-abortion care to patients. Although all three doctors conducted abortions, the majority of them were done by the senior male doctor who lived on the hospital premises. He performed 15 of the 27 abortions, while the two female doctors together did the remaining 12.

As indicated earlier, a total of 33 women were provided abortion services at a government hospital in the six months for which the women were recruited. Abortions were conducted in the hospital's labour room and registered in the maternity register. There was no specific consent form for MTP. Every patient who came in for an abortion had to pay a nominal fee of Rs 5 or Rs 50 if they needed to stay overnight. The hospital did not supply medicines or food, which had to be bought from outside.

Most women said that they chose the government hospital because they could not afford to go anywhere else. However, follow-up data indicated that there were also other reasons. Many cited convenience, saying that the hospital was close to their homes (the majority of the women were from the town itself or from nearby villages). Some women (seven) used the hospital because they knew the staff. Almost all said that they were too poor to pay for private services. One woman said that she felt comfortable with the female doctors in the hospital. According to another woman, the fact that the hospital was located very far from her home made it possible to keep her abortion secret.

Six of the women were not asked to sign any consent form. In terms of services, pre-abortion cleaning and medication were provided to most of the women. However, none of them were asked to undergo a blood-grouping or haemoglobin-percentage tests. Clean perineal pads and bed linen were provided to only four women. While most women expressed satisfaction with the abortion procedure and medication, they were not happy that they had to get medicines and food from outside. Lack of water was a major problem and all women complained about the poor cleanliness standard of the hospital.

Initially, most women expressed satisfaction with the behaviour of the staff—doctors, nurses, dais and others—and said that they had been treated with dignity and respect. However, on further probing, more than half (15 out of 27) admitted that they had not been treated with dignity. One woman was not happy with the behaviour of the doctor, three did not like the behaviour of the nurse and five did not like the behaviour of the dai. In fact, one woman was not happy with the behaviour of any of the hospital staff. She was much too poor to pay for anything, not even for a rickshaw: she had come walking to the hospital despite being in pain. Instead of being sympathetic, the staff had insisted that she pay the hospital charges. Finally, her mother had to borrow money to pay the hospital and the dai.

Discharge Advice and Information

Most women were informed about the medications they were required to take, the need for rest, symptoms of post-abortion complications, and the need for a review visit (Table 7.8), but very few were told about perineal care, diet and sexual activity. Only eight women were told about contraception use after abortion. Of these, only three began using contraception by the end of six months. Three women were counselled about sexual activity.

Table 7.8: Health advice before discharge

Follow-up advice given before discharge	Frequency
Explained about medication	26
Explained about review visit to hospital	22
Warned about post-abortion complications	19
Advised adequate rest	16
Explained importance of perineal care	11
Advised about diet	9
Motivated for family planning	8
Counselled about sexual activity	3

Follow-up Visit to Hospital

A total of 21 women made follow-up visits to the government hospital after abortion. Of these, 17 said they went because they had health problems such as weakness, bleeding, abdominal pain and fever. Four said they went on the advice of the doctor. Another woman's mother, who worked in the hospital, took her there when her bleeding wouldn't stop. Of the six who did not go to the hospital for follow-up, most were unmarried girls who wanted to avoid unnecessary exposure. In the case of one unmarried girl, her sexual partner got her some medication for abdominal distension from a private clinic.

In the community study, six of the 13 women had their abortion at home while seven went to the hospital after bleeding had started. All seven said they received immediate treatment but only five said they were treated respectfully by the hospital staff. Six women had to undergo scanning. Three said that the doctor informed them about the necessity for abortion but they were not told about its implications. Eight of the 13 women said that they had approached a service provider (government or private) at least once, either before or after abortion. Only one reported that she preferred the village practitioner (dai) because she was more easily accessible.

Post-Abortion Services Provided by ANMs

Only three of the 27 women were visited by an ANM within two weeks after abortion (Table 7.9). In one case the ANM gave her medicines

Table 7.9: **Home visits by ANM**

Home visits by ANM	Within 2 weeks	Within 2 months	Within 6 months
Yes	3	4	2
No	24	23	25

and asked her to visit the health centre. Another ANM accompanied a woman to the hospital when she approached the ANM for advice before seeking abortion.

Women's Awareness about ANMs

Nearly half the women who had abortions said that they were familiar with the ANM. Eight women did not know her at all and seven knew her but not her name. Among the eight who did not know her at all, five were from an urban area where ANMs did not make regular home visits. Of the other three, two belonged to a very low socio-economic group and one had not had occasion to interact with the ANM since she did not have any children. Of the seven women who were aware of the ANM but did not know her name, three were unmarried and therefore had no need to interact with her. Two belonged to an urban area which ANMs did not visit often. Two had no reason to interact with the ANM earlier since this was their first pregnancy; and some women did not approach her because they felt they could not reveal their pregnancy that was the result of premarital or extramarital relationships or rape.

Of the 13 women identified in the three villages, three said that the ANM had known about their abortion and had provided them with services. Three women did not know the ANM at all, five knew her but did not know the sort of services she provided, and one said that the ANM had a good reputation. Three others were not happy with the village ANM who, as one of them said, was 'more interested in family-planning operation cases and she visits houses only for that purpose'. Another woman said that she had gone to the ANM for help but the ANM had refused to take up abortion cases.

Post-Abortion Service Provided by ANM

Three of the 27 who had their abortion at the government hospital were visited by an ANM within the first two weeks after abortion, four between two weeks and two months, and two between two and six months after the abortion (Table 7.9). Only one woman was visited thrice. They all said that the ANMs checked them for fever, vaginal discharge, abdominal pain, bleeding and burning micturition. They were happy that the 'sister' had enquired about their well-being, given them a physical check-up and reassured them. One ANM offered to get the medicines prescribed by the hospital, another gave advice about post-abortion care, diet and rest, and one advised the woman she visited about family-planning methods. The experiences of some women who received post-abortion care are presented in Box 7.8.

Box 7.8: Post-abortion services from ANMs

GM received regular post-abortion follow-up care because her neighbour was an ANM. Although the ANM did not serve the area in which she lived, GM consulted the ANM because she did not get her period after she gave birth to a baby girl 7 months earlier. The ANM confirmed her pregnancy and spoke to her about the problems of poor spacing. GM and her husband decided to have an abortion. The ANM accompanied GM to the government hospital and visited her regularly after the abortion. Later, she referred GM for an IUD.

When ZB's fourth child was less than a year old and she was 10 weeks pregnant, the ANM gave her some tablets and said that she would start bleeding. When ZB started bleeding, the ANM accompanied her to the government hospital and facilitated the abortion. The ANM gave her B-Complex tablets and advised sterilisation, but ZB declined the advice since this was against her religion and instead decided to take herbal medicines.

AM was pregnant for the first time. She started bleeding at 16 weeks and went to the government hospital. She did not approach the village ANM. But when the ANM heard about the abortion during her visit to the village, she met AM and provided her with follow-up care and advice.

Perceptions, Practices and Problems of Service Providers

A total of 17 service providers were interviewed: four doctors, nine ANMs, three staff nurses and one health visitor. All providers were either from the hospital where abortions were conducted or the PHC where the community survey was done.

Of the four doctors, two had completed a post-graduate diploma in gynaecology, one had had MTP training and the fourth had experience in assisting abortions in a private hospital.

Providers' Awareness about Abortion and MTP

None of the ANMs were trained to provide MTP/abortion-related care. Five had been providing abortion care for the last six to seven years, they had picked up the skills along the way. Five service providers said that they had received reproductive and child health (RCH) training during last five years. Two staff nurses had undergone in-service training in clinical skill enhancement. One ANM had attended health visitor training as well as double puncture laparatomy and integrated skill development training during the last five years. Four service providers were not even aware that there are different types of abortion. Only seven seemed to know of this, while eight were only aware about the indications for conducting an abortion.

All service providers (except one) were aware of the instruments required to conduct an abortion. Only four were aware about the package of services to be included in post-abortion care. They mentioned checking for bleeding, fever and white discharge, giving advice on personal hygiene, and recommending complete rest and family-planning methods as post-abortion services.

Awareness of the MTP Act was shown by 11 out of 13 non-medical service providers; the two ANMs did not know anything about the Act. Only two doctors could list the indications for MTP according to the Act. Three out of the four doctors did not know whether MTP services are included in the RCH programme.

Attitudes of Service Providers

The 17 service providers were asked key questions about their attitude towards women who approach them for abortion treatment and care. The questions dealt with HIV, the need for the positive or single women, husband's consent, abortion as a spacing method, etc.

Two of the four doctors said that since the women who come for abortion cannot afford an HIV test, doctors take their own precautions. One doctor said that if they knew that a particular woman was HIV positive, they would not provide her with any service. The fourth doctor did not make any comment.

Only five service providers said some women—such as unmarried girls, promiscuous women and women with alcoholic husbands—come alone for an abortion. Only four said they would conduct the abortion even if a woman came alone. Among them, three were doctors and one was an ANM. The ANM said she would accompany the woman to hospital. Ten service providers said that they would not conduct an abortion if the woman came alone.

The majority of service providers (11) said they would not conduct an abortion for single women, including separated/widowed/unmarried women. They said that an abortion might block the fallopian tubes and the woman may not be able to conceive again. Others said that if they did not perform the abortion, the women would just go elsewhere.

Most service providers said that they insisted on obtaining the husband's permission for the abortion to avoid any trouble with family members later on. Only four said that it was enough for a woman to be accompanied by a responsible person.

Almost all service providers said that abortion was not an appropriate spacing method. About half (8) of them said abortion could be used as a spacing method once or twice but not repeatedly. Three said that abortion was a more convenient method of family planning than the other methods available.

The majority of service providers (14), including doctors, said abortion should not be permitted if a sex-determination test has been done. But three said that this test should not be used to deny abortion services to women.

Women's Rights, Choice and Access

Ten service providers, including doctors, did not perceive abortion as a women's right. However, all four doctors said that the MTP Act had given women the freedom of choice. They felt that the Act had reduced the number of illegal medical practitioners and hence the number of complications. Two doctors said that the MTP Act had facilitated abortion services for women. However, another doctor said that it had raised the number of illegal abortions.

On further discussion, almost all service providers admitted that women could not access MTP services easily mainly because of the high financial cost involved. Women's access to safe abortion services was also hindered by other factors such as ignorance, social and economic instability, large family size, illiteracy, poverty, reservations against using family-planning methods, health problems, preference for male children, prenatal sex determination and domination by husbands. Three out of four doctors agreed that women should have legal access to abortion, as well as the right to sue in case of complications. Two doctors pointed out that, other than rape victims, the MTP Act did not mention other valid cases for abortion, such as separated women, widows or unmarried girls. As such, it had not really helped all women.

Six out of 17 service providers said women do not prefer to access MTP services at the first referral unit (FRU) because they want to maintain confidentiality about abortion. Five service providers said that PHCs do not have adequate MTP facilities. Only two recommended that abortion services be provided at the PHC level.

Role of Non-allopathic and Mid-level Service Providers

None of the service providers was in favour of non-allopathic practitioners offering abortion services. Seven said that since such providers were not trained to conduct abortions, availing their services might lead to infection and risk to life. Two service providers said that the government should ban non-allopathic, non-medical and local medical practitioners from conducting abortions.

Many service providers (13 of 17) said that ANMs should be trained to provide MTP services as they were closest to the com-munity and could be accessed by women very easily. Four (two nurses and two ANMs) said that only doctors should conduct abortions. Another four said that if, along with ANMs, dais were also trained to conduct early abortion, abortion services would be more easily acces-sible to women in villages. About half of the non-medical service pro-viders said that the nurse's main role was to assist the doctor during abortion and provide the patient with post-abortion care.

Abortion-related Practices

Our findings indicated that some government doctors who were neither gynaecologists nor trained in MTP, provided abortion services in their private clinics and their charges depended on the pregnancy duration of the clients as well charged higher when secrecy had to be maintained as in the case of unmarried girls.

Box 7.9: The medical doctors

Dr UK was a gynaecologist with 16 years' experience. Besides working in the government hospital, she ran a private clinic at home and was a visiting doctor in a nursing home. She did not think that abortion was a woman's right; it was just a necessity at times. She had conducted eight of the 27 abortions followed up in this study.

Dr SH had seven years' experience as a doctor. She was neither a gynaecologist nor had undergone MTP training. She ran a private clinic at home besides working in the government hospital. She conducted abortions for cases up to 20 weeks of gestation in her private clinic. She had conducted four of the 27 abortions followed up in this study.

Dr RN was a senior male doctor. He lived on the hospital premises and, although not a gynaecologist, conducted deliveries and abortions regularly. He had conducted 15 of the 27 abortions in this study. His fee ranged from Rs 300 to Rs 1,500. He insisted on being paid before conducting an abortion and even refused to do a D&C until his fee was paid in advance. He charged less (Rs 300) if the woman was referred by other doctors. However, his fee was higher for unmarried women.

The majority of the providers of abortion services preferred the D&C method to that of vacuum aspiration, although the latter is easier to perform and does not require giving anaesthetics to women (see Table 7.10). This is partly because those who have received training were trained in D&C. Vacuum aspiration as a method of abortion has developed more recently and the doctors are not yet comfortable using it.

Abortion-related Practices of ANMs

Only four of the nine ANMs said they knew of women who had undergone abortion at the hospital during the study period. Eight had made follow-up visits. Six ANMs said they had provided follow-up to all women and two said that they had followed up only those women who had consulted them for abortion. During their visits, ANMs usually checked the woman's temperature and BP, and also checked for bleeding and abdominal pain. Only two ANMs provided advice on sanitation and hygiene. One ANM even conducted an abortion after giving injections and charged for the procedure. All of them claimed that maintaining confidentially was a major problem: since ANMs are associated with antenatal care, people become suspicious

Table 7.10: Abortion services provided by doctors

Issues	Responses of doctors (N = 4)
Preferred method of abortion	D&C up to 12 weeks' of gestation: 3 doctors. Vacuum aspiration: 1. Intra-amniotic induction method at 13–20 weeks' gestation: 4.
Medication for inducing abortion	Use of Prostaglandin injection: 3 doctors. Syntocin tablets: 1. Curettage after abortion to check for completeness of abortion: 4.
Use of anaesthesia	Local anaesthesia, irrespective of the duration of gestation: 4 doctors. General anaesthesia used only when necessary. Doctors who said that they themselves administer local anaesthesia with the help of a nurse: 3.
Tests done before abortion	Doctors who prescribe HB and urine tests and, if the patient can afford it and is willing, also blood cell count, grouping, HIV and blood sugar tests: 4 doctors. Doctors who conduct the HB test before discharging the patient: 3. Doctor who checks the PV: 1. Checking for passage of urine and effect of sedation: 1.
Drugs prescribed after abortion	Antibiotics for 1 week to prevent infection: 4 doctors. Antispasmodic and anti-inflammatory drugs: 4. B-complex tablets for 1 week to help the patient regain strength: 2. Analgesics and Streptovit tablets to help women expel leftover clots: 1.
Follow-up care	Advice to women, before discharge, regarding personal hygiene and regular use of medicines: 4 doctors. Advice about family-planning methods: 3. Advice to women not to have sexual intercourse for 5 days after abortion: 1. Advice for follow-up within 1 week: 4. They said that 90 per cent or more women come for follow-up if asked.

if a non-pregnant woman is seen with them. ANMs also said that women did not speak freely with them even though they were willing to listen and provide services.

The Dai as an Abortion Service Provider

In another village, an experienced dai conducted abortions on a regular basis. She did not give any injections but used her hands to gently massage the abdomen. Many women came to her for abortions because they believed that she had special skills. One woman whom we followed up for six months went to this dai for five consecutive abortions. But the dai refused to help her after the fifth abortion. She suggested a family-planning 'operation' instead.

Conclusions

Our research comprised a qualitative, multi-component assessment of the perceptions, problems and experiences of 40 women who had had abortions (27 from a government hospital and 13 women from three villages) and 17 service providers. The women who had abortions at the government hospital were followed up several times for six months after the abortion, in order for us to record their post-abortion experiences and elicit information about the follow-up services they received from public health service providers. Interviews were held with 13 women from three villages serviced by a nearby PHC; these women had had abortions during the 12 months preceding the study. We selected 17 service providers working in the selected hospital and PHC and interviewed them for their perceptions and practices.

While our sample size was too small and the area covered by our research too limited to allow any generalisations, our findings do indicate that there is

- low utilisation of government facilities for MTP by women,
- an extremely low record of post-abortion follow-up by public health staff (ANMs),
- extensive use of abortion as spacing method, and
- a fee for abortion even in government hospitals.

In view of these findings, there is clearly a need to re-examine and expand the role played by mid-level and peripheral service providers in the provision of abortion and abortion-related services. It appears that the most common difficulty that service providers face is maintaining confidentiality and the reluctance on the part of women to express their problems freely. To overcome these problems, and strengthen the efficacy of the public health system in this area, there is need to focus on the following tasks:

- Increase awareness among women and men about the availability of safe and free abortion services in the public health sector
- Increase access to abortion services at the FRU level through better-quality services and control of unofficial fee-collection

- Organise better linkages between the hospital and its outreach services so that each woman is visited at least twice after abortion
- Increase awareness among adolescents regarding reproductive health and safe sex to prevent socially unwanted pregnancies
- Improve access to contraceptives for all, irrespective of marital status
- Sensitise couples towards family planning
- Recognise the sexual rights of single women
- Factor confidentiality into the provision of abortion services by the public health system
- Improve management of post-abortion complications in facilities where abortion services are provided
- Plan and implement an effective and sustained strategy for the promotion of spacing methods
- Provide service providers with training oriented towards making them more sensitive to women's needs

References

Barge S., N. Kumar, G. Philips, R. Sinha, S. Lakhanpal, J. Vishwakarma, S. Kumber, U. Khan, G. Kumar and V. Uttekar. 1997. Situation Analysis of Medical Termination of Pregnancy Services in Uttar Pradesh. Baroda: Centre for Operations Research and Training.

Chhabra, R. and S. C. Nuna. 1994. *Abortion in India: An Overview*. New Delhi: Veerendra Printers.

Chhabra, S., N. Gupta, Anita Mehra and Arti Shende. 1988. 'Medical Termination of Pregnancy and Concurrent Contraceptive Abortion in Rural India'. *Studies in Family Planning* 19.

Greenslade, F. C., H. McKary, M. Wold and K. McFaurin. 1994. *Post-Abortion Care: A Women's Health Initiative to Combat Unsafe Abortion. Advances in Abortion Care*. Carrboro, NC.: Ipas.

Gupte, M., Sunita Bandewar and Hemlata Pisal. 1997. 'Abortion Needs of Women in India: A Case Study of Rural Maharashtra'. *Reproductive Health Matters* 9.

ICMR (Indian Council of Medical Research). 1989. *Illegal Abortion in Rural Areas: A Task Force Study*. New Delhi: ICMR.

Jejeebhoy, S. J. 1998. 'Adolescent Sexual and Reproductive Behaviour: A Review of the Evidence from India'. *Social Science in Medicine* 46.

Johnson, Heidi Bart. 1999. Draft on Abortion and Post-Abortion Care in India: A Review of the Literature. Carrboro, NC.: Ipas.

Kerrigan, M., L. Gaffikin and R. Magarick. 1995. 'Post-Abortion Care Services in Uttar Pradesh State, India'. *JHPIEGO* 28.
Maitra, N. 1998. *Unsafe Abortion: Practices and Solutions, Abortion Facilities and Post-Abortion Care in the Context of the RCH Programme*. New Delhi: Centre for Operations Research and Training.
Mathai, S. T. 1998. Review of Incomplete and Septic Abortions in India with Particular Reference to West Bengal. Department for International Development, 50.
Sinha, R., M. E. Khan, B. C. Patel, S. Lakhanpal and P. Khanna. 1998. *Decision-Making in Acceptance and Seeking Abortion of Unwanted Pregnancies: Abortion Facilities and Post-Abortion Care in the Context of the RCH Programme.* New Delhi: Centre for Operations Research and Training.
United Nations. 1993. *Abortion Policies: A Global Review*. New York: United Nations.
WHO (World Health Organisation). 1991. *Maternal Mortality: A Global Fact Book*. Geneva: World Health Organisation.

VIII

Induced Abortion: A Study of Rural Tamil Nadu

P. Balasubramanian, T. K. Sundari Ravindran
and U. S. Mishra

Abortion was legalised in India by the Medical Termination of Pregnancy (MTP) Act of 1971. Since then, a number of studies have been published on the incidence of abortions within and outside approved medical facilities, the nature, distribution and quality of abortion services, the characteristics of women seeking abortion services from approved and unapproved sources, and abortion-related morbidity. A review of literature shows that most abortion seekers were in the 20–34 age group, married, and had not used a method of contraception prior to the pregnancy that was sought to be terminated (Agarwal 2000; Johnson 1999).

Only a small number of studies have ventured into areas beyond mortality and morbidity, contraceptive use and demographic profiles of abortion seekers, to examine the decision-making process to terminate pregnancy among married women. The findings suggest that it is invariably the woman concerned who makes up her mind to terminate a mistimed or unwanted pregnancy. She then consults her husband and a joint decision is taken by both to seek induced abortion (Gupte et al. 1997; Parivar Seva Sanstha 1999; Singh and Singh 1991; Sinha et al. 1998). The abortion is usually kept secret from the in-laws. In one study (Singh and Singh 1991), over 50 per cent of the women who had induced abortions had also consulted friends and relatives before making a final decision. Sinha et al. (1998) found that the husband's approval played a significant role in whether or not a woman was able to terminate an unwanted pregnancy. However, several women above 30 years of age, who had experienced repeated pregnancies and did not have their husbands' support, had gone ahead secretly with the abortion.

In all these studies, women were using abortion to space births or prevent an additional birth. Many of those who did not want any more children underwent sterilisation along with the abortion. However, those who had terminated a mistimed pregnancy rarely accepted a reversible method of contraception after the abortion.

Why do women undergo induced abortions rather than use contraceptives to space or limit births? Could it be that, rather than being an indicator of women's exercise of their reproductive rights, induced abortions signify their lack of reproductive and sexual rights? This would certainly be the case when women are disallowed from using contraception and cannot say no to sexual intercourse. But it is also possible that women may be using the threat of an unwanted pregnancy as a bargaining chip to negotiate space within which they can accept or refuse sex.

There may also be a number of simpler explanations for the low use of reversible methods, such as women's lack of adequate knowledge about their safety, and the limited availability of methods and information through the government's family-planning services. Another reason could be that women may have stopped using reversible methods following adverse side effects and were therefore forced to rely on induced abortions for spacing. Or again, they may have been using ineffective methods, or effective methods may have been used incorrectly, leading to contraceptive failure.

We know relatively little about the reasons and processes that lead to women's choice of induced abortion to space births. We also do not know whether changes in indicators of women's status, or the wider social acceptance and high levels of use of birth control measures over the past decades, have made any difference to the extent of reliance on abortion for birth spacing. Such information is vital for the planning of interventions to prevent unwanted pregnancies, if such interventions are to have any significant positive impact on women's health.

It is in this context that, in 2002, we decided to explore the extent to which induced abortions are a result of women's lack of power to control sexual and reproductive decisions within marriage, and of the gender power dynamics between the couple. In the light of the dramatic decline in fertility levels and the widespread social acceptance of contraception that has come about over the last two decades, we also decided to explore the changes, if any, which may have taken place in women's ability to prevent unwanted and mistimed pregnancies.

The research was carried out by the Rural Women's Social Education Centre (RUWSEC). Based in the Kanchipuram district of Tamil Nadu, RUWSEC is a grassroots women's organisation that has been working on women's reproductive health and rights issues since 1981. One of our activities is to promote contraceptive choice, by disseminating information to women and men on a range of reversible methods whose use has remained very low in spite of an increase in levels of female education, women's assertiveness and their access to information through the media. Women apparently continue to use induced abortion either for regulating or limiting children. Further, the decrease in the number of children desired is perhaps contributing to a greater demand for abortion services.

Objectives, Research Questions and Methodology

Our study was therefore initiated to explore the factors and processes that underlie an induced abortion, with the ultimate goal of designing community-based interventions to prevent unwanted pregnancy, based on the in-depth understanding of the processes leading to married women's choice of abortions to space birth. The main questions we focused on were:

- How do gender power relations within married relationships influence the choice of induced abortion to space births?
- How has this role changed during the course of a generation of major changes in the social, economic and demographic context?
- Are there differences in gender power relations between couples who are 'ever-users' of induced abortion, and those who are 'never-users' of induced abortion?

'Gender power relations' within marriage were defined to include

- the nature of communication between couples—whether the relationship is a sharing, friendly one or one where the husband is the 'superior' partner;

- women's freedom of movement;
- women's role in making everyday decisions related to the running of the household and in relation to their children;
- the role women play in decisions regarding money matters;
- the freedom women have in deciding whether and when to have sexual relations, the number and spacing of pregnancies, and the use of contraception; and
- women's freedom from violence or the threat of violence.

'Changes' during the span of a generation in gender power relations and their role in the use of induced abortion were sought to be captured by including, as study participants, two generations of married couples.

Geographical Location

Our research covered 98 hamlets in the Thiruporur and Thirukazhukundrum blocks of Kanchipuram district, Tamil Nadu, which also constitute the project area served by RUWSEC.

Despite relatively high rates of female literacy and female work participation in Tamil Nadu, indicators from NFHS-II (1998–99) suggest that women in Tamil Nadu do not necessarily enjoy a high status or autonomy. For example, the proportion of women suffering from anaemia in Tamil Nadu (56.5 per cent) is higher than the national average of 51.8 per cent, and 14 per cent of pregnancies do not end in a live birth, as compared to 9 per cent for India. Almost 40 per cent of the women do not take decisions related to their own health. Also, 40 per cent of the women in Tamil Nadu reported being beaten or physically mistreated since the age 15, and 16 per cent said they had experienced the same in the 12 months prior to our survey; all these figures are above the all-India averages (IIPS 2000).

According to estimates based on NFHS-I (1992–93) data, Tamil Nadu had the highest rate of abortions (spontaneous and induced) among Indian states. As against 6.3 per cent of all pregnancies ending in abortion (induced and spontaneous) in the country as a whole, in Tamil Nadu this figure was more than double: 13.1 per cent. It is believed that a significant proportion of induced abortions are either reported as spontaneous or not reported at all. If true, this would mean that the induced abortion rate would be quite high

(Mishra et al. 1998). The widespread use of abortion as a method of birth spacing was evident in a study on fertility transition in Tamil Nadu (Ravindran 1997).

Kanchipuram district, where our research was based, is a coastal district located very close to the state capital Chennai and accounting for 5 per cent of the state's population, and is quite similar, on many indicators, to the state. Nearly 95 per cent of the rural population of the district receives full antenatal coverage, with little variation by caste (scheduled caste (SC)/scheduled tribes (ST) and others) or level of education. Although the knowledge of modern methods of contraception, including the condom, oral pill and IUD, is nearly universal, barely 7 per cent of the couples in the district use reversible methods of contraception.

As pointed out earlier, our research covered 98 hamlets in two blocks that are part of the project area served by RUWSEC. These hamlets are predominantly Dalit, with some hamlets comprising the poorest and 'most backward castes'. Low-income and socially marginalised, over three-fourths of the households were landless, with agricultural wage work being the main occupation for both men and women. Housing conditions were very poor, with nearly three-fourths of the households residing in mud huts with thatched roofs, 36 per cent without electricity and 93 per cent dependent on public water sources for drinking (taps, open wells and irrigation pump-sets). Only four households had toilet facilities within their homes. The literacy rate for the population aged seven and above was 59 per cent for males and only 40 per cent for females.

Sample Selection

Using in-depth interviews as our main research tool, we decided to draw our research sample from RUWSEC's database created on its project villages in 1996–97. Using a systematic, random-sample design, 2 groups of women and their husbands were selected for the study:

a. Older women: Ever-married women who had completed childbearing (were either menopausal or had undergone sterilisation) and had adult children (above 18 years).

b. Younger women: Ever-married women below 35 years who had not undergone sterilisation as yet.

Within each group, we selected equal numbers of 'ever-users' and 'never-users' of abortion. There were 1,491 'young' and 656 'older' women who were never-users of abortion. We selected a 10 per cent sample for the younger and a 20 per cent sample for the older women, and prepared a village-wise list of women to be interviewed in the 'never-users' category. Ever-users of abortion were identified through several methods. One, RUWSEC had in its database the names of women who, during routine data collection drives, had voluntarily reported having had an induced abortion. RUWSEC's village health workers and some of the ever-users who consented to be interviewed also suggested names of others who were willing to be interviewed. Husbands of women selected for the study were interviewed with the consent of the women.

In all, we had intended interviewing 60 women and 40 men. The 60 women were to include 30 'young' and 30 'older', divided equally between 'ever-users' and 'never-users' of induced abortion. Fewer men than women were included in the sample to allow for the possibility that not all women would agree that their husbands be interviewed, or have husbands currently living with them. The final sample consisted of 66 women and 44 men.

Research Tools

The research team, consisting of four males and five females, had considerable experience conducting research, workshops and trainings on gender, and reproductive health and rights issues within the community.

Interview guidelines for the in-depth interviews were developed through an interactive process. We led with a brainstorming meeting with the coordinators and project officers of RUWSEC, in order to identify major questions to be included in the guidelines. Based on this meeting, eight different interview guidelines were developed, one for each group of study participants: ever- and never-users of induced abortion; and men and women in the two age categories.

The guidelines were reviewed and revised several times after discussions with the field investigators and a few external reviewers. They were then pilot-tested with 15 persons. Finally, the research team had a meeting with the ethics committee members to finalise the guidelines and methodology for the study. The final guidelines had eight major sections:

1. The socio-demographic characteristics of participants
2. Marriage
3. Household decision-making
4. Sexual relations within marriage
5. Pregnancy and childbearing
6. Contraception: knowledge and practice
7. Views on abortion
8. Experiences of abortion users

Fieldwork

Fieldwork began with orientation and training in methodology and ethical issues. Data collection was spread over four months, during which we met once every fortnight to plan fieldwork, share issues and get clarifications.

Each interview followed three steps:

Step 1: The women field investigators went in pairs to a particular village with a list of never-user women to be interviewed, and met them in their homes. In the case of ever-users, the field investigators met the RUWSEC's village health worker, who contacted the women and obtained their permission for the investigators to meet them.

Step 2: After ascertaining their willingness to participate in the study, a time and place for the interview was fixed with each participant as per her/his preference.

Step 3: Field investigators met study participants as per their appointment and carried out the interview.

Ethical Considerations

A special ethics committee, comprising five people—two social scientists, two social activists and one public health specialist—was set up to guide the research. Information on the identity of those who had undergone abortions was not shared with anyone. All efforts were made to obtain written informed consent from all participants, also giving them the option to withdraw from the study at any stage. For those with limited literacy skills or those who could not read, investigators read out the contents of the consent form, including a description of the study and its aims and objectives. If a person was willing to participate in the study but unwilling to sign the form, the signature of a witness was obtained attesting to the participant's willingness.

Respondents' identities were protected through the use of codes for identifying them. No person or village was named in the transcripts, thereby ensuring that no person other than the interviewer knew their identity. Data entered into the computer were similarly protected.

Women were interviewed first. After completing each woman's interview, the husbands were interviewed, if the woman and the husband had consented to be interviewed. Women and men were interviewed at different places and at different times, the women by female investigators and the men by male ones. There was thus no possibility of the information given by one partner being inadvertently communicated to the other.

These norms were followed very strictly. No name was recorded anywhere in the study or the transcripts. To ensure privacy most interviews were conducted in isolated places in the community or in participants' homes.

Despite these precautions, there were one or two incidents where respondents got upset with the research team. In one village when we approached a respondent (who was a never-user of abortion) based on the sample list, she shouted at the investigator saying: 'Who gave you my name to interview? I am not a "such" a person to answer your questions.' The reference may have been to the aims and objectives of the study, which are first shared with a potential respondent in order to obtain her/his consent to participate in the study. In another village when, during an interview, the investigator asked questions relating to sexuality, the respondent suddenly got angry and withdrew her participation, tearing up the notes taken by the investigator. There were four women who withdrew from the study halfway through their interviews. A few men and women said: 'Sexual matters are something very personal. How can we share them with you?' However, there were also women, including those who had undergone induced abortions, who approached the investigators and volunteered to be interviewed.

FINDINGS

Socio-Demographic Characteristics of Participants

There were 110 respondents in all—66 women and 44 men. They included 44 couples and 22 women who did not want their husbands to be interviewed. All 44 men were husbands of women interviewed.

Of the 66 women, 34 had had one or more induced abortions in their lifetime (ever-users) and 32 had never had an abortion (never-users); and 23 of the 44 couples were ever-users, while 21 were never-users.

A total of 55 respondents—23 men and 32 women—belonged to the 'younger' category, which included women who were 35 years old or less (and their husbands) and had not yet stopped having children. The other 55 participants—34 women and 21 men—belonged to the 'older' category, which comprised women above 35 years (and their husbands) with adult children.

Table 8.1 summarises the socio-demographic characteristics of the participants. The majority were Hindus; only eight participants were Christians and all but seven belonged to the dalit community. Of the total, 38 per cent (42) came from households that owned some land, while 62 per cent were from landless households. The average household size was 5.51, and was 5.38 and 5.64 respectively for the younger and older group of respondents. Around 60 per cent (66/110) lived in nuclear families, with the remaining 40 per cent living in joint families.

The mean age of women respondents was 26.3 years and 40 years for the younger and older groups respectively. For men, the mean age was 30.9 years and 48.2 years respectively. The mean difference in age between couples was a little less than five years for the younger age group and a little more than eight years for the older age group.

There was a wide sex difference in the proportion of persons with schooling. Only 56.3 per cent of younger women and 38.2 per cent of older women had had some schooling. Among the men, 82.6 per cent of the younger and 62 per cent of the older groups had attended school.

The majority of participants, both women and men, were agricultural labourers. They usually averaged three to six months of regular work in a year and their daily wage ranged between Rs 25 and Rs 40

Table 8.1: **Socio-economic characteristics of participants**

Characteristics	Young women			Old women			Young men			Old men		
	*EU**	*NU**	*TOT**	*EU*	*NU*	*TOT*	*EU*	*NU*	*TOT*	*EU*	*NU*	*TOT*
Mean age	27.44	25.06	26.25	39.17	40.94	40.00	32.58	29.00	30.87	49.09	47.30	48.24
Religion												
Hindu	13	16	29	16	16	32	10	11	21	10	10	20
Christian	3	0	3	2	0	2	2	0	2	1	0	1
Caste												
Dalit	15	16	31	16	14	30	12	11	23	10	9	19
Other	1	0	1	2	2	4	0	0	0	1	1	2
Land-owning status of household												
Landed	3	8	11	6	5	11	4	7	11	4	5	9
Landless	13	8	21	12	11	23	8	4	12	7	5	12
Family type												
Nuclear	7	8	15	14	12	26	6	4	10	8	7	15
Joint	9	8	17	4	4	8	6	7	13	3	3	6
Household size												
Total persons	94	80	174	108	80	188	63	59	122	69	53	122
Average	5.88	5.00	5.44	6.00	5.00	5.53	5.25	5.36	5.30	6.27	5.30	5.81
Schooling												
No schooling	6	8	14	9	12	21	2	2	4	4	4	8
1–5 years	5	3	8	8	2	10	4	6	10	4	4	8
6–8 years	1	2	3	1	2	3	3	2	5	1	1	2
9–12 years	3	3	6	0	0	0	2	1	3	2	1	3
Degree	1	0	1	0	0	0	1	0	1	0	0	0

Occupation												
Agricultural wage labour	8	12	20	12	12	24	5	4	9	8	5	13
Own farm work	1	3	4	4	2	6	3	1	4	0	3	3
Other wage labour	1	1	5	0	0	0	0	5	5	0	0	0
Not working outside home	4	0	1	1	2	3	0	0	0	0	1	1
Others**	2	0	2	1	0	1	4	1	5	3	1	4
Average age at marriage	18.56	17.56	18.06	16.56	16.25	16.40	22.58	22.36	22.48	22.82	20.30	21.62
Pregnancy												
Total pregnancies	65	41	106	113	72	185	—	—	—	—	—	—
Average	4.06	2.56	3.31	6.28	4.50	5.44	—	—	—	—	—	—
Children ever born												
Total children ever born	41	29	70	83	66	149	—	—	—	—	—	—
Average	2.56	1.81	2.19	4.61	4.13	4.38	—	—	—	—	—	—
Total respondents	16	16	32	18	16	34	12	11	23	11	10	21

Notes: * EU = Ever users of abortion; NU = Never users of abortion; TOT = Total

** Include salaried employment, trading and vending.

for women and Rs 50 and Rs 100 for men. When agricultural work was not available, they sought work as unskilled manual labourers. Although two-fifths of the participants owned some land, though the size of landholding was very small and income from cultivation was not enough to sustain a household. Members of households with small landholdings were often engaged in other occupations in order to supplement their income.

There was approximately a year's difference in the average age at marriage between the younger and older age groups. The average age at marriage was 18.06 and 16.41 for younger and older women respectively, and 22.48 and 21.62 for men.

The average number of pregnancies among younger women was 3.31, and 5.44 among older women. Similarly, the average number of children ever born to younger women was 2.19, and to older women 4.43. Ever-users of abortion had a slightly higher average number of pregnancies as well as children ever born in both age groups. In the younger age group, abortion users had an average of 4.06 pregnancies and 2.56 children ever born, compared to an average of 2.56 pregnancies and 1.81 children ever born to women who had not used abortion. In the older age group, the comparative figures were 6.28 pregnancies and 4.61 children ever born among abortion users, and 4.5 pregnancies and 4.13 children ever born among never-users of abortion.

Marriage

In rural areas in Tamil Nadu, the majority of marriages are arranged by families, usually with the consent of prospective bride and groom. Among our participants, 35 of the 44 couples had had 'arranged' marriages. There were also nine 'love' marriages—seven in the younger age group and two in the older group.

Of the 44 couples, 14 were related to each other before marriage. Among the 35 arranged marriages, eight women and two men reported being forced into the marriage. In one marriage, neither party had wanted to marry the other. One man had been compelled by his family to marry a bride of their choosing. The remaining seven women said that they had not consented to the marriage, whereas their husbands did not say this.

'Love' marriages took place in varying circumstances. In three instances, the couple were related to each other, and although their families were initially against it, they had married with their parents' consent. Five couples had eloped and got married without family support, and in three of those, the woman was pregnant at the time of marriage. One marriage was between a widow with two children and a friend of the family.

Dissatisfaction with the state of their marriage was expressed by 12 wives (but not their husbands), one husband (but not his wife) and one couple. All those who had reported a forced marriage were unhappy even after several years. Two women who had married for 'love' also said that they had an unhappy marriage.

Household Decision-making

Overall, men took all the important decisions in the family. Some husbands consulted their wives when taking major decisions, but in no instance could a wife take independent decisions except on trivial matters. The most commonly heard response regarding household decision-making was: 'Men decide on money matters and women decide on household matters' (16/44). There were several (9/44) instances where the wives and husbands interpreted the women's roles differently, with the wives expressing dissatisfaction at their lack of decision-making power.

Of the 16 couples that claimed that the husbands took all the major decisions, 10 were in the younger age group. Among them, the women could decide on some day-to-day matters such as buying flowers, clothes and groceries. As reported by a husband:

> In my household I take decisions about money matters and important matters like the purchase of dresses and jewels during festivals, etc. My wife can decide on her own to buy things of daily need for the household, and about the children's health.

However, this was not simply a matter of division of responsibilities. Women could not spend money on any major purchases without their husbands' permission. They certainly could not go out on their own. In some cases, but not all, they could take their children to health facilities without being accompanied by anyone. Many women and men mentioned that the wives never went anywhere without the husbands' permission, conveying to us that this was appropriate and approved behaviour. Participation in the public sphere by women was not possible without their husbands' permission and was often disallowed.

> I have to get his permission to go out. Otherwise he will beat me. I was interested in joining the village self-help group. He was not there, and I went to the meeting without telling him. He beat me terribly for this, so I did not join the group. (YWNU–13)

Unilateral decisions by the man in all matters was reported by both husband and wife in 11 (five younger and six older) of the 44 couples. In these instances, the women had no say in running the household.

> I take decisions in my family. I will not allow her to take any decisions. She cannot have any money of her own, if she has I take it away. I have beaten her for her wrong decisions. So, she never takes any decisions. (YMNU–7)
>
> He decides all matters in my household. I never say anything. What is there to say? He is my husband, he decides. (OWNU–6)
>
> He takes all decisions. I didn't even buy a sari for myself during the five years of my marriage. One day, when I took my son to hospital without his permission because he was not there, he abused me: 'You, who turn your back on me like a donkey, how dare you?' I have to ask him to accompany me even for small things, like going to the bathroom at night. Otherwise he calls me a prostitute. (YWNU–4)

One young woman narrated how her father-in-law was the decision-maker in all matters.

> In my family, my father-in-law takes all decisions. Even for my personal things, he takes the decisions (things like jewels, money, dress, flowers, etc.). Once, when I objected, he scolded me and shouted, 'Shut your mouth and be a woman.' (YWEU–2)

Two women, one in the younger and one in the older age group, said that it was they who took all the important decisions: their husbands were alcoholics and did not support the family.

In nine couples (four younger and five older), men and women viewed their decision-making roles differently. While the men said that they always consulted their wives and that decision-making was done jointly, the women felt that they did not have an equal say in any matter. The wives also resented the restriction on their mobility and the need to seek their husbands' permission for almost everything. For example, according to one husband:

> In my household we both take decisions jointly with due consultation. She can buy flowers, dresses and other things for herself. Regarding borrowing or lending money, we both take the decisions.... We both jointly make decisions about the children's health and future. (YMEU–2)

However, his wife said that:

> Usually he takes decisions in my family. He never considers my view in the decision-making process. I have to accept his decisions even to buy things for myself like flowers or clothes. He never bothers about the children's future and education. For example, yesterday I borrowed some money from my mother and bought notebooks for the children. He never thinks about it. (YWEU–5)

Likewise, according to a man who has been married for 23 years:

> We both take decisions jointly, with mutual consultation, particularly on matters like purchasing land, taking loans, buying household items, etc. We never take decisions unilaterally. (OMEU–4)

But his wife had a different tale to tell:

> I can't take any decision because he is a drunk and shouts at me if I decide anything without his knowledge. I have to get his permission to even go to places like my natal or relatives' homes. (OWEU–5)

As mentioned earlier, only 5 couples of the 44 (3 younger, 2 older) interviewed said that they took joint decisions. One husband said:

> In my household, I ask for her consent in all of my decisions. Similarly, she seeks my opinion in her major decisions. But about purchasing household things and small matters she decides on her own. We both decide on matters relating to the children's health and our future. (YMNU–4)

His wife agreed:

> We both jointly decide all matters. But I am the implementing authority of all decisions. I can buy things for the household and myself and decide money matters also. I can go out without his permission. (YWNU–7)

Similarly, a 50-year old man, who has been married for 25 years, said:

> I never take any decision without my wife's knowledge. Usually, we both discuss them before finalising decisions relating to money and property matters. (OMEU–10)

His wife corroborated this:

> We discuss even money matters jointly and come to a common agreement/conclusion. (OWEU–12)

Overall, a slightly smaller proportion of younger (5/23) than older couples (6/21) had men taking unilateral decisions. There were also fewer younger (4/23) than older (5/21) couples where the wife reported that she was not being consulted in decision-making, while her husband said that decisions were made jointly.

Sexual Relations within Marriage

Talking about Sex and Expressing Desire

The vast majority of women (54 out of 66) stated that they did not talk about sex with their husbands, or express their sexual desire in other ways. Contrary to women's statements, 29 out of 44 men in the study said that they openly spoke about sexual matters with their partners. Only four couples out of 44 said that they were able to talk freely about sexual matters, and all but one of them were younger couples.

Most women gave the stereotypical response: 'How can women talk about sex?' Except for the seven women who had had 'love' marriages and had experienced sex before marriage, all the others had learnt about sex within marriage. One older woman said she did not know anything about sex even after several months of marriage:

> I didn't know about sex before marriage and I have never spoken about sex with him. Even after marriage we hadn't 'joined' [had sex] for six months because I was fearful and shy. (OWEU–2)

Most women said that they had sex whenever their husbands wanted. Some said that they felt shy even to look at his face the morning after a night of sex. This was true even for women who had had 'love' marriages and those who had become pregnant before marriage:

> We were lovers and had sex before marriage. As a result of that I conceived before marriage. I don't talk about sex with him; this is something secret and happens only in the night. So how can we talk about these things openly? (YWEU–12)

But there were a few women who not only felt free to talk about sex but also to express their desire to their husbands:

> I didn't know about sex before marriage. But I can now talk about sexual matters openly. If I have the desire, I tell him. He accepts and we have it [sex]. Sometimes when I call him he says, 'I am not interested now; we will have it tomorrow.' Similarly I can tell him if I am not interested. We respect each other and do things that we like. (YWNU–7)

As has been mentioned earlier, most men reported that they felt free to talk about sex and express their desire to their wives. All but three of 44 men said that they were able to do this. One of the men who could not was an older man who said that since he was no longer employed he did not have the authority to call his wife for sex. Another older man said:

> I never speak about sex with her because we both feel shy about it. Whenever I have the sexual urge, we have it [sex]. (OMEU–1)

The third was a younger man who did not think that talking about sex was appropriate:

> I don't talk about sex with her. How can we speak of these things in a village? Whenever I have the feeling I have it [sex]. She never says no. When I call her she pretends that she is not interested. But she is happy when we have it. She never expresses her sexual desire. (YMNU–2)

Many of the older men complained, however, that their wives no longer liked their husbands talking about sex and desiring sexual relations.

> I like to speak openly about sex. I used to speak those days but now she does not like it because we have an adult son and adult daughters. (OMNU–5)

Non-consensual Sex

Non-consensual sex was highly prevalent in the area. In 56.8 per cent of the couples (25/44), the women (17) or both partners (8) stated that the woman could not refuse if her husband desired to have sex. Six men also talked about their inability to take no for an answer when it came to sexual matters. Many of the women whose husbands were not included in the interviews (15/22) had experienced non-consensual sex. Overall, 40 women reported non-consensual sex, with their experiences ranging from being nagged into submission to outright sexual violence. A commonly heard comment from most women was that if they refused, the men abused them verbally and asked: 'If not me, who do you want to sleep with?' This appeared to be a routine threat to cow women into submission.

In its mildest form, non-consensual sex led to the woman feeling humiliated and resigned. Several women reported that 'they would lie like an inanimate object, like a piece of wood, while he went ahead'. There were other instances reported involving physical abuse. A woman who had been married for 18 years said:

> Sex is a regular event for him—a regular habit like chewing betel leaf. If I object, then he will hurt me by saying, 'Do you have someone else? If not with me, whom do you have it [sex] with?'

If he decides to have sex, he won't leave me. He will have it no matter what—even during my menstrual periods.

If I don't want to have sex I have to act as if I am not well (lie in bed, call out in pain). Then he accepts. I can use this technique only on rare occasions. I don't love him; I have only fear and hate. (OWEU–1)

Women were also forced into having sex under threat of their husbands seeking sexual pleasure elsewhere. Nine men (of 44 couples) had one or more sexual partners besides their wives.

Sex is a regular event for him; he has it daily before he goes to sleep. Whenever I say no, he beats me and says, 'I will go in search of another woman.' (YWNU–5)

He has extramarital relations and I once rejected his desire because of fear of getting infection. That time he beat me badly. He had sex by force and said that even if he had sex with a thousand women, he got something different from me. (OWEU–14)

In several instances where the wives reported sexual coercion, the men concerned tended to report being considerate and always engaging in consensual sex. But there were a few men (9) who admitted that they would not accept 'no' for an answer. According to them:

She doesn't object to sex usually, and I have it as I wish. If she objects when she is not well or when she is menstruating, I accept it. But if she objects for other reasons I don't accept it and will have it by compulsion without her desire. I beat her in two situations. One is when I am drunk and the other is when she says no to sex. (YMEU–2)

My wife would often express her reluctance because she was afraid of getting pregnant. I wouldn't accept her rejection because I was unable to control my feeling. I would force her into sex saying, 'What is wrong if you conceive again?' Mostly, I was under the influence of alcohol and that affected my judgement, but I would feel bad in the morning for my harsh behaviour. (OMEU–7)

Sexual Violence and Other Forms of Partner Violence

Sexual violence within marriage is embedded within the larger context of the use of physical violence or the threat of such violence to keep women submissive. Of the 25 women who reported non-consensual sex, 19 spoke of regular or routine sexual violence. There were an additional 11 women who reported other forms of intimate partner violence, bringing the total number of couples where the woman reported sexual or other forms of violence to 36 (out of 44). Of the 66 women interviewed, 47 reported experiencing violence: 40 reported sexual violence and seven reported other forms of intimate partner violence.

There were some interesting differences between the reporting of violence by women and men. Some partners of women reporting sexual violence admitted to both coercive sex and physical violence. However, in almost every case, the men portrayed the reason for violence as a domestic disagreement relating to the wife's inadequate performance of her duties:

> She doesn't care about children's neatness. I beat her for that, and for not preparing the food when I am hungry and sometimes for not cleaning the house. (YMEU–3)

> I beat her because she quarrels with my mother. (YMNU–8)

Further, unless it was extreme, women tended to under-report violence that was not sexual. For example, in eight of the 11 couples reporting non-sexual violence, it was the husband who reported that he often beat his wife when he was drunk or because 'she answered back'; the wife did not report experiencing any violence from her husband. The sort of non-sexual violence that women did report had to do with quarrels relating to the husband's extramarital affairs, routine drunken abuse and extreme forms of cruelty.

> He beat me with his shoes. I had delivered only two weeks ago, and he was angry that I had delivered a third girl child. (YWNU–13)

Within such a context of violence, a couple can hardly be expected to communicate or relate to each other on any equal or easy terms.

This lack of communication plays out in the extent to which women can regulate their fertility.

Sexual Rights

Despite the reality in which they live, there were few women who believed that men had a right over women's sexuality. But they regretted that for many women, it is not possible to exercise their sexual rights.

> Women should have the right where and when to have sex. I am a slave. How can I exercise my rights? (YWNU–5)

> It would be good if women have decision-making powers regarding sex. But this is not possible in my life. (YWEU–6)

> No man would accept the notion that women have the right to decide whether and when to have sex. It will not work in a majority of women's lives. (OWNU–13)

> I have the right to decide whether, when and where to have sex. But generally men view women as childbearing machines. (OWNU–10)

Pregnancy and Childbearing

The Pregnancy Experience

The average number of pregnancies among the younger women was 3.31, while it was 5.44 for those in the older age group. However, this does not necessarily indicate a generational change in the number of pregnancies, because not all women in the younger age group had completed childbearing, whereas those in the older age group had.

The majority of women (42 of 66 or two-thirds) received *some* support or help during their pregnancies in carrying out household tasks, *but not for heavy work* such as fetching water and fuel. This was equally true for both younger and older age groups. More than half the women worked in the farms as agricultural labourers late into their pregnancy. 'I worked in the fields till evening, and delivered the baby at home the same night', was a not uncommon assertion. However, only about a third of the younger women reported working in the fields during their pregnancy, as opposed to three-fourths of the older women.

In 41 cases (62 per cent), women said that their husbands had been supportive. They had accompanied the women to the health facilities, provided financial support for care seeking and sometimes even helped with some of the daily chores 'whenever' they were at home. The husbands we interviewed corroborated this, saying that they had been happy to learn about their wives' pregnancy and had supported them. Most of them were in nuclear family situations, where no other source of help was available, and they felt that it was their responsibility to pitch in when they could.

In some instances (13/66), men who had been supportive during earlier pregnancies were annoyed and even irritated with the later ones. Two women talked about being beaten by their husbands because of repeated female births and of being neglected throughout the pregnancy. In 12 cases, the men just ignored the pregnancy and carried on as if it was none of their business.

Care Seeking During Pregnancy and Delivery

The majority of women (49 women of 66) claimed having had antenatal care for all their pregnancies; only three women did not have antenatal care for any pregnancy, and 14 women had antenatal care for some of their pregnancies. Two of the three women who did not have antenatal care for any pregnancy were from the older age group. In the younger age group, there was only one woman who did not have antenatal care for her last pregnancy, which she said was unwanted. Thus, there has been a major shift in care seeking during pregnancy. Women have begun seeking antenatal care not only from the village health nurses (VHNs) who run antenatal clinics in the community once or twice a month, but also from the primary health centre (PHC). Many even go to the Medical College Hospital in Chengalpattu for 'testing' their pregnancy, for immunisation, and for 'scans' in the case of complications.

As many as 17 women (26 per cent) had delivered all their children in a health facility: most had used the services of the medical college hospital, though some had used the government's block-level hospitals. However, 24 (36 per cent) had delivered only some children—usually the first and the last—in the hospital, where they also got themselves sterilised after the last delivery. The remaining 25 women (38 per cent) had delivered all their children at home. Given that almost all women had antenatal care, the decision to have home deliveries appears to have been motivated more by economic considerations and availability of social support than lack of information. Once again, there was a distinct shift towards deliveries in health facilities in the younger age group: 38 per cent of younger women had all their deliveries at the hospital, while only 29 per cent had all their deliveries at home.

Unless probed, most women, including those who had complicated deliveries, did not think it important to report pregnancy-related morbidity as part of their pregnancy experience. Only two out of 66 women reported pregnancy-related morbidity spontaneously. One woman reported having eclamptic fits that resulted in a premature delivery, while another reported night blindness during several pregnancies, to which no one in her household paid any attention.

However, several women experienced miscarriages as well as complicated deliveries resulting in early infant deaths. Out of 291 pregnancies, 18 (6.91 per cent) resulted in miscarriages and stillbirths (6) and 26 babies of the 219 live births (11.87 per cent) died in infancy. The most common causes reported included reaching the health facility several hours after the 'bag of waters' had burst, delivering en route to the hospital and twin pregnancies. Despite the increased tendency among younger women to seek health care, natural pregnancy losses suffered by them were disproportionately high. Approximately 12.26 per cent of their pregnancies ended in miscarriage or stillbirth as against 5.95 per cent for the older women. Similarly, women in the younger age group experienced a much higher level of infant loss than the older age group, despite not having completed childbearing. For younger women, 13 out of 70 (18.57 per cent) live births ended in infant deaths, most of them immediately after or within the first week of birth. For the older age group, the comparable figures were 13 out of 149 (8.73 per cent).

Contraception: Knowledge and Practice

Knowledge of Contraceptives

Not many of our respondents knew much about reversible methods of contraception. Only 29 of 66 women (44 per cent) knew about permanent as well as reversible methods in some detail. Another 13 knew about permanent methods and had 'heard' about reversible methods. About a third (21 women: 32 per cent) knew only about sterilisation and vasectomy, and three said that they did not know about any method. A slightly higher proportion of men (25 of 44 or 58 per cent) than women knew about reversible as well as permanent methods of contraception, seven (16 per cent) had only a vague idea about reversible methods but knew all about permanent methods, and 11 (25 per cent) were only aware of sterilisation. One man said that he knew only one method for spacing births, which was induced abortion. For both women and men, knowledge of reversible methods was much more common among the younger than the older age groups.

But 'knowing' about a particular method of contraception did not mean that they ever used it. Quite likely their knowledge about reversible methods was based on hearsay, whereas that of sterilisation was based on the lived experience of women for well over a generation.

Reasons for Not Using Contraception

Among older couples, lack of knowledge about any method except sterilisation was an important reason for non-use of any spacing method. While about half the women had got themselves sterilised after completing childbearing, the other half had not done so. The reasons given for this included fear of the operation; the woman's poor health because of which she was refused sterilisation by the doctor; lack of help to cope with household tasks after the surgery; fear that surgery would make it difficult for the woman to work as an agricultural labourer; and being denied permission by husband or in-laws. One woman said that she had successfully avoided conception through the use of a herbal preparation that she had been taking for several years.

> I would have had the operation a long time ago, but my mother-in-law did not allow it. Recently I went to a doctor for sterilisation, but he said that I was too weak. (OWEU–3)

> We did not go for sterilisation because there was no one to help my wife after the operation. We did not have sex frequently. Now, 13 years after the last birth, she has not conceived. (OMNU–6)

My wife wanted to have sterilisation after her fourth delivery. But I objected, saying we need one daughter. So we are not using any method. (OMEU–3)

There were times when the husband and the wife had different perspectives on non-use of contraception:

We practised only abstinence. No other method was necessary. (OMNU–1)

Can't use any spacing method with this man who always suspects my fidelity. He does not want an operation either. (OWNU–1)

Another reason why couples did not use any contraceptive method despite not wanting any more children appears to be related to the belief (usually among men) that there is no risk of conception unless one has sexual intercourse everyday for a week or more. Since they did not have sex frequently, they believed that there was no need to use contraception.

Reasons for Not Using Modern Reversible Methods

The most commonly stated reasons for not using reversible methods like condoms, pills and the Copper-T were a fear of side effects and an embarrassment related to the lack of privacy in using contraceptive methods. The Copper-T was especially distrusted because women and men had heard that it could cause serious problems, such as perforation of the uterus, white discharge and weight gain. Such fears were common even among younger men and women.

If we use the Copper-T, it will go into the stomach, damage the intestine and cause white discharge. (YWEU–1)

Many preferred to have all the children they wanted and then opt for sterilisation because, according to them, reversible methods were only appropriate for urban and upper-class women who did not have to engage in hard manual labour.

We don't use any contraceptives. Even if we get them free, we won't use them because modern contraceptives [spacing methods] lead

> to various health problems. Women's health is affected and we have to spend money for that. So, I think an operation is better. After having the next child I will undergo the operation. (YWNU–2)

> Temporary contraceptives are not suitable for us because we do hard manual work in the field all round the year, and there is no rest. So these methods lead to various problems. I think after getting two or three children it is better to go for sterilisation. (YWEU–3)

It was also believed that if a woman had a long interval between her first two pregnancies, the same interval would continue for later pregnancies, and that no specific contraceptive method needed to be used.

As for condom use by men, many non-users stated that they did not want to use it because it would interfere with sexual satisfaction. There were also situations where men felt embarrassed to use it because of lack of privacy.

A significant number of couples, especially in the younger age group, had used at least one reversible method of contraception at some point in the past, although a very small number of them were current users. The numerous barriers to the effective use of reversible methods included side effects, lack of privacy, irregular availability of free supplies, and the cost incurred when purchasing them from pharmacists.

> We used oral pills and injections to prevent conception after my second child. But my wife didn't use the pills regularly. She was breastfeeding the baby and was afraid that it might affect the infant's health. (YMEU–1)

> I had used the Copper-T for one and a half years to space the births. But we removed it because I became weak and had a white discharge and nausea. I will have an operation after having my next child. (YWNU–11)

> My wife took tablets to space the first and second births. We got them from Chengalpattu Medical College Hospital. She had developed a vomiting sensation and a poor appetite and so she stopped taking them. I use a condom whenever I have it. But I feel

dissatisfaction in sex while using it. Also I have teenage children so I find it difficult to use the condom regularly. (YMEU–5)

Views on Abortion

A majority of never- and ever-users of abortion felt that abortion is wrong and has many negative health consequences like excessive bleeding, severe backache and abdominal pain, uterus damage and, in extreme cases, death. Many said they knew women who had died from septic abortions. But they also felt that with qualified doctors performing them, abortions had become safer and more accessible in recent times. Some women who had undergone abortions thought that it was better to have an abortion than an unwanted child. Similarly, they did not think of abortion as a sin. Interestingly, many men whose wives had had an abortion felt that abortion is a sin.

> Abortion is wrong and it is equal to a murder. It has wider health consequences. I know that a woman has died of it. I have also heard that women develop severe stomach-aches and acidity after the abortion. (YMEU–5)

A woman who had an abortion said:

> Considering the risks of bearing and rearing an unwanted child, abortion is good. (YWEU–5)

A woman who had four children and had experienced one induced abortion said:

> Earlier, I used to think that abortion is a sin. But now, after my own experience, I also realise that it is hazardous to women's health. So I will never take such a risk in future. [The implication here seems to be that the woman now feels that the ethical dimension of abortion is not the sole reason to avoid it; health concerns are also an issue.] (YWEU–6)

Table 8.2 lists the range of views about abortion expressed by men and women who have had an abortion as well as those who have never had one.

Table 8.2: Perceptions of abortion

Perceptions	Women*		Men*	
	Ever-users of abortion	Never-users of abortion	Ever-users of abortion	Never-users of abortion
Abortion is a serious health hazard	18	22	13	14
Better to have abortion than an unwanted birth	7	0	0	0
Abortion is a sin	2	8	6	8
Abortion is a sin but sometimes necessary	3	2	0	0
Abortion is not wrong	4	2	0	0
There is no health problem if abortion is done under safe conditions	5	3	1	1
The choice of abortion depends on individual circumstances: economic circumstances, health situation (there can be no single view on it)	2	4	4	2
Abortion is a means to have a small family	0	0	1	0

Note: * More than one view expressed.

A few reasons given by almost everyone to explain why couples opted to terminate a pregnancy were:

- The earlier child was still an infant
- Children were grown up
- The foetus was female
- They could not afford another child
- The woman's health was poor
- The astrological time was not right: it was inauspicious to have a birth in the month of *Chitirai* (May, the hottest month of the year)

More than a quarter of the women (19/66), both users and non-users, said that unwanted pregnancy was caused by the 'non-cooperation of the husband' who compelled women to have sex. Only 13 women held non-use of contraception as responsible for unwanted pregnancy. Clearly, the women believed that they would be able to avoid unwanted pregnancy only if men abstained from sex when a pregnancy was not immediately desired.

Experiences of Abortion Users

Of the 34 women who were ever-users of abortion, 16 belonged to the younger and 18 to the older age category. Nearly two-thirds of them (22) had had one abortion, eight had undergone two abortions, and two had undergone three and four abortions respectively, making a total of 52 abortions. In four instances, the women had attempted to have an abortion in a previous or subsequent pregnancy but the method used had not been effective and they had carried the pregnancy to term. Most abortions (36 of 52) had been terminated in the first trimester, and a further seven within the first 20 weeks, the legally permitted period. Some women (13) had had abortions during the sixth (10) and even in the seventh month (3) of gestation. There were no differences between the younger and older women in the distribution of the number of abortions per woman or the period of gestation when abortion took place.

About one-third of the pregnancies terminated were of a lower order—three and below—and one-fourth were of the order of six and above. Of the 18 who terminated a pregnancy of the order of three or below, only three were older women, and of the 13 who terminated higher-order pregnancies, only two were younger women.

Occasionally, the number of abortions reported by wives and husbands did not match. The confusion was perhaps in perception. In one case, what the wife reported as a stillbirth her husband viewed as a late abortion. In another instance, a woman reported having had two abortions, whereas her husband reported four. In a third case, a woman admitted to having had an abortion, but the husband called it a miscarriage.

Decision-Making on Abortion

In two-thirds of the 52 abortions (34), the decision to terminate pregnancy had been taken by the women concerned. In a little less than half of these instances (15/34), the women had not been able to get their husbands' support but had gone ahead regardless. Such instances were far more common among women in the older age group (11/27) than among younger women (4/25).

> I already had five sons and my husband was not co-operating with me. His second wife also had two children. Taking all this into account, I decided to abort and informed him of my decision. But he didn't agree. Then I went to my mother's home and had the abortion. My parents paid for all the expenses. (OWEU–14)

In 11 cases the decision was a joint one. The support of mothers/mothers-in-law was also often sought:

> At first, I suggested terminating the pregnancy. Initially he rejected my suggestion, but I convinced him later. My mother also agreed. (YWEU–8)

Two women had undergone late abortions (in the seventh month of gestation) under medical advice, while five women had been compelled by their husbands and/or in-laws to have an abortion, in some cases because it was believed that the particular pregnancy was inauspicious, and in some because the pregnancy came at an inconvenient time when the family could not afford to have the woman 'confined'.

> I was not interested in terminating the pregnancy, but my in-laws and husband compelled me to. When I objected, they scolded me and tried to send me to my natal home. I then decided to go for abortion. (YWEU–2)

> When I told him about the pregnancy, he was silent for some time. Then he asked me to go to my mother's home and abort the pregnancy. (OWEU–1)

> My abortions—I had two—were for economic reasons. When I told him of my pregnancy he said, 'You have become pregnant in the high season for business, what can we do?' We run a shop and both of us have to work. I would not be able to stand all day in the shop during my pregnancy and that would affect the sales and our income. So he asked me to terminate the pregnancy and I did. (OWEU–18)

Reasons for Having an Abortion

Women gave several reasons for terminating pregnancy. Predictably, the most common amongst them were the need to limit the family, either because the desired family size had been achieved or for economic reasons, and to have a longer interval between births.

The most common reason for abortion among women in the older age group was 'to limit family size' (11 abortions). A concomitant reason for some of them was that since their children had now become teenagers or adults, they felt acutely embarrassed to continue with the pregnancy. A few said that they wanted to limit family size because they could not afford any more children.

> We terminated my fifth pregnancy to limit family size. My previous born child was already 18 years old. So I didn't want to continue with the pregnancy. He suggested that I deliver the baby and have the operation. But keeping in mind my 'mature' [attained menarche] daughters, I didn't want to continue with the pregnancy. (OWEU–13)

> I conceived 10 times and aborted 4 pregnancies, mainly to limit my family. I was the only earning member in my household and I could not afford more children. (OWEU–15)

In contrast, the most common reason given by younger women was 'economic circumstances' and 'poverty' (nine cases). A concomitant reason given by some of them was that there was no one to support them either during or after the pregnancy.

> I aborted three pregnancies: my third, fourth and fifth ones. My family's economic situation was very bad at that time, and I was also not keeping well. My husband knew about the pregnancy and didn't say anything. But I decided. Only I knew the pain and the worries. (YWEU–5)

> I aborted my first pregnancy because of my family's economic crisis. We were in a nuclear family and very poor. We took the decision with a heavy heart. There was no way we could have this child because we had no money and no family support. (YWEU–18)

> During my second pregnancy, the elders with whom we were living decided that we should set up home separately. We were in a dilemma. Our first-born was a daughter and we were hoping that the second would be a son. He convinced me to have an abortion,

> saying that we could not manage in a nuclear family without anyone to help me and with only one person working. (YWEU–17)

Another important reason given, especially by the older age group (two out of 9 abortions) was that the previous child was too young. The saying was: 'To save the baby in hand, let go off the baby in the womb.' But this was usually said when the previous child was a male infant. There appeared to some anxiety that the pregnancy might jeopardise the health and survival of the male child—hinting at the existence of son preference even among Dalits. However, there were only a few instances (two) when abortion was used to avoid a female birth. Both women had had several previous pregnancies that had resulted in female children and they did not want to risk having one more daughter. The woman who reported being beaten by her husband for delivering a third female child, for example, aborted the next pregnancy. In one tragic case, the woman aborted her fifth pregnancy after three daughters in a row:

> When I was leaving for the hospital my husband said, 'It could be a male, don't abort it.' Even in the hospital the nurse tried to change my mind, but I was stubborn. When I regained consciousness after the abortion, they told me it was a male foetus. I felt devastated, like I was going mad. I wept a lot and it took me several months to feel normal. I lied to my husband and told him it was a female foetus. I never had a male child: even the next one was female and after that I had some problems and my uterus was removed. (OWEU–4)

Two women had undergone late abortions (in the seventh month of gestation) under medical advice. In one instance, a scan revealed that the foetus was seriously deformed and termination was advised. This was a first and wanted pregnancy. In the other instance, the foetus had to be removed because it had been damaged when the woman met with an accident. Both were younger women.

In two cases, pregnancy was terminated because the unborn child was thought to be inauspicious:

> When I became pregnant for the second time, my husband injured his leg in an accident. He consulted an astrologer, who said that the (unborn) child may be inauspicious and suggested that we terminate the pregnancy. My in-laws and husband compelled me

by saying, 'Is your unknown baby's life worth more than your husband's?' (YWEU–2)

In our family, it is believed that the third-born child does not survive. So they compelled me to terminate my pregnancy. (YWEU–4)

Sometimes, women gave reasons that defy all logic. For instance, a woman who had had two previous C-sections had been advised to avoid getting pregnant for the next few years. She did get pregnant, but the couple terminated four consecutive pregnancies 'for health reasons' because they felt that she would die if she continued with them.

Women Accompanied to the Service Provider

In 30 out of 52 abortions, the husbands accompanied the women and, in five of them, mothers or mothers-in-law also went along. Younger women were accompanied by their husbands and mothers/mothers-in-law in 21 of 25 abortions, and by their mothers for two abortions. Only one woman went with a neighbour and one went alone. The older women, on the other hand, were accompanied by their husbands and mothers-in-law in only 9 out of 27 abortions. They had to seek help from their mothers, neighbours, sisters-in-law and sisters, the local *dai* or distant relatives. In the case of three abortions, women reported they had gone alone. This suggests that husbands among younger couples were far more involved with decisions relating to abortion.

Choice of Abortion Provider

As many as 40 of the 52 abortions (77 per cent) were performed by rural medical practitioners who were neither trained nor qualified to conduct abortions. Contrary to the popularly-held view that rural women prefer to seek the services of women doctors, most of these practitioners were men, According to the women, some of the practitioners were assisted by their wives.

Only 7 abortions were performed in government health facilities, despite the fact many of the survey villages are well connected by buses to Chengalpattu Medical College hospital and some PHCs that provide abortion services. This may have been due to the fact that availing the services of a government facility is a time-consuming process, which few women seeking abortions can afford:

> I told my husband about my decision to terminate my fourth pregnancy. He just nodded and went away, the good-for-nothing man. I took my child, who was just a year and a half, and walked from my village to the government hospital which is 4 km away. I went back and forth four to five times, but they kept asking me to come later. I would go and wait for hours and return home without the abortion being done. Finally, I went to the private [untrained] doctor, paying Rs 100 per month of gestation. I took a relative's daughter with me to mind my baby, and gave the excuse that the baby was not well. (OWEU–7)

An obstetric gynaecologist performed only one abortion, although there were two or more of them (albeit unlicensed) available in the towns where the unqualified practitioners were located. However, the use of traditional abortion providers was not common. Only two older women, accounting for four out of 52 abortions, had gone to traditional providers.

The most common method used for pregnancy termination was Dilation and Curettage (D&C). However, nine women reported having been given 'injections' that required them to make two visits, after which they had had the abortion at home. Since the women could not provide us with any more information, it was not clear whether some of the local practitioners were using RU-486. Unlike medical practitioners, traditional providers usually inserted the stick of a particular tree into the cervix to induce abortion.

Quality of Care and Abortion-related Morbidity

Not many women commented on the quality of abortion services they received, except in instances when things had gone wrong. They also often mixed up issues relating to quality of care with abortion-related morbidity; 21 out of 34 women reported morbidity, with the younger and older age groups almost equally represented (11 and 10 respectively).

Excessive bleeding was the most commonly mentioned problem, reported by 17 of the 21 women. The other problems were lower abdominal pain and backache, though two women also mentioned wheezing and stomach-burn as being a consequence of abortion.

> The doctor gave me an injection for becoming unconscious. But it didn't work. Then he cleaned the uterus with an instrument. The pain was killing, and I could not get up for nearly three hours after the abortion. For the second abortion I went to another hospital because I was afraid to go back to the earlier one. This time also the medicine to lose consciousness didn't work. I was conscious and felt the pain when the abortion was being done. It was unbearable. I cursed myself for being born a woman. I cursed God. I was bedridden and bled for 20 days. I thought I would die. In the end I had to be hospitalised. (YWEU–6)

> [After the abortion of the sixth pregnancy] I had bleeding for a long time; when it wouldn't stop, we went to the government hospital. They refused to treat me, and told me to go to the same doctor who had performed the abortion. After five months of bleeding everyday, we went to a private hospital. The doctor found that there were some remaining pieces in my uterus. I was in the hospital for seven days. I still have several problems and am often under treatment. (OWEU–3)

> Initially the doctor refused to do the abortion because I was more than three months pregnant. When I begged, he agreed. He gave me an injection and asked me to come the next day, when he 'cleaned' my uterus. I became quite ill. After that I conceived and delivered the next child. I wanted to have the operation, but the doctor said I was too weak and refused. This led to my fifth pregnancy. I approached the same doctor who had done the earlier abortion. He refused, saying if something happened he would be in trouble, because of the problems I had the last time. I assured him that no one would come with a complaint even if something happened to me.... I was very weak for many months after that. (YWEU–5)

Abortion Use and Gender Power Relations within Marriage

Part of our research was devoted to exploring the differences, if any, between ever-users and never-users of abortion in significant aspects of gender power relations within marriage. We elicited abortion users' own perceptions of the role gender power relations play in their exposure to the risk of unwanted pregnancies and in their use or non-use of abortion. We focused on the following questions:

- Were marriages with the consent of both (more equal power relations) as against the woman being forced into the marriage (unequal)?
- Did women experience unhappiness and dissatisfaction with the marriage (unequal)?
- What was the women's role in decision-making within marriage: joint (more equal), some decisions (less equal) or no decisions (unequal)?
- What was the extent of women's freedom of movement and freedom to act independently?
- What was the extent of non-consensual sex, sexual violence and any other intimate partner violence?
- What was the level of husbands' co-operation in pregnancy prevention?

Type of Marriage and Satisfaction in Marriage

Overall, there did not seem to be any major differences between abortion users and non-users either in terms of consent to marriage or in terms of satisfaction with the marriage. However, as indicated earlier, the number of love marriages was higher among younger than older couples.

Role in Decision-Making

A noticeable difference between abortion-users and non-users in terms of women's role in decision-making can be seen (Table 8.3) in the numbers who reported a traditional division of decision-making authority—with men deciding on all money matters and women deciding on household matters—and those who did not. Ten out of 23 in the abortion-users group reported a traditional division as compared to only 5 out of 21 in the non-users group. On the other hand, the number of couples where men made *all* decisions was approximately the same for both groups. We could discern no clear or definite differences in decision-making roles, except that more women in the abortion-users group reported the stereotypical, traditional division, wherein their decision-making roles were confined to such household matters as buying vegetables and groceries for daily use and buying items like flowers for themselves.

Table 8.3: Status of couples in decision-making

	Ever-users of abortion couples		Never-users of abortion couples	
Decision-making	Younger	Older	Younger	Older
Both say that decisions are jointly made.	1	1	2	1
Both say: 'Men decide money matters and women decide household matters.	6	4	3	2
Both say that the man makes all decisions.	3	2	2	4
Discordance: Wife says husband is decision-maker, husband says joint decisions.	2	3	3	3
Decisions made by in-laws, neither the husband nor the wife has much of a say.	0	0	1	0
Total	12	11	11	10
Need husband's permission to go anywhere	11 of 16 women	11 of 18 women	10 of 16 women	5 of 16 women
Need husband's permission to go to natal home	11 of 16 women	11 of 18 women	9 of 16 women	6 of 16 women

Women's autonomy was also assessed in terms of freedom of movement. As shown in Table 8.3 more than half of the women required the husband's permission every time they wanted to go somewhere. Further, they reported that they could not go anywhere without an escort, except perhaps to the health facility if the children were sick. Visiting the natal home appeared to be a particularly sensitive issue. Several women, especially in the younger age group, reported that they were only infrequently permitted to visit their parents and that too if accompanied by their husbands, and were not allowed to spend the night there. While women generally viewed regular contact with the natal home as an empowering factor, the men viewed it as a threat to their authority.

In addition, there was a difference in the degree of freedom enjoyed by abortion users and non-users, both among younger and older women. Most of the older women in the never-user group reported that they had greater freedom of movement now than in the past.

The amount of freedom they enjoyed clearly increased with age. But this pattern did not seem to hold in the ever-user group. It is therefore safe to suggest that there are differences in the autonomy and freedom enjoyed by women who experience an abortion and those who don't. This hypothesis gains further ground when we examine the next set of indicators related to non-consensual sex and sexual violence (Table 8.4).

Table 8.4: Sexual and other forms of violence against women

	Ever-users of abortion couples*		Never-users of abortion couples*	
	Younger	Older	Younger	Older
Non-sexual violence	12	10	9	7
Non-consensual sex	8	10	7	5
Sexual violence	9	8	7	3
Total	12	11	11	10

Note: * Some women suffered more than one form of violence.

Non-consensual Sex, Sexual and Other Forms of Violence

Overall, the presence of violence was more common in the abortion users' group. While non-sexual violence was more common in the non-users group, non-consensual sex and sexual violence were more common among the abortion users. By allowing women little control over their sexuality, non-consensual sex and sexual violence exposed them to the risk of unwanted pregnancy. Many of the women considered unwanted pregnancy and abortion to be a direct consequence of non-consensual sex, often accompanied by violence if the woman resisted.

> I could have avoided my abortions but he didn't co-operate with me [did not accept her refusal to have sex]. (OWEU–18)

Some women reported that their husbands compelled them to have sex, saying that they would pay for the abortion in case of pregnancy.

> If I reject his desire to have sex, he says, 'It is me who will be meeting the expenses. If you conceive you can go for an abortion.'

But he doesn't realise the problems associated with abortions. (YWEU–17)

We heard numerous stories of women's unsuccessful attempts to avoid unwanted pregnancies, pregnancies which often ended in abortion and sometimes unwanted births. The men, on the other hand, tended to blame their wives for getting pregnant frequently.

An older woman who became pregnant for the fifth time, said:

> He is working outside the village and comes home once in two or three days. In that situation I am not able to say no [to sex], even if it is during the day. I have to accept it. If, I object, he shouts, 'When I am not at home, who comes here?' If I don't accede to his desire, I have to face beating and shouting. This is something that happens to most women.
>
> If I give fear of pregnancy as a reason, he won't leave me alone. He says conception doesn't take place frequently. I am pregnant now. Everyone is talking about my getting pregnant after having grandchildren. I am ashamed…I wanted to abort this pregnancy, but the doctor refused, saying I was very weak. Also, I did not realise I was pregnant until the sixth month, because my periods were not regular anyway. If I get sterilised I can live without fear. But he says, 'You are physically weak, don't do it'. But I am stubborn; I have experienced two unwanted pregnancies [one was terminated] and I am ashamed of it (OWEU–17).

A young woman of 25 years who was also pregnant for the fifth time said:

> I have aborted two pregnancies—the second and fourth. I was very worried. I first considered ending my life, but then I boldly decided to go for abortions. There was no other way. He said, 'You get pregnant with a single touch.' Fear and embarrassment in asking for spacing methods and his compulsion for sex have led to three unwanted pregnancies and two abortions.
>
> Even though men are responsible for pregnancy, people generally say that it is the woman's fault. They say, 'Men are good, but women are foolish, emotional and looking for body pleasure.' I felt very

bad when some people teased me saying that I don't leave my husband alone for a minute and that my stomach is always bulging. (YWEU–6)

Contraceptive Use

If the women were so keen to avoid pregnancy, why did they not use any method of contraception? When we compared contraception usage by abortion users and non-users, we found that women with a history of abortion had also used some contraceptive method at some time in their lives. This trend is corroborated by NFHS data, which shows an association between a current unwanted pregnancy and ever use of reversible methods of contraception (see Table 8.5).

Table 8.5: Contraceptive use among women

	Ever-users abortion		Never-users abortion	
	Young	Old	Young	Old
Ever used one or more modern reversible methods	11	8	6	1
Ever used one or more natural methods (safe period, abstinence, *coitus interruptus*)	4	7	3	5
Ever used sterilisation	0	9	0	11
Never used any method of contraception	4	4	8	4
Total	16	18	16	16

As discussed earlier, the most commonly used contraceptive was the condom, which the men discontinued or used irregularly for reasons such as irregular supply, interference with sexual satisfaction and expense. Reasons for discontinuing the pill and the Copper-T were usually related to their side effects.

Husbands' opposition to the use of any method of contraception was more common among older women, although some of the younger women also mentioned it.

Only he is responsible for the abortion, because first he prevented me from having an operation and then he beat me when I was reluctant to have sex. So again it led to another unwanted pregnancy and abortion. (OWEU–2)

Currently I am pregnant. I had decided to abort this also, whether I survived or not. But he and my father convinced me to have this child and then go in for sterilisation. [After the previous abortion] the doctors did not say anything about preventive methods [contraceptives]. When I asked my husband to find out whether there was any way to avoid getting pregnant, he said, 'Am I having sex with a prostitute that I have to ask about preventing pregnancy?' (YWEU–6)

He didn't want us to use any contraceptives and that is why it [the abortion] has happened in my life. (YWEU–15)

Average Number of Pregnancies and Live Births

As can be seen in Table 8.6, there appear to be interesting differences between women who had had an abortion and who had not, in the average number of pregnancies experienced, pregnancy losses and infant deaths.

Table 8.6: Pregnancy outcomes and infant deaths

	Ever-users of abortion women		Never-users of abortion women	
	Younger	Older	Younger	Older
Average number of pregnancies	4.06	6.28	2.56	4.50
Average number of live births	2.56	4.61	1.81	4.13

The average number of pregnancies and live births was higher in the ever-users' group than in the never-users' group. When viewed in conjunction with the higher reporting of sexual violence and non-consensual sex among ever-users of abortion, we can see that the factor which distinguishes women who have had abortions from women who did not, was the exposure to repeated, unwanted pregnancies because of non-consensual sex.

Conclusions

We started out with asking whether and how gender power relations affect the choice of abortion to space or limit births, and whether these relations have changed across generations. We had also wanted to examine the differences between never-users and ever-users of abortion in terms of how gender power relations played out within marriage.

Our findings reveal that, in general, women—even the younger ones—have limited decision-making power within the household. Men control most of the decisions. Women may have physical mobility, but only for specifically sanctioned purposes such as taking children to the health facility or going to the market. Women also cannot participate in any public activities without their husbands' prior permission. In this respect, there is not much difference between women in the younger and older age groups. If older women appear to have more autonomy, it is very likely because, as they grow older, they are viewed less and less as 'sexual beings'. That freedom is a variable associated with age was evident from the fact that the older women reported that they were much more restricted when they were young compared to the current younger generation which seems to enjoy more autonomy.

Discussion and communication on sexual matters is rare, but when it does happen, it is among the younger couples. On the other hand, non-consensual sex and sexual violence are also more common in the younger than in the older age group.

Non-consensual sex and sexual violence appear to underlie the need for abortions among many couple, both young and old. Although women are well aware of their sexual rights and believe that men ought to take responsibility for preventing pregnancy, the ground reality is very different. Women go through one pregnancy after another —terminating them when they can, and carrying them to term when they cannot.

There are many differences between younger and older couples who have used abortion. Older women often have to make the decision by themselves; many have little support from their husbands and have to take the help of their mothers, sisters and neighbours. They also have to seek abortion from providers that are affordable, including traditional abortion providers. Among younger couples, the decision to abort is supported by the husband, who accompanies the wife to the abortion facility and pays for the services. This is despite the fact that the pregnancy might well have been the consequence of sexual coercion on his part. Testimony by some women indicates that men may be taking abortion very lightly—as something they can pay for and be done with. The frequent mention of poverty and economic considerations as reasons for abortion in the younger age group, as also instances of younger women being compelled to terminate their pregnancies, are rather disconcerting developments.

What are the differences between never-users and ever-users of abortion, especially in terms of gender-power relations within marriage? Our data on contraceptive use suggests that non-users of abortion are as exposed to the risk of unwanted pregnancy as abortion users, or perhaps more so, other things being equal. One feature that distinguishes the two groups is that among the 'never-users', more husbands 'co-operate' in preventing unwanted pregnancies, taking responsibility for fertility control even though they do not use condoms. This explains the lower average of pregnancies experienced by the 'never-users' group, and also its lower reporting of non-consensual sex and sexual violence.

In the abortion users group, while some initiative is taken by men to use condoms, their use is inconsistent and irregular. Women are unwilling to use the pill and the Copper-T because of side effects. Many women are also hesitant to use any form of contraception without their husbands' explicit approval, because they fear that in the event of side effects, the men may not pay for their health care. When efforts to prevent pregnancy through contraceptive use fail, and men are unwilling to abstain from sex, women have to rely on abortions to prevent unwanted births. They do this at considerable risk to their health.

The most noticeable difference between 'ever-users' and 'never users' of abortion is the preponderance of non-consensual sex and sexual violence among the former. Thus, most unwanted pregnancies are usually the consequence of unwanted sex and women's inability to refuse their husband's sexual demands. Many men seem to believe that sex within marriage is their right and that the women have no say in the matter.

Interventions to prevent unwanted pregnancies would have to address the issue of sexual violence within marriage as well as intensify efforts to make reversible contraceptives acceptable and available free of cost regularly to young couples. One way would be to hold regular sexuality and reproductive health-education workshops for young and/or newly married couples. This would provide young women and men an opportunity to learn more about sexuality and reproduction, as well as serve as a forum to clarify and understand better women's and men's differing perspectives on these matters.

It appears that a more proactive approach to promote reversible methods of contraceptives would be welcomed by both women and men, who feel embarrassed to ask volunteers or nurses for them. Also, a campaign addressing the unacceptability of sexual coercion within marriage would be another important intervention that needs to be implemented urgently.

Notes

We would like to take this opportunity to express our most sincere and grateful thanks to the HealthWatch Trust, New Delhi, for funding the study. Out thanks, also, to all the ethics-committee members for their valuable and proactive suggestions throughout the project.

We also express our gratitude to all the women and men who so willingly gave of their time and shared their views and their life-stories with us. Thanks also to the RUWSEC staff, who helped us in many different ways at different points during the course of the study.

Throughout the chapter, each respondent is identified by a number; also quoted material by respondents is referenced by abbreviations, as follows:

Older woman, ever-user: OWEU
Older woman, never-user: OWNU
Younger woman, ever-user: YWEU
Younger woman, never-user: YWNU
Older man, ever-user: OMEU
Older man, never-user: OMNU
Younger man, ever-user: YMEU
Younger man, never-user: YMNU

References

Agarwal, Sapna. 2000. *Annotated Bibliography on Abortion in India*. New Delhi: HealthWatch Trust.

Gupte, M., S. Bandewar and H. Pisal. 1997. 'Abortion Needs of Women in India: A Case Study of Rural Maharashtra', *Reproductive Health Matters* 5 (May): 77–86.

IIPS (International Institute for Population Sciences), ORC Macro. 2000. *National Family Health Survey* 2, 1998–99: India. Mumbai: Indian Institute of Population Studies.

Irudaya Rajan, S., U. S. Mishra and T. K. Vimala. 1997. 'Role of Abortion in the Fertility Transition in Kerala'. Paper prepared for the seminar Socio-cultural and Political Aspects of Abortion from an Anthropological Perspective. Trivandrum: International Union for the Scientific Study of Population (IUSSP).

Johnson, Heidi Bart. 1999. 'Abortion and Post-abortion Care in India: A Review of Literature, Draft 3'. North Carolina: IPAS.

Kulkarni, P. M., S. Krishnamoorthy and N. Audinarayana. 1996. 'Review of Research on Fertility in Tamil Nadu'. Monograph. Coimbatore: Department of Population Studies, Bharathiyar University.

Mishra, U. S., M. Ramanathan and S. I. Rajan. 1998. 'Induced Abortion Potential among Indian Women', *Social Biology* 45 (3–4): 278–88.

Parivar Seva Sanstha. 1999. *A Study on Abortion in Varanasi, Uttar Pradesh*. New Delhi: Parivar Seva Sanstha.

PRC (Population Research Centre), Gandhigram Institute of Rural Health and Family Welfare Trust and International Institute of Population Sciences. 2001. 'Tamil Nadu: Reproductive and Child Health Project: Rapid Household Survey 1998–99'. Trivandrum: Centre for Development Studies.

Ravindran, T. K. S. 1997. 'Women's Status and Fertility Transition in Tamil Nadu: An Inquiry into the Inter-linkages'. Report of the UNDP Project on Human Development in India. Trivandrum: Centre for Development Studies.

Singh, K. P. and R. Singh. 1991. 'A Study of Psycho-Social Aspects of MTP'. Report. Chandigarh: Population Research Centre, Department of Sociology, Punjab University

Sinha, R., M. E. Khan, B. C. Patel, S. Lakhanpal and P. Khanna. 1998. 'Decision-making and Acceptance in Seeking Abortions of Unwanted Pregnancies'. Paper presented at the international workshop on abortion facilities and post-abortion care in the context of the RCH programme. Baroda: Centre for Operation Research and Training (CORT).

IX

Pregnancy Wastage among the Poor in Coastal Karnataka

K. Susheela and K. Nagaraj

The main thrust of this study was twofold. One was to broadly estimate the extent and components of pregnancy wastage including abortion, which is an important reproductive health as well as rights issue, amongst two poor occupational groups, i.e., agricultural labourers and *beedi* workers in the Udipi district, a relatively advanced region in coastal Karnataka. The second was to understand the social, economic and cultural, as well as the medical underpinnings of this issue in these two groups. While some pregnancy wastage is inevitable, the right to induced abortion is not often a free choice for women but operates in the context of power relations.

About the Region

Udipi, in which this study was carried out, is a coastal district of Karnataka. The coastal part of the district is relatively more advanced than the interior parts or the *ghat* region lying to its east. Our survey village is located in the interior more backward part of the district. Along with high-value cash crops (like cashew and coconut), paddy cultivation, forest produce and fisheries are primary sources of livelihood for a majority of the population. In spite of abundant and assured rainfall, the topography of the region and the absence of agricultural modernisation has led to unemployment and underemployment, necessitating the adoption of alternative survival strategies like migration—permanent or seasonal—and non-agricultural activities, such as beedi-rolling.

The district's tertiary sector, which comprises banking, trade and transportation, is well developed. The literacy level among both men and women is also quite high. The district has a large number of educational institutions, including many professional ones. There is also a fairly well-developed system of health care. A recent study on district-wise human development in the country (Geetha Rani 1999: 30) ranks the erstwhile (composite) Dakshina Kannada district, from which Udupi was carved out in 1998, first in the country. Nevertheless, access to health care and education is uneven, with the poor in the region not always able to access these facilities.

At the same time, the high level of infrastructure and social development, the 'mobile' character of the population and rural–urban linkages, the high level of rural non-farm employment and the exposure to mass media like the television and radio lead to a situation where the transference of urban lifestyles and values to the rural population, including the poor, is quite high. As a result, people's aspiration levels are high. It is this disjunction, between poor living conditions on the one hand and high aspiration levels on the other, that underlies another basic phenomenon with important consequences for pregnancy wastage among the poor in the region—i.e., rapid fertility transition.

Fertility Decline

During the last decade, the district witnessed a rapid decline in fertility rate, which today, at 1.5, is below replacement level. In fact, it is one of the lowest among all districts in the country (Guilmoto and Irudaya Rajan 2002: 665–72).[1] While high female literacy may be a factor underlying the low fertility rate in the district, we believe that it constitutes only a partial explanation. A plausible explanation for the low level of fertility may lie in the high and increasing aspiration levels of the people. Inability to meet the aspirations leads to 'aspiration gaps', particularly among the poor. And one way of bridging this gap is through family limitation or social capillarity.

Further, while better access to health care facilities facilitates reduction in pregnancy wastage, it may also lead to a more liberal or permissive attitude towards induced abortion and hence increase its incidence. Rapid fertility transition based almost solely on family limitation can also affect pregnancy wastage in a number of ways. Reduction in the total number of pregnancies can lead to reduction in pregnancy wastage and, depending on the relationship between pregnancy wastage and birth order, it can also affect the rate of pregnancy wastage. On the other hand, non-use of spacing methods of contraceptives would lead to shorter birth intervals and an increase in pregnancies-at-risk, and hence to an increase in pregnancy wastage. The desire to limit family size can also increase the use of induced abortions. These linkages between socio-economic development indicators and fertility transition on the one hand and pregnancy wastage on the other will be taken up for discussion in later sections.

Female Autonomy

There is one more socio-economic and cultural dimension that needs to be considered, the issue of female autonomy. Given its obvious consequences for decision-making by women on matters relating to reproduction, health care and abortion, it is an issue that has important implications for pregnancy wastage.

For a number of historical, socio-economic and cultural reasons, the extent of gender discrimination in Udipi, as well as in Karnataka state, is much lower than in India as a whole. This is evident from three indicators—sex ratio, literacy and work participation rates for males and females shown in Table 9.1.

In addition, specific to this region is the matrilineal system of inheritance which is still prevalent to a significant degree. In this system, known as *aliya santhana*, ownership rights are with the women of the household and are inherited through the female line; the right to manage the property, however, is in the hands of the oldest male member of the joint household, though it devolves not on his own, but his sister's son. The system is matrilocal in the sense that after marriage the woman stays back with her children in her parental home, where the husband visits her. The oldest female member of the household is considered the head of the household.

This system of inheritance was once widely prevalent and practised by the landholding caste, the toddy-tappers and the fishermen. The Dalits, who are largely agricultural labourers, also followed the system, but the Brahmins, Muslims and Christians did not. This system has weakened in recent years in the more advanced coastal belt but is still practised in the relatively backward interior parts of the district.

Table 9.1: Gender discrimination in Udupi, Karnataka and India

Region	Sex ratio, 2001		Literacy rate, 2001			Work participation rate, 1991		
	For 0-6 the age group	For the whole population	Male	Female	Index for female with male = 100	Male	Female	Index for female with male = 100
Udupi district	955	1127	86.6	74.0	85	51.7	35.1	68
Karnataka state	949	964	76.3	57.5	75	54.1	29.4	54
All-India	928	933	75.9	54.2	71	51.6	22.3	43

Note: Work participation rate data for 2001 are not yet available; the 1991 data given here refer to the erstwhile (composite) Dakshina Kannada district from which Udupi was carved out in 1998. The sex ratio is the number of females per 1000 males.

Source: Census of India 1991 and 2001.

It is a moot point whether this system led to the empowerment of women. In spite of females inheriting property it has been the male members who manage and take decisions related to land and property.

Among the poorer sections of the peasantry, however, the matrilineal system, which is also matrilocal, does provide considerable leeway and authority to women within the household. The woman is considered the head of the household, and remarriage—of widows as well as divorcees—is permitted. Coupled with a woman's access to employment (particularly to cash income from non-farm employment), the system provides her space within the domestic sphere and an important role in decision-making in matters such as health-seeking behaviour for herself and her children, which has important implications for maternal health and hence for pregnancy wastage.

Apart from providing women with some autonomy, the system affects pregnancy wastage in two other ways. First, since the continuation of the family lineage depends crucially on female offspring, there is a premium on the girl child; thus both sex-selective abortion and female infanticide are practically unknown in the region. Second, the rules governing the family in aliya santhana make for a reasonably liberal milieu in relation to marriage and male–female relationships.

However, in recent years, the process of elite-emulation or Sanskritisation on the part of the lower castes and the poor is increasingly visible in the region. Thus, for example, the practice of bride price is being replaced by dowry among communities that follow aliya santhana.

Research Design and Methodology

Choice of Village

The study village was one of two villages surveyed by us in 2001 as part of a study on beedi workers in the region. Choosing one of these two villages had certain advantages: we already had a good database for both villages, comprising a detailed house listing; a village-level enquiry on beedi workers; and a detailed survey of 100 beedi worker households (in both villages). We had also established good rapport with the residents of the two villages. But while the earlier survey provided us with some basic information on the health status of female beedi workers, more detailed information on pregnancy wastage was collected in the present study to bridge the gap in our understanding.

The study village, compared to the other village, is relatively more interior and backward with a sizeable workforce engaged in agricultural labour, enabling us to do a comparative study of pregnancy wastage among them and the beedi workers.

Research Design and Tools

Quantitative Survey

To start with, a quantitative method was used to list all the households in the village, where information on the occupation status of all workers in the households was collected, to enable us to later identify the beedi and agricultural-labour households. A beedi household was defined as one where at least one female worker was a beedi worker, while an agricultural-labour household was identified as one with at least one female agricultural labourer. The house listing was also used as a sample frame for further in-depth study of beedi and agricultural-labour households.

A random sample of 100 each of beedi and agricultural-labour households was selected for a detailed household-level enquiry. Since we had already obtained information on beedi-worker households during the earlier survey (in 2001), we mainly focused on agricultural-labour households.

From the selected households, ever-married women were interviewed to collect information on their health and pregnancy wastage. Where a household had two or more ever-married women, the oldest and the youngest among them were interviewed in order to capture inter-generational differentials. In all, we surveyed 211 women, of whom 69 were beedi workers, 110 agricultural labourers and the remaining 32 were 'secondary' or 'marginal workers', who generally identified themselves as 'housewives'.

Qualitative Enquiries

Using a checklist, some key informants were interviewed to get a perspective on the beedi industry and beedi workers and on the agricultural economy and agricultural labourers in the village. Also, discussions were held with auxilliary nurse midwives (ANMs), the doctor in the village health centre and some older women on the general health status of the village women, the health facilities available and aspects of pregnancy wastage. Discussions were also held with some private doctors in the nearby *taluka* headquarters, who generally provided abortion services. Talks were also held with members of the older generation, especially on the aliya santhana system. In addition, in the quantitative inquiry, responses to some open-ended questions provided valuable insights and details.

Ethical Issues

Pregnancy wastage is a very sensitive, personal issue, particularly when it is induced. The most important ethical issue was therefore the need to maintain strict confidentiality and to obtain respondents' informed consent. However, written consent was not always practical since more than two-thirds of the women were illiterate. However, women were informed at the outset that they were free to refuse to answer any question or even call off the interview at any point. The interview had to be called off in only one case. The women were also assured that their names and that of the village would be kept secret. When the purpose of the interview was explained to them, they had no hesitation in answering our questions.

However, it was difficult to maintain privacy and kept the 'gatekeepers' at bay. In order to overcome this problem, we tried to time the interviews either in the late morning or later in the afternoon, when male adults were likely to be away at work. Also, some of the sensitive questions were asked only when privacy could be ensured. When it became difficult to ensure privacy, the interview was abandoned.

Socio-Economic Profile of Respondents

The respondents were engaged either in beedi-rolling, agricultural labour or reported themselves as home workers. Beedi workers worked from home after getting the necessary inputs from the depot maintained by a contractor, and delivered the rolled beedis back to him. For this they received a cash wage. Beedi rolling is a relatively recent activity and came to the village in the early 1970s. Agricultural landless labourers, who form the poorest strata of the village, generally received their wages in kind. All those women who reported themselves as home workers looked after their kitchen gardens and occasionally worked as agricultural workers on their own farms.

They did not receive any wages—in cash or kind. About a third of the women in our sample were beedi workers and more than half were landless labourers (Table 9.2). Nearly four out of 5 women belonged to the matrilineal households. A little less than half the women were categorised as old; the criterion used for the purpose was those who had had their last pregnancy before 1992. The young were those whose first pregnancy was after 1990.

Table 9.2: Socio-economic distribution of women

Criterion of classification	Socio-economic group		Number of respondents	Percentage of respondents
Occupation	Beedi workers		69	32.7
	Agricultural labourers		110	52.1
	Home workers		32	15.2
	Total		211	100.0
Family system and occupation	Matrilineal	Beedi workers	41	19.4
		Agricultural labourers	106	50.2
		Home workers	19	9.0
		Total matrilineal	166	78.7
	Patrilineal	Beedi workers	28	13.3
		Agricultural labourers	4	1.9
		Home workers	13	6.2
		Total patrilineal	45	21.3
Age and occupation	Young	Beedi workers	31	14.7
		Agricultural labourers	16	7.6
		Home workers	14	6.6
		Total young	61	28.9
	Old	Beedi workers	16	7.6
		Agricultural labourers	71	33.6
		Home workers	11	5.2
		Total old	98	46.4
	Others	Beedi workers	23	10.9
		Agricultural labourers	23	10.9
		Home workers	6	2.8
		Total others	52	24.6

However, while poverty was a general feature in the status of all the women in our sample, they did vary in terms of other socio-economic factors, some of which are presented in Tables 9.3 and 9.4.

As is evident from Table 9.3, the matrilineal system has weakened considerably over the years: today, only about 40 per cent of the women live in their parental homes. The tendency towards nucleation appears to be quite strong. Close to half the women reported that

Table 9.3: **Some demographic and socio-economic characteristics of women**

Basis of classification	Social group	Average age in years	Marital status (%) Married	Widowed	Deserted	Divorced/separated	Average age at marriage	Literate (%)	aliya santhana (%)	Pattern of residence (%) Parental home	In-laws' home	Separate home	Female headed households (%)	Per cent who reported Bride price paid (%)	Dowry paid (%)
Occupation	Beedi workers	34.7	91.3	4.3	4.3	Nil	18.7	57.8	59.4	36.2	10.1	53.6	36.2	11.6	56.5
	Agricultural labourers	46.6	68.5	22.5	8.1	0.9	17.3	13.5	96.4	47.3	4.5	48.2	40.0	56.0	25.7
	Home workers	36.0	86.6	13.3	Nil	Nil	18.4	50.0	58.1	25.8	29.0	45.2	32.3	3.3	53.3
Family system	Matrilineal	41.6	77.7	15.1	6.6	0.6	17.9	27.1	100.0	50.3	4.8	44.8	40.0	42.3	35.6
	Patrilineal	40.0	81.8	15.9	2.3	Nil	17.7	59.1	Nil	6.7	28.9	64.4	28.9	2.3	48.9
Age	Young	28.8	91.8	4.9	3.3	Nil	20.3	49.2	77.0	59.0	16.4	24.6	36.1	6.6	73.8
	Old	56.5	60.8	28.9	9.3	1.0	15.8	20.7	90.9	33.7	7.1	59.2	43.2	56.8	18.2
	Others	38.5	96.2	1.9	1.9	Nil	18.8	42.3	75.0	35.3	7.8	56.9	34.6	31.4	39.2
All respondents		41.2	78.6	15.2	5.7	0.5	17.9	33.3	78.6	40.5	10.0	49.5	37.6	33.8	40.1

Source: Village survey (2002).

they did not live with either parents or in-laws, but had set up their own (possibly nuclear) households. The proportion of female-headed households, at around 38 per cent, was much lower than the percentage claiming to follow aliya santhana, indicating that there was no strict adherence to the system. The increasing replacement of bride price by dowry also points to this.

Further, only about a third of the women in our sample were literate; their average age at marriage was 17.9 years. But their exposure to mass media—both radio and TV—and hence also to urban influences, appeared to be quite high (see Table 9.4).

While this is the general picture, considerable variation existed across different social groups in terms of these attributes. For instance, beedi workers were considerably younger than the women who worked as agricultural labourers; they were also more literate and more exposed to the mass media. On the other hand, just about a seventh of the agricultural labourers were literate; their exposure to the mass media and urban influences was also lower compared to that of the beedi workers.

Given the criteria used for selecting young and old women, it is not surprising that the average age of 'young' women was 28.8 years and of the 'old' 56.5 years. The young were also much more literate, and their average age at marriage, at 20.3 years, was 4.5 years higher than that of the old. The incidence of matriliny was also lower among the young. The relatively high prevalence of matrilocality among the young is very likely indicative of a 'life cycle effect'. Upon marriage, girls continue to stay in their maternal home for some time and set up their own home after a few years, possibly when the children have grown up.

Decision-making in the Household

The questions on decision-making pertained to decisions on routine daily matters and those on which decisions have to be taken once in a while, such as those relating to marriage and 'purchasing consumer durables for the household'.

The responses of women indicated that the 'day-to-day' decisions within the domestic sphere appear to be essentially their preserve in the household, regardless of their socio-economic background. But they had much less autonomy when it came to matters such as choosing a life partner. Out of a total of 211 women, only two reported

Table 9.4: Exposure to mass media

Category	Social group	% who read newspaper/magazine at least once a week	% who listen to radio at least once a week	% who watch television at least once a week	% who watch a film at least once a week	% who are members of some social or political organisation
Occupation	Beedi workers	16.4	62.7	56.7	7.5	9.0
	Agricultural labourers	2.8	60.4	32.1	5.7	0.9
	Home workers	12.9	54.8	45.2	Nil	Nil
Family type	Matrilineal	9.4	67.1	45.6	6.3	4.4
	Patrilineal	7.0	39.5	25.6	2.3	Nil
Age	Young	15.3	59.3	37.3	3.4	5.1
	Old	7.6	57.6	37.0	4.3	1.1
	Others	4.0	70.0	50.0	10.0	6.0
All respondents	Persons with low	9.0	61.2	42.8	5.5	3.5
All-India (rural	standard of living	4.1	20.3	18.5	8.2	NA
and urban) 1998–99	Population as a whole	20.8	36.5	45.7	10.6	NA
Karnataka (rural and urban), for the population as a whole, 1998–99		27.9	60.9	58.4	19.7	NA

Note: NA = Not Available.

Sources: 1. Village survey (2002). 2. For all-India and Karnataka figures, NFHS-II 1998–99.

taking the decision about whom to marry—one with the consent of parents and elders and the other without. In 30 per cent of the cases, the marriage was arranged without even consulting the girl.

The degree of autonomy with respect to major decisions varied considerably across social groups. The extent of autonomy enjoyed by beedi workers—who were younger, more literate, had higher exposure to mass media and urban influences, and had access to cash wages—was significantly higher than that enjoyed by agricultural labourers. Similarly the young—who again were more literate and comprised a higher proportion of beedi workers with access to cash income—had much more autonomy compared to older women. Evidently, access to cash, exposure to mass media, etc., were much more important than the living arrangements or the aliya santhana system.

Pregnancy Wastage

Measures of Pregnancy Wastage

Table 9.5 presents some gross measures of pregnancy wastage for our sample as a whole. The measures used by us are: a) the gross rate of pregnancy wastage, which is defined as the number of pregnancy wastages per 100 pregnancies; b) the net rate of pregnancy wastage, which is the number of pregnancy wastages per 100 live births; c) the number of pregnancy wastages per woman; and d) the incidence of pregnancy wastage, which is defined as the percentage of women in the group (or any sub-group) who have undergone pregnancy wastage.

The data in Table 9.5 show that nearly a third of the women suffered pregnancy wastage at some time or other in their reproductive span, and nearly a tenth of their pregnancies were wasted. This figure is higher than that reported by NFHS 1998–99 for Karnataka state (rural and urban combined), which was 7.2 per cent. At the same time, we have reason to believe that our estimate of pregnancy wastage is likely to be lower than it should be because it excludes premarital and extramarital pregnancies from our survey, and because our sample consists of only poor, largely illiterate working women and does not cover the better-off, better-educated women in the village, among whom induced abortions are likely to be higher. Also, our estimates relate to lifetime pregnancies and pregnancy wastages and are not current rates. If there is a tendency for abortion rates to increase over

Table 9.5: **Some measures of pregnancy wastage**

Category of respondents	No. of respondents in each group	Total no. of pregnancies in each group	Total no. of pregnancy wastages in each group	Gross rate of preg-nancy wastage (per unit)	Net rate of pregnancy wastage (per cent)	No. of pregnancy wastages (per cent)	Incidence of pregnancy wastage (per cent)	No. of preg-nancies per respondent	No. of live births per respondent
Those with any pregnancy wastage	73	448	108	24.1	31.8	1.49	100.0	6.14	4.65
Those without any pregnancy wastage	138	568	Nil	Nil	Nil	Nil	Nil	4.12	4.12
All respondents	211	1016	108	10.6	11.9	0.51	34.6	4.82	4.31

Source: Village survey (2002).

time (and this seems to be true for induced abortions) our rate would be an understatement of the current rate.

It may be noted that the number of pregnancies per woman, or the rate of pregnancy, was significantly higher among those who experienced pregnancy wastage, than among those without any pregnancy wastage. When a number of pregnancies get wasted, the number of live births or children ever born (CEB) per woman also get reduced; consequently, the fertility gap between the two groups becomes narrow. Thus, while the pregnancy rate for those who experienced pregnancy wastage was nearly 50 per cent higher than those who did not experience any pregnancy wastage, the corresponding difference in the children ever born among them was just 13 per cent. In a context where fertility transition is taking place, 'voluntary wastage' or induced abortion may be a means to achieve the small family norm. On the other hand, where fertility transition has not taken place, a high rate of pregnancy may in fact be a response to a high rate of 'involuntary pregnancy wastage', such as spontaneous abortions and stillbirths. Pregnancy wastage thus plays a role similar to that of infant mortality. But while the role of infant mortality in fertility transition is well recognised and established, the role of pregnancy wastage in fertility behaviour has not received adequate attention.

Further, it appears that pregnancy wastage gets clustered in relatively small groups. This is evident from the fact that only a third of the women accounted for all the wastages. This phenomenon of clustering is even more striking because 14 per cent of all women who experienced multiple pregnancy wastage accounted for nearly 60 per cent of the total number of pregnancy wastages (Table 9.6). Part of the reason for this was their high 'vulnerability' to pregnancy itself. Such clustering of pregnancy wastage among highly vulnerable groups has an obvious policy implication, and identifying such clusters and exploring the socio-economic and medical causes underlying such clustering would help in targeting measures to reduce wastage.

Components of Pregnancy Wastage

There are three different types of pregnancy wastage, viz., induced abortions, spontaneous abortions and stillbirths. The latter two are involuntary forms of pregnancy wastage. In our study they accounted for nearly 80 per cent of all pregnancy wastage. Compared to those reported having experienced single pregnancy wastage, women with

Table 9.6: Pregnancy wastage for different groups of women

Category of respondents		No. of respondents	No. of pregnancies	No. of pregnancy wastages	No. of pregnancies per respondent	No. of live births per respondent
Those with any pregnancy wastage	Those with single pregnancy wastage	44 (20.9)	232 (22.8)	44 (40.7)	5.27	4.27
	Those with multiple pregnancy wastage	29 (13.7)	216 (21.3)	64 (59.3)	7.45	5.24
	All—those with any pregnancy wastage	73 (34.6)	448 (44.1)	108 (100.0)	6.14	4.65
Those without any pregnancy wastage		138 (65.4)	568 (55.9)	Nil (0.0)	4.12	4.12
All respondents		211 (100.0)	1016 (100.0)	108 (100.0)	4.82	4.31

Note: 1. The relative index of vulnerability to wastage for a group is defined as: (percentage contribution of the group to total wastage x 100) / (percentage contribution of the group to total number of respondents).

2. Figures in brackets give column percentages.

Source: Village survey (2002).

multiple pregnancy wastage had significantly higher rates of wastage for all the three types of wastage. The differential was particularly sharp in the case of involuntary wastage; spontaneous abortions among those experiencing multiple pregnancy wastage were four times higher than among those who experienced only single pregnancy wastage.

Pregnancy wastage for a group of women (as a whole) depends on: a) the size of the affected group (those who experience pregnancy wastage) or the 'cluster'; b) the rate of wastage within the affected group; and c) the pregnancy rate for the affected group. In fact, the rate of pregnancy wastage for the group as a whole (R) can be expressed as follows:

R_g = $I_n \times r_g \times p_r$ where
R_g = the gross rate of pregnancy wastage for the group as a whole;
I_n = the incidence of wastage, i.e., the percentage of women within the group who have undergone any pregnancy wastage;
r_g = the gross rate of pregnancy wastage considering only the affected group (this gives the intensity of wastage within the affected group); and
p_r = the relative pregnancy rate, i.e., the pregnancy rate for the affected group divided by the pregnancy rate for the group as a whole.

Similarly, the net pregnancy wastage rate for the group as whole (R_n) can be expressed as:

R_n = $I_n \times r_n \times f_r$ where
I_n = the incidence as defined above;
r_n = the net pregnancy wastage rate for the affected group; and
f_r = the relative fertility rate as given by the ratio of CEB per woman for the affected group to CEB per woman for the group as a whole.

The component analysis can provide us with some clues about the factors underlying variations in pregnancy wastage. However, without presenting the details of the analysis, the salient findings are as follows:[2]

- The young and the old women differed greatly in the type of pregnancy wastage they experienced. The rate of spontaneous abortion and stillbirths was significantly lower among the young women but the rate of induced abortion among them was almost three times that experienced by the older women. Clearly, induced abortion was used by the younger women for family limitation.
- The rate of induced abortion among beedi workers was nearly twice compared to that among agricultural labourers. In fact, induced abortion among young beedi workers accounted for nearly 60 percent of the total pregnancy wastage.
- Among the young agricultural labourers, the incidence of stillbirths accounted for high pregnancy wastage; this group did not resort to voluntary abortion as a means for family limitation to the same extent that the beedi workers did. Among the older agricultural labourers, a high pregnancy rate was a response to high levels of pregnancy wastage.
- Overall, both pregnancy and fertility rates were found to be much more sensitive to the socio-economic factors that facilitated fertility transition in the region than to the factors associated with the nature of the family system.

We turn now to examine the data on induced abortion more closely to discern the extent of its use for spacing of births or for limiting family size by various socio-economic groups in the region.

Induced Abortion

In our sample of 211 women, 17 had undergone induced abortion. Between them, they had experienced 26 pregnancy wastages, 21 induced abortions, two spontaneous abortions and three stillbirths. In this section we deal with four basic issues: a) attitudes towards induced abortion; b) the characteristics of the 17 women and whether they differ from the rest in any significant ways; c) the decision-making process and the reasons stated by the women for undergoing induced abortion; and d) the abortion care available to them.

Attitudes towards Induced Abortion

Three basic questions on which attitudinal data were collected from all respondents were: One, did women know that abortion is now legal and, if they did, were they aware of the reasons for its legalisation? Two, what were the circumstances under which women felt justified in resorting to induced abortion? Three, what was their perception of the accessibility of abortion services? While the majority knew that abortion is legal, very few knew why it was legalised. A few thought that it had been legalised to 'control population growth'.

From the responses (Table 9.7), it is evident that more than 85 per cent knew that abortion is legal, and almost all of them did not want it to be banned and approved of it under various circumstances, *including* pre- and extramarital pregnancies. Women approved of abortion for reasons of health (both of the mother and child), as well as for pregnancies due to rape. It is possible that the aliya santhana system, which enabled women to develop a liberal attitude in relation to marriage, man–woman relationships, and pre- and extramarital relationships, also enabled them to develop liberal views on induced abortion. In the words of some of the women:

> It may be true that the girl has committed a mistake, but her life should not be ruined because of that mistake.

> Life in this society for an illegitimate child is a very difficult one—and one should think of such a child's future life.

> I have seen illegitimate infants abandoned immediately after birth; it is better to abort them than subject them to such treatment.

But despite holding liberal views, most women still believed that access to abortion should be restricted. While they approved of abortion in the case of contraceptive failure, very few advocated it as a method of contraception. Less than a tenth wished for free access to abortion. The reasons for wanting to limit access to abortion were the fear that free access would encourage premarital and extramarital relations, which were still unacceptable and seen as 'mistakes'; and that free access would encourage repeated recourse to induced abortions, which in turn would impact poorly on the mother's health.

The important question is: Do the 17 women who underwent one or more induced abortions also hold similar views? As expected, *all* those who had undergone induced abortions knew that abortion is legal. They also opined that there should be no ban on abortions; only one of the 16 women on whom we have data wanted unrestricted

Table 9.7: Women's attitude towards induced abortion

Scheme of classification	Social group	Percentage who knew abortion is legal (before discussion)	Percentage who agreed that abortion is acceptable in the following circumstances						Percentage who advocated that abortion should be		
			Mother's health is in danger	Foetus is abnormal	Rape	Preferred method of contraception	Failure of contraception	Pre-marital or extra-marital pregnancies	Banned	Available at low cost	Available on demand at any time
Occupation	Beedi workers	94.1	98.5	98.5	98.5	22.4	94.0	92.5	1.5	52.2	10.4
	Agricultural labourers	84.7	94.8	94.8	94.8	21.6	94.8	93.8	1.0	44.3	7.2
	Home workers	83.9	94.7	94.7	93.8	10.5	89.5	89.5	Nil	31.6	5.3
Family system	Matrilineal	86.1	95.9	95.9	96.6	21.6	94.6	93.9	0.7	45.3	6.8
	Patrilineal	93.2	95.5	95.5	95.5	15.9	88.7	86.4	2.3	43.1	11.4
Age	Young	93.8	96.7	96.7	96.7	18.0	93.4	90.2	Nil	44.3	4.9
	Old	80.2	93.0	93.0	93.1	24.1	79.3	89.7	2.3	49.4	11.5
	Others	94.0	100.0	100.0	100.0	15.9	100.0	100.0	Nil	38.6	6.8
All respondents		86.7	96.2	96.2	96.2	20.8	94.0	92.9	1.1	44.8	8.2

Source: Village survey (2002).

access to abortion and only eight wanted abortions to be available at a lower cost. And while all but one believed that abortion is justified in cases of contraceptive failure, only a third saw it as a preferred method of contraception. The moral and maternal health considerations that characterised the absence of permissiveness in the other women also seemed to motivate those who had undergone induced abortion.

Characteristics of Those Who Have Undergone Induced Abortions

Of the 17 women who had induced abortions, 7 were beedi workers, eight agricultural labourers, and two home workers. Those who had induced abortion were younger in age, currently married, and more literate. This was evident among both beedi workers and agricultural labourers. The women were also more exposed to mass media such as radio and films and to the urban way of life. Interestingly, exposure to television was almost uniform across all women in this region, although the younger women bear a heavier burden in terms of child-care which prevents them from watching a lot of television.

The Decision-making Process and Reasons for Abortion

The question before us was: Did higher literacy, greater exposure to mass media and urban influences, and access to non-agricultural employment such as beedi-rolling and providing cash income), translate into a relatively higher degree of autonomy for women, such that they could decide on abortion themselves? The responses of women who underwent abortion suggest that all 17 women take decisions on seeking health care, on buying consumer durables for the household as well as on marriage. Thus, these women seemed to enjoy a higher degree of autonomy compared to the rest.

However, as is event from Table 9.8, on the decisions related to abortion—whether to undergo abortion, and if yes, in which facility, etc.—only half the women reportedly made the decision themselves.

But it is noteworthy that in all 16 cases for which we have data, the women were party to the decision-making process: in 6 cases with their husbands, and in 2 with the help of other family members, including a married daughter in one case.

Along with decisions related to undergoing abortion, decisions regarding the choice of facility were also taken by the women in half

Table 9.8: Decision-making with respect to induced abortions

Decision-maker(s)	Decision to undergo induced abortion		Decision regarding choice of facility	
	Number	Percentage	Number	Percentage
Respondent alone	8	50.0	8	50.0
Respondent's husband alone	Nil	Nil	1	6.3
Respondent with her husband	6	37.5	4	25.0
Respondent with other members of the family	2	12.5	3	18.8
Total	16	100.0	16	100.0

Note: We could not obtain the data for one respondent; so the total number of observations is 16.
Source: Village survey (2002).

the cases, in consultation with husbands in 7 cases and by the husband alone in one case where the wife was illiterate, and did not know of any abortion facility.

As we have noted earlier, all the women said that induced abortions should not be used as a method of contraception. However, this stated view seems to contradict an earlier finding that abortion is in fact used as a method to limit family size in the context of rapidly declining fertility. What then are the reasons women stated for opting for induced abortion? Table 9.9 provides a brief, qualitative summary of the reasons given by each of the 17 women who had undergone induced abortion.

It is evident that each case is unique and the reasons for deciding on abortion are varied and compex. However, the most important proximate cause for opting for abortion is clearly family limitation or spacing. There appears to be a disjunction between what women opined that induced abortion should not be used as a method of family planning because of its negative impact on maternal health and yet, in practice, several of them used abortion as a method of family planning.

In this context, it is useful to remember that fertility reduction in Udipi district has been brought about by very heavy reliance on sterilisation with virtually no use of spacing methods or increase in age at marriage, as has been the case in Tamil Nadu and Andhra Pradesh. There has been very little effort on the part of the state or the public health establishment to educate the public on the various options available for family planning. Consequently, the level of public awareness of alternative means of controlling fertility appears to be rather low. In fact, in our sample as a whole, only about 18 per cent of the live births were followed by *any* instruction regarding health education or family planning practices. This poor knowledge of contraceptive methods appears to be one of the reasons why the use of spacing methods was low, or why the failure rate was high even when spacing methods were adopted.

Consequently, women who wanted to but could not limit family size by adopting sterilisation resorted to induced abortions. This was also true for those who wanted to adopt a spacing method but either could not do so or used it improperly. And, as the Table 9.9 makes clear, there were a number of reasons why some women who wanted to undergo sterilisation or adopt spacing methods in fact could not do so.

Women cited poor maternal health, even lack of permission from the local deity as reasons for not using sterlisation in spite of their wanting to stop family increase. Instead they took recourse to induced abortion in most such instances.

The case studies also indicate that girls get married at a fairly early age in this region and most couples attempt to complete the desired family size—mostly comprising two children—soon after marriage and by the time the girl is barely 20 years of age. In such instances, when doctors refuse to conduct tubectomy, abortion is used to terminate the unwanted pregnancy. Similarly, when couples want a child of a particular sex—male in most instances—they opt for abortion without even undergoing sex determination test, fearing that a girl will be born again. Also, a sense of shame prompts a woman to opt for abortion when she becomes pregnant when her daughter has also started producing children.

The case studies also suggest that there are some misconceptions prevailing in the region in spite of improved education among women. One woman believed that she would not conceive for some time after delivering twins; another believed that tubectomy can be performed only after a delivery. Women also had fears and apprehensions about some of the spacing methods, such as the fear that IUDs can cause harm. The fear of 'operation' was reported. Lack of knowledge about how oral pills should be used was also evident, leading women to using them as abortifacients with adverse consequences for maternal and foetal health.

Table 9.9: Reasons for induced abortions

Socio-economic characteristics of the respondent	Reason(s) for undergoing induced abortion(s) and general remarks
Young Hindu beedi worker, matrilineal system	The respondent wanted only 2 children and, after the second child, wanted to undergo tubectomy. But for this she had to take the permission of the family deity—Naga Devaru, the serpent god—who makes its appearance through the community priest. However, before she got the permission, she became pregnant and decided to have an abortion. After the abortion she did not undergo tubectomy, because she thought that a tubectomy could be done only after a delivery. She had to have 3 induced abortions because of this belief.
Young Hindu beedi worker, matrilineal system	Because of her poor reproductive health, the doctor refused to perform a tubectomy or insert an IUD either before the conception (of the unwanted child) or after the abortion.
Young Muslim beedi worker, patrilineal system	Married at the age of 16 and having given birth to 2 children before 18, she wanted to undergo tubectomy at 20 years of age. But the doctors refused. She was scared of using the loop and oral contraceptives were inconvenient. Her third pregnancy was aborted. At the time of the interview she was pregnant for the fourth time and was planning to have a tubectomy. This time around she expects the doctor to oblige.
Old Hindu beedi worker, matrilineal system	She had given birth to 1 male and 2 female children. But the male child had died. She conceived for the fourth time, hoping to get a male child. But after conception she was haunted by the fear that either the child would be female or, even if it were male, might again not survive. So she got the pregnancy aborted and underwent sterilisation.
Old Muslim home worker, patrilineal system	After the desired family size of 4 children, she did not undergo sterilisation because of fear of 'operation'. She had 5 more pregnancies and, after the ninth delivery, she wanted to have a tubectomy, but developed some serious complications after the delivery and the doctors refused to perform a tubectomy. She had 3 more pregnancies and, at the time of her last pregnancy, her eldest daughter was already married. She felt too ashamed to continue with the pregnancy and so terminated it and started using the loop.
Old Hindu agricultural labourer, matrilineal system	After attaining the desired family size, she used oral contraceptive pills irregularly for about 6 months but conceived. She got the pregnancy terminated and has since been using pills regularly. She would prefer her husband, an alcoholic, to undergo vasectomy, but he refuses.

Old Hindu agricultural labourer, matrilineal system	Her repeated attempts to obtain permission from the family deity (Naga Devaru) to undergo tubectomy failed. After having 3 children, she got the fourth pregnancy terminated, but the fear of the deity prevented her from having a tubectomy. She also had a fear of the IUD. She had the fourth child because the doctor refused to abort 2 successive pregnancies. However, she aborted the next pregnancy. After that she used oral contraceptive pills for 6 months, supplied by the ANM. When the ANM stopped her visits and she could not afford to buy the pills from the market, she conceived again twice—the first one she delivered and the next one was a stillbirth. Tired of repeated pregnancies, induced abortions and stillbirths, she decided to have the tubectomy done without the deity's permission.
Old Hindu agricultural labourer, matrilineal system	After having been deserted by her husband for 6 years, she did not want to have any more children. But she did not know of any family-planning method and conceived at a time when her own daughter had had a tubectomy. So she and her husband felt ashamed and decided to terminate the pregnancy.
Agricultural labourer, 'other' age group*, Hindu, matrilineal system	After having had 3 children, she could not get permission from the family deity to undergo tubectomy. She was also afraid of using an IUD. During her fourth pregnancy she consumed several oral contraceptive pills to abort the foetus. When it did not work, she worried about the adverse consequences of the pills on the foetus and had an induced abortion.
Agricultural labourer, 'other' age group, Hindu, matrilineal system	After her third delivery, she was motivated by the ANM to undergo sterilisation. But she developed an abscess after the delivery and could not have a tubectomy. Later, she migrated to a village where there was no health worker. She aborted her next 2 pregnancies.
Young Muslim home worker, patrilineal system	She did not know much about family-planning methods and by the time she decided what method to use, she had 3 pregnancies in 2 years. She aborted the third and subsequently had loop insertion.
Home worker, 'other' age group, Hindu, matrilineal system	She was under the impression that after delivering twins she would not conceive for some time and hence did not use any family-planning method. She was also afraid of using the IUD. But she conceived again immediately after delivering twins. She felt it would be very difficult to look after 3 babies and decided to have an abortion. She had 1 more delivery and then had a tubectomy.
Young, Hindu beedi worker, matrilineal system	Early in her first pregnancy, she suffered a fracture and was hospitalised. The doctors did not know of her pregnancy. When they learnt about it, she was referred to an obstetrician who

(*Table 9.9 continued*)

(*Table 9.9 continued*)

Socio-economic characteristics of the respondent	Reason(s) for undergoing induced abortion(s) and general remarks
	advised termination of pregnancy as it was feared that the drugs used to treat her would have an adverse effect on the foetus.
Young, Hindu beedi worker, matrilineal system	She suffers from muscular dystrophy. When she got married, the disease was in remission. But it recurred during her first pregnancy and hence she went in for abortion.
Old Hindu beedi worker, matrilineal system	During her third pregnancy, she developed a third-degree prolapse of the uterus and the doctors in the government hospital advised her to undergo MTP. She had an induced abortion at 14–16 weeks of pregnancy and then had a hysterectomy.
Agricultural labourer, 'other' age group, Hindu, matrilineal system	She delivered 7 daughters while waiting to have a son. During her eighth pregnancy, fearing that it might also be a female, she experienced a lot of psychological stress. So she consumed 60 oral contraceptive pills given to her by an ANM to abort the foetus. She developed severe side effects, and was shifted to a hospital where the pregnancy was terminated. She later became pregnant, delivered a son, and underwent tubectomy.

Note: *'Other' age: women who had their first pregnancy before 1990 and their last one after 1992.

The analysis raises a question: Is the decision to abort an unwanted pregnancy a result of a free, preferred choice or does it have a constricting effect because it rules out other choices? In other words, the right to abortion has to be viewed as part of the larger set of reproductive rights, taking into account the socio-economic and cultural contexts that facilitate or constrain this larger set of rights. The issue needs deeper thought, data and analysis to unravel its implications.

Access to Abortion and Abortion Care

Perhaps the most striking aspect regarding the nature of service providers in Udipi district was the almost total absence of informal providers. Our general enquiries revealed that this group of providers disappeared from the region quite a while ago. None of the 16 women for whom we have the relevant data reported that they had made use of the services of any informal provider; all of them had gone to a registered medical practitioner.

The other striking feature about the service providers was the overwhelming presence of private facilities. Of the 16 women, only one had gone to the government hospital in the taluka headquarters; the others had all used private medical practitioners in the vicinity of the village. There appear to be three major reasons for this preference for private providers:

- The public facility was available only in the taluka headquarters, which is about 20 km away from the village. The private facilities—small 'nursing homes'—are more numerous and closer to the village.
- In the government hospital, most abortions are conducted under local anaesthesia, whereas in private facilities they are done under general anaesthesia. Many women preferred the latter pain-free procedure.
- After abortion in the government facility, women are generally asked to adopt some family-planning method. There is no such demand made in private facilities.

However, one adverse consequence of the almost total reliance on private providers is that it leads to a considerable amount of running around when some private providers refuse to conduct MTP if they fear that it will impact negatively on the mother's health, if it the first pregnancy or if it is of more than 20 weeks' duration. Of the 16 women, three reported that the search for a provider who would agree to abort was quite extensive. No private provider was willing to do an MTP on a woman suffering from muscular dystrophy. She had to finally get it done at the government hospital. Another 2 had wanted to abort their successive pregnancies and, when the providers refused to conduct repeat abortions on the same woman, they had to search for new providers for their second and subsequent abortions.

The Use of Oral Contraceptive Pills as an Abortifacient

The practice of using oral contraceptive pills as an abortifacient was reported by some women. In all, eight women had resorted to taking several pills at one time, predictably without success. Later, five of the eight decided to get the abortion done medically—one after developing severe side effects, and another because she was afraid that the pills she had consumed would adversely affect the foetus. The remaining three continued with the pregnancy.

It is not clear why and how the idea of using oral pills as an abortifacient has gained currency in the area. Perhaps it had something to do with the fact that contraceptive pills are commonly used to regulate menstruation. It is also possible that the perceived 'advantages' of this method—anonymity, absence of surgical procedure, etc.—have played an important role in its spread. The local chemists might also be responsible for spreading such a myth. Of the eight women who resorted to this practice, seven purchased the pills from the local chemists. When there are no regulatory mechanisms to oversee the sale of drugs—even prescription drugs—and where chemists often double up as doctors, it is not surprising that they make most drugs available to people.

With just one exception, no woman reported any post-abortion complications. The one woman reported that she had continuous bleeding for five days after the procedure. However, it may be kept in mind that all the women in our sample belong to the poorer strata of society who often stoically accept minor discomforts. Further, post-abortive morbidity, as any other type of morbidity, has a strong, subjective bias built into it, and the poor often tend to understate its occurrence. In fact, as many as 10 of the 16 women who underwent induced abortion did not even have a post-abortion medical check up: eight did not see the need for it, and two did not avail of it for financial reasons. (For more details on abortion care, see Table 9.10.)

Finally, from the perspective of abortion care, involuntary abortion needs some discussion and attention because of its plausible linkage with occupational health. Table 9.11 provides data on the distribution of involuntary wastages by the gestation age of the pregnancy, separately for each of the three occupation groups. It may be noted that beedi workers reported a higher rate of early wastage (first trimester spontaneous abortions), whereas agricultural labourers and home workers reported a much higher rate of late wastage (i.e., second trimester spontaneous abortions and stillbirths).

The pertinent question is whether these distinct patterns are linked to the conditions of work in each of the occupations. While establishing these links beyond any reasonable doubt would need considerably more research, there are reasons to believe that such links do exist. Generally speaking, first trimester spontaneous abortions outnumber those that occur later. The preponderance of second-trimester spontaneous abortions among agricultural labourers is likely to be related to their working conditions, which involves tasks like carrying

Table 9.10: Some aspects of induced abortions: access, nature and care

	Aspect dealt with		No. of observations
Unmet demand for induced abortion	Respondents who wanted to have abortion but did not		6
	Reason for wanting abortion	For family limitation	3
		For spacing	2
		Because of premarital pregnancy	1
Latent demand	Those who would have abortion if conceived again		3
	Reason: Because the desired family size is complete		3
Nature of service provider	Respondents who went to an informal provider for abortion		Nil
	Those got the abortion done by a qualified doctor		16
	Public/private nature	Those who went to a public facility	1
		Those who went to a private facility	15
Gestation age of abortions	In first trimester	Total in first trimester	18
		Within 6 weeks	3
		In second trimester (total)	3
Pregnancy order	Abortion of first pregnancy		2
Abortion and post-abortion care	Those who did not have any post-abortion care		10
	Reason for not having post-abortion care	Not necessary	8
		Did not have money	2
	Medical complications due to induced abortion		1 (bleeding)
Search	Those who had to search a lot for a provider		3
Use of oral pills as abortifacient	Those who used contraceptive pills as abortifacient		8
	Those who bought the pills from the chemist		7
	Those who had to undergo MTP after consuming pills		5

Source: Village survey (2002).

Table 9.11: Gestation age at involuntary pregnancy wastage

Occupation group	No. of pregnancies	No. of involuntary pregnancy wastages: Spontaneous abortions: I trimester	II trimester	Total	Stillbirths	Total involuntary wastage	Gross rate of involuntary pregnancy wastages: Total (for all involuntary wastages)	For spontaneous abortions: I trimester wastage rate	II trimester wastage rate	Total spontaneous abortion rate	Rate of stillbirths	Early wastage rate	Late wastage rate	1st trimester wastage as a per cent of total spontaneous abortions	Late wastage as a per cent of total involuntary wastage
Beedi workers	275	8	1	9	11	20	7.3	2.9	0.4	3.3	4.0	2.9	4.4	88.9	60.0
Agricultural labourers	596	10	26	36	16	52	8.7	1.7	4.4	6.1	2.7	1.7	7.0	27.8	80.8
Home workers	145	2	9	11	4	15	10.3	1.4	6.2	7.6	2.8	1.4	9.0	18.2	86.7
All respondents	1016	20	36	56	31	87	8.6	2.0	3.5	5.5	3.1	2.0	6.6	35.7	77.0

Source: Village survey (2002).

heavy loads, transplanting and harvesting, which have to be performed standing up in a forward-bending posture. In the second trimester, these may lead to increased intra-uterine pressure, which in turn may lead to spontaneous abortion. Such tasks may also put pressure on uterine blood circulation, leading to utero-placental hypoxia and abortion.

Among beedi workers also, the impact of working conditions cannot be completely discounted. The effect of smoking or exposure to tobacco on what are called euploid abortions, which generally occur in the first trimester and peak around the thirteenth week, is well documented in the literature. *William's Obstetrics* reports that for women smoking more than 14 cigarettes a day, the risk of euploidic abortion is approximately twice that for those who do not smoke. That continuous exposure to fine tobacco dust—often in a small, enclosed space with no proper ventilation—has very likely a similar effect. This hypóthesis is supported by the fact that, among the beedi rollers in our sample, those with spontaneous abortions had spent more years rolling beedis compared to those who suffered other types of pregnancy wastage. The average number of years spent in beedi-rolling was 12 years for those with induced abortions, and 20.2 years for those with spontaneous abortions.

Thus it appears that work conditions do have some influence on the extent and nature of involuntary pregnancy wastage. While this supports our broad generalisation that pregnancy wastage is a phenomenon that has strong social roots, measures to ameliorate the working conditions of women and removing some of the work related health hazards must receive priority.

Conclusion

We have made two broad contentions—that pregnancy wastage is embedded in the social context of the region, and that it is linked to fertility transition. If true, then, like fertility transition, pregnancy wastage should also display a wide degree of variation across space and social groups. Our research has shown that, like fertility, pregnancy wastage is also locally rooted and varies across social groups even in the same locality. Given this, attempts to comprehend the phenomenon of pregnancy wastage would be as futile as searching for general laws of population. Marx's famous dictum that 'a universal law of population exists for plants and animals only' is perhaps equally relevant for pregnancy wastage and underscores the futility of a uniform, universal policy regime to deal with it.

Notes

1. There are only three districts in the country which have a fertility rate of less than 1.5: Chennai (1.3), Kolkata (1.4) and Leh (Ladakh) (1.3). The first two, it may be noted, are completely urban. Only three other districts—all in Kerala—have a fertility rate of 1.5: Alappuzha, Ernakulam and Pathanamthitta.
2. Considering the subgroups by occupation and family system and excluding the patrilineal agricultural-labourer group (i.e., with n=5), the coefficient of variation (CV) for gross percentage rate is 12.4; for net wastage rate 13.8; for incidence 24.0; and for the vulnerability index 33.1. The corresponding values for classification by occupation and age (with 8 observations, excluding home workers in the 'other' age group) are 31.8 per cent, 35.0 per cent, 36.8 per cent and 52.4 per cent. The CV for pregnancy rate is 22.8 per cent for the first group of classification and 38.8 per cent for the second. The CV for fertility rate is 21.6 per cent and 39.2 per cent.

References

Census of India. 1961. *Naravi Village: Village Survey Monograph No. 3. Volume XI: Mysore (Part VI)*. New Delhi: Office of the Registrar General, India.

———. 1991. *Availability of Infrastructural Facilities in Rural Areas of India: An Analysis of Village Directory Data*. New Delhi: Office of the Registrar General, India.

———. 2001. *Provisional Population Totals, Paper I of 2001, Supplement: District Totals*. New Delhi: Registrar General and Census Commissioner, India.

Centre for Monitoring Indian Economy. 2000. *Profiles of Districts*. Mumbai: CMIE.

Geetha Rani, P. 1999. 'Human Development Index in India: A District Profile', *Artha Vijnana* XLI (1).

Guilmoto, Christophe Z. and S. Irudaya Rajan. 2002. 'District Level Estimates of Fertility from India's 2001 Census', *The Economic and Political Weekly* XXXVII (7), February 16–22.

International Institute for Population Studies. 1995. *National Family Health Survey (NFHS–1), 1992–93, India*. Mumbai: IIPS.

International Institute for Population Sciences and ORC Macro. 2000. *National Family Health Survey (NFHS–2) 1998–1999, India*. Mumbai: IIPS.

Williams S. and Gary Cunningham. 2001. *Williams' Obstetrics* 21st edn. New Delhi: MacGraw Hill.

X

Informal Providers of Abortion Services: An Exploration

Bela Ganatra and Leela Visaria

Abortions have been around forever. At different points of time in history they have received attention for differing reasons, some in support of them, but often against them. Abortion is primarily a health concern of women but it is increasingly being governed by patriarchal interests, which more often than not curb the freedom of women to seek abortion as a right.

With the present focus of the concern for women's health being entirely on her reproduction in terms of either preventing or terminating pregnancy, abortion practice has become a critical issue. Given the official perspective of understanding abortion within the context of contraception, it is important to review abortion and abortion practice in India, particularly the role played by abortion providers—both formal and informal. Informal providers of abortion services exist in varying degrees throughout India and, though their use may be declining in some settings, inefficient public systems, inadequate or expensive private options and the social stigma associated with abortion ensure that they continue to play a role in the provision of abortion services at least in some circumstances. But while there is a substantial amount of literature available on formal providers of abortion, informal providers remain inadequately explored.

Despite abortions being legal in India on wide-ranging grounds, it is well known that those performed outside the legal framework outnumber those within it. The only legal providers are obstetric gynaecologists (Ob-Gyns) or MBBS (generalist) doctors with specialised training in Medical Termination of Pregnancy (MTP). Public hospitals are by default authorised to provide abortion services: all others need to be certified. While illegal abortions are sometimes performed by legal providers practising at uncertified sites, a range of informal providers also provide abortion services in a scenario where public services are unevenly distributed and not always functional, and formal private facilities often too expensive.

The term 'informal provider' has been variously used to refer to illegal providers, untrained providers, home-based providers, non-physician providers and/or sometimes to those working outside a formal (organised) health system, whether public or private. The varying use of the term limits comparisons over time and across regions.

In the northern parts of India, where recognised abortion facilities are few and far between, informal service provision continues to play a major role (Barnes 2003; Johnston et al. 2004). The facility surveys undertaken as part of the larger Abortion Assessment Project, India[1] in three northern states (Rajasthan, Madhya Pradesh and Haryana) and in Orissa showed that informal providers (the term used to refer to all providers who are not registered or formally trained to conduct abortions) of abortion services not only existed but also often outnumbered formal providers (CINI 2004; George 2003; Iyengar and Iyengar 2004; SORT 2004). Most informal providers admitted to treating a host of reproductive health problems including delayed menstruation. Some admitted to treating incomplete abortion and a few also spoke of using invasive methods to induce an abortion.

In recent years, a few qualitative studies in the southern and western parts of the country have suggested that, in these areas, the use of informal providers for abortion services may actually be declining (Ganatra and Hirve 2002; Ramchandar and Pelto 2002). A recent facility survey in Kerala found few informal providers (Ramanathan et al. 2003) in its mapping exercise, although focus group discussions (FGDs) in the community did reveal the presence of both older women in the community and local pharmacists who functioned as informal providers for early abortions (Ramanathan et al. 2003). But in these situations too, there is evidence that socially or economically marginalised women—the unmarried, those who do not get support from their husband or married adolescent girls with lack of mobility and control over resources—are more likely to use the services of informal providers (Ganatra and Hirve 2002; Radkar 2003; Varkey et al. 2000).

Thus, while the degree of use may vary, as also the methods used, informal providers do exist and are involved in health seeking for unwanted pregnancy at various levels. They exist because they meet the felt needs of at least some women in certain situations. Understanding when and in what circumstances they are used and how they practise is crucial for the formulation of policy and programmes. Safe and unsafe practices need to be distinguished and the ability of these providers to meet clients' needs studied.

Research Questions, Tools and Methodology

It is in this context a collaborative study was undertaken, to examine the role that informal providers play in the provision of abortion care in different geographic contexts. Although not a part of the original qualitative abortion studies, it was felt that abortion services provided by informal providers was an under-researched area. Therefore, HealthWatch and Ipas proactively decided to sponsor, design data instruments and identify organisations to undertake an exploratory study of informal providers in the regions where they were actively working on a range of health issues. Thus, research in different geographical locations was conducted by seven partner non-government organisations (NGOs).[2] The NGOs were:

- ARTH, Udaipur
- Bharat Vaidyaka Sanstha (BVS), Nashik
- Centre for Health and Social Sector Studies (CHSSS), Secunderabad
- Karuna Trust, Karnataka
- Shramik Bharti, Kanpur
- SORT, Vadodara
- Swaasthya, New Delhi

This chapter is prepared as a synthesis report based on the individual study reports and discussions with the researchers.[3] At most sites, data collection began by November 2002[4], based on a common set of research questions that were developed jointly through brain-storming meetings. All partners agreed that the key questions to be explored were:

- Who are the providers that communities recognise as informal providers of abortion services?
- What sorts of services do they provide? How do they secure their practice in the community? How flexible are they in terms of place and cost of abortion services?

- When and under what circumstances are services of informal providers preferred over those of formal providers?
- How does the formal health system view and interact with them?

In addition, most partners decided to probe additional issues like the sequence of events from the recognition of a missed period to care seeking for an unwanted pregnancy, decision-making and the role played by men in the decision-making process.

Research Sites

The research sites, which were located in seven different states, represent a diverse range of geographic settings, ranging from rural (tribal as well as non-tribal) to peri-urban and urban. In some areas communities had easy physical access to formal abortion services; in others they did not.

Several of the partner NGOs chose the site of their field operations as their research site because they were familiar with the area and had already built a rapport with the community or communities concerned. Some organisations deliberately chose a location that was distinct from their area of field interventions. For example, ARTH felt that an exploration of informal providers in the area where ARTH itself provides legal abortion services would not yield meaningful results. SORT and CHSSS located their research in a smaller subset of the same geographic area where they had recently completed a facility-based survey of abortion service providers.

A description of the research areas chosen by the different organisations is given in Table 10.1.

Table 10.1: Research locations

NGO partner	State	District	Type of area	Access to formal abortion service providers
ARTH	Rajasthan	Udaipur	Rural 7 villages	CHC* provides irregular services Public and private facilities in nearby towns (30–50 km) & Udaipur (100–120 km)
BVS	Maharashtra	Nashik	Rural–Tribal 5 villages	CHC in the area. Several legal private providers
CHSSS	Madhya Pradesh	Ujjain Sidhi	Rural 18 villages	District Hospital; CHC & 1–2 legal private facilities. 2 public sector hospitals

Karuna Trust	Karnataka	Chamraj-nagar	Rural–Tribal 30 villages, 16 of which were tribal	No formal providers within easy access
Shramik Bharti	Uttar Pradesh	Kanpur	Peri-urban	A few legal private providers Public and private facilities in Kanpur (35 km)
SORT	Haryana	Jind	Rural 2 villages	Public and private hospitals in nearby town (10 km) and in the district headquarters (20–30 km)
Swaasthya	New Delhi	—	Urban Resettlement colony	2 large private hospitals situated within 2–3 km of the colony

Note: *CHC: Community Health Centre.

Data Collection

While all researchers agreed on the bare minimum of issues that they would address, there was enough flexibility to allow partner organisations to choose the qualitative tools that they felt would work best in their individual contexts. Table 10.2 highlights the research methods used by the partner NGOs.

After considerable discussion, partners agreed on a working definition of informal abortion service providers that included all providers of abortion services *except* Ob-Gyns, MBBS doctors and those qualified in Indian Systems of Medicine (ISM). The exclusion of ISM practitioners from the working definition of informal providers was much-debated, given that such practitioners are not legally allowed to provide abortion services. But while the partners agreed to this broad definition, they retained the flexibility to modify it based on their local context and field experiences.

Informal providers in the community were identified through key informants and through mapping exercises done with community members. CHSSS and SORT used the enumeration and listing of formal and informal providers done for the Abortion Assessment Project of India (AAP–I) facility survey as a base from which they identified informal providers for in-depth interviews. A purposively selected sub-sample of identified informal providers was interviewed. The degree of rapport and familiarity with the providers, and ethical concerns were important considerations that determined the number and range of interviews conducted.

Table 10.2: Data collection methods

Organisation	FGDs with community members Women (N)	Men (N)	Interviews with key informants[a] (N)	Interviews with informal providers[b] (N)	Interviews with women with an abortion experience[c] (N)
ARTH	4	2	No information	5	Nil
BVS	4	Nil	No information	7	Nil
CHSSs	19	11	No information	20	Nil
Karuna Trust	7	6	21	32	44 (through a household survey)
Shramik Bharti	3	1	10	6	7
SORT	5	2	1 FGD with ANMs*	7	4
Swaasthya	6	Nil	4	2	Nil

Notes: [a] While key informants were contacted by all organisations, not all were interviewed in-depth at all sites and not all organisations reported on the numbers of key informants they contacted. SORT conducted 1 FGD with the ANMs.

[b] Providers identified to be providing abortion services by the community or other providers or key informants. Not all of them admitted to providing services when interviewed.

[c] Some of these were with unmarried adolescent girls.

*Auxilliary nurse midwives.

Partner organisations differed in the types of field investigators they used to collect data. Some, like Swaasthya, used fieldworkers who had been involved for several years in their field intervention activities; others, like the Karuna Trust used ANMs while still others used field investigators familiar with the context and subject matter but external to the communities being researched. Most investigators were female, though at some sites male investigators were also used to conduct FGDs with men or to interview male informal providers. All organisations developed their own interview guidelines and included, for their fieldworkers, a component of training in the collection of qualitative data.

Ethical Dilemmas

Each partner NGO appointed its own local ethical committee or had an Institutional Ethics Committee that vetted the proposed research framework and made, where necessary, context-specific recommendations for changes in the framework or methodology to be used.

While the oral consent of all respondents (both community members and informal providers) was obtained, a number of ethical concerns and questions came up during the course of the research, not all of which could be fully resolved. Many of these were larger ethical issues requiring broader debate and discourse:

- Should the real purpose of the research be camouflaged from the informal providers who were to be interviewed in the larger interest of obtaining more accurate information?
- If harmful practices were identified, would the researchers be obliged to do something about them?
- Did researchers have an obligation to identify/report illegal providers?
- Would researchers face any potential danger, either during the course of the research or later, from the providers or others trying to protect the providers' interests and practices?
- Was there a possibility that despite precautionary measures, the identity of women who used these providers for reasons of secrecy be accidentally revealed?

All organisations decided that it was important to maintain the confidentiality of the informal providers they interviewed in terms of both their identity and the place where they practised.

Most individual ethical committees vetoed the idea of interviews with clients who had used the services of informal providers. While the informal providers were apprised of our research objectives, the focus on abortion was diffused by framing questions relating to it in the broader context of understanding a range of services that informal providers extend for general as well as for reproductive health, including delayed menstruation.

Salient Findings

Since our research essentially comprised small case studies carried out in purposively selected geographic areas and among purposively selected respondents and was very exploratory in nature, the findings should be interpreted with caution and in the context of the population to whom they apply. While some patterns do exist, broad generalisations or quantitative comparisons across the seven research sites areas would be inappropriate.

WHO IS REGARDED AS AN INFORMAL PROVIDER?

Researchers found that definitions of informal providers varied greatly among the respondents and bore little relation to the working definition with which they had started.

Box 10.1: How common are informal providers?

While the research was not designed to determine the actual numbers of informal providers in the community, the sites in both Haryana and Madhya Pradesh were located within the same area where SORT and CHSSS respectively had just completed an enumeration of formal as well as informal abortion providers. Similarly, ARTH in Rajasthan had done a mapping of all providers in a district not too far from the site of the present research.

In all the three areas, informal providers constituted more than 60 per cent of all providers identified through the mapping exercise. All the interviewed informal providers in Madhya Pradesh and about two-thirds of those interviewed in Rajasthan and Haryana admitted to providing treatment for delayed menstruation.

Note: (For more details see George 2004; Iyengar and Iyengar 2004; SORT 2004.)

Thus the informal providers identified by the respondents were a vast, amorphous group that included herbalists, faith healers, traditional birth attendants, and a wide range of rural medical practitioners or RMPs (popularly known as '*jhola chhap* doctors' in Uttar Pradesh and as 'Bengali doctors' and 'Gujarati doctors' in rural Rajasthan).

Informal providers were seen as those who were readily available in the village or nearby, although government clinics (like primary health centres or PHCs), even if located in the same village, were recognised by respondents across all seven research sites as formal service providers. Neither qualification nor training had any correlation with who was perceived as an informal provider. Indeed, determining who was trained or qualified proved an impossible task, compounded by the fact that a person, despite being formally trained in health service provision (e.g., an MBBS doctor), may not be trained to provide abortion services. Some providers categorised by communities as informal abortion service providers (e.g., nurses and auxilliary nurse midwives or ANMs) were also formal health service providers at the local primary health centre (PHC). Providers trained in ISM were also seen by communities as belonging to the category of informal providers. In several cases, even the occasional provider who claimed to be an MBBS degree holder was perceived by the community to be an informal provider.

The same categories of providers were often viewed differently in different locations. For example, in Haryana the *dai*s who provided services for delayed menstruation were perceived as informal providers distinct from doctors, while respondents in a resettlement colony in Delhi categorised a trained dai, practising as an informal provider, as a doctor. In fact, in this community, all abortion service providers were distinguished on the basis of their being 'doctors' or 'non-doctors'. A person identified as a 'doctor' did not need to have a medical degree or training within the formal health system. Any piece of paper framed and displayed as a 'degree' or 'certificate' was enough to earn her/him the label of a doctor.

> They have a board outside the clinic on which their qualifications are displayed. That is how they can be recognised. (FGD with women in New Delhi resettlement colony [Swaasthya])

Socio-Economic and Demographic Profile of the Informal Providers

The sex composition of informal providers varied greatly from region to region. In Karnataka, the majority of informal providers were females; in fact, 31 out of the 32 providers identified and interviewed were women. The reverse was seen in Madhya Pradesh where, of the 20 providers enumerated in the two blocks that comprised the research area, 18 were men. At all other sites both men and women were reported as informal providers.

Across sites, most women who practised as informal providers were either illiterate dais or trained paramedical workers (ANMs, nurses), although among the respondents in Rajasthan there was one male nurse who was reportedly a popular abortion service provider. On the other hand, most RMPs were men, though female RMPs were also occasionally mentioned, especially in Karnataka. It appears that the profession is not restricted to members of one sex. The preponderance of either men or women in a particular region may have historical reasons or may be due to the passing of skills from one generation to another depending upon the local tradition.

In both Chamrajnagar (Karnataka) and Nashik (Maharashtra), most herbalist informal providers were illiterate; their main source of income was through daily-wage labour or agriculture, and treating delayed periods or inducing abortion was usually a subsidiary activity. Several of them also doubled up as dais. In Karnataka, most of the providers who used herbal remedies to induce abortion were reported to be women, while in rural Maharashtra both men and women were practitioners.

How Do Informal Providers Practice?

As can be seen from Table 10.2 above, between the seven sites, 79 providers identified by the relevant communities were interviewed, although several of them refused to admit that they provided services for either inducing abortion or for treating delayed periods. Thus information about informal-provider practices also came from key informants and members of the community.

Knowledge and Use of Abortion Methods

The methods used by informal providers existed along a continuum ranging from home remedies to concoctions to instrumentation using Dilatation and Curettage (D&C) and even Electric Vacuum Aspiration (EVA). Providers often shifted in the continuum depending on the circumstances or nature of the case. Nevertheless, for purposes of further discussion, the interviewed providers have been divided into the following three broad categories based on the methods they used most commonly to treat delayed periods or perform abortions.

- Herbalists using oral herbal preparations
- Those using 'oral' allopathic/*ayurvedic* medicines and/or injections
- Those using invasive procedures with traditional or 'modern' methods

While this classification is artificial and the distinctions not always clearcut, it may be a useful way of categorising providers for future interventions and advocacy efforts.

Herbalists

Although not categorised as providers by any of our respondents, family members, especially elderly women in the family, use traditional knowledge passed on through the generations to perform a function similar to that of the informal providers. Most limit themselves to advising the use of concoctions (*kadhas*) and foods that are supposed to increase body heat and thereby induce bleeding. As is evident from Table 10.3, while there are many regional variations, jaggery appears to be widely recognised as a key ingredient in most concoctions.

Table 10.3: Menstruation-inducing substances mentioned by respondents

NGO	Substances used by respondents
Karuna Trust, Karnataka	Strong coffee with jaggery, no milk or sugar; horse gram with pepper; garlic boiled in water; fresh ginger with jaggery
Shramik Bharti, Uttar Pradesh	Jaggery; ground carrot seeds; sour foods like vinegar; bamboo leaves; tea leaves
SORT, Haryana	Dry fruits (dates, almonds, currants); ginger; old jaggery boiled in water; seeds of roots like carrots and radish; spices like cardamom and clove; carom seeds (*ajwain*), strong hot tea
Swaasthya, Delhi	Ginger (raw or in powdered form); sesame; jaggery; asafoetida (*hing*); carom seeds cumin, clarified butter

Interviews with key informants and FGDs with the community members in the tribal area of Nashik (Maharashtra) revealed that most informal providers in the area induced abortion using locally available herbs. Six of the seven providers interviewed also followed this practice. While the actual names of the herbal remedies could not be obtained, most of them were made with local plants and herbs which the providers themselves collected regularly. In rural Karnataka, too, a herbal preparation (referred to as green medicine or *kashaya*) was the most commonly used formulation to induce abortion and most informal providers (21 out of 32) who were interviewed confirmed the exclusive use of kashaya in their own practice. These practitioners generally restricted the use of traditional medicines to 'oral' preparations or to pastes meant for external application on the abdomen. Sometimes the use of herbs was accompanied by chanting *mantras* (prayers). One herbalist reported giving alcohol to her clients in addition to the herbs. The knowledge of the use of local plants was acquired through information passed down from generation to generation.

In Haryana too, the dais who worked as informal providers limited their advice to suggesting *kadhas* (liquid concoctions made of 'hot' foods and spices) or other heat-inducing foods like strong tea or 'hot *halva*(pudding-like dessert)'. As one said during an FGD:

> Why would she want to dig her own grave? Obviously it is the doctor who will do it [perform the abortion]. The dai only tells you about the kadha. It is up to you to decide whether you want to take the kadha that she has recommended. (FGD with women [SORT, Haryana])

However, while dais in other settings like Delhi and Uttar Pradesh also used herbal remedies, they did not restrict their practice to just traditional oral methods. The same is true of Madhya Pradesh, where it was reported that herbalists and herbal remedies do not enjoy much popularity.

Providers Using 'Modern' Medicines and Injections

A few providers who had been formally trained in ayurvedic medicine restricted their practice to the use of ayurvedic preparations like *ashokarista* and *churnas* (powders) made with turmeric and other ingredients (George 2003). While many other providers also used ayurvedic preparations, they supplemented their use with allopathic drugs. The majority of informal providers identified in Haryana, and about half of those identified in Madhya Pradesh used allopathic drugs and injections. Interestingly, many of these drugs were hormonal preparations that bring on withdrawal bleeding only if the woman is not pregnant; their use is specifically contraindicated in the case of a pregnant woman due to the risk of foetal deformity. Use of the antimalarial drug, chloroquine, was commonly mentioned in both Madhya Pradesh and Haryana, but none of the interviewed providers mentioned either mifepristone or misoprostol (generic or trade names).

In addition to oral drugs, some providers also used 'hot' injections, usually as a second line of treatment. Prostodine injections were not uncommon in Madhya Pradesh and Haryana. Providers who used these injections were aware that they could produce severe side effects, but used them nevertheless.

All the interviewed practitioners who prescribed allopathic medicines and used injections were more educated than the herbalist providers. Many had Bachelors' degrees and several were trained paramedical workers. Some were qualified ayurvedic practitioners as well.

Most of them had acquired knowledge of menstruation-inducing medicines through their past training or through their contacts with formally trained providers.

Chemists also fell into the category of informal providers. In Haryana, in the peri-urban areas of Uttar Pradesh and in the resettlement colony of Delhi, FGDs revealed that chemists were often consulted as a first line of treatment for a suspected unwanted pregnancy. One local chemist interviewed in Delhi admitted to providing a variety of tablets and capsules to women with delayed periods or those seeking abortion. He chose the appropriate drugs based on the ability of the client to pay and also decided on the dosage. If the medicines did not work the first time, he repeated them in higher dosages.

Providers Using Invasive Procedures

While an overall 5 per cent of informal providers admitted that they use invasive methods to induce abortion, none of those interviewed in Haryana did so. The use of invasive methods was found to be much higher among the providers interviewed in Madhya Pradesh (46.5 per cent). In Maharashtra, one of the seven providers interviewed admitted to inserting medicated roots into the vagina. In Delhi too, key informants and community women mentioned that local dais sometimes performed abortions by inserting herbs into the vagina.

Community women in Madhya Pradesh mentioned that abdominal massage was commonly used by dais in the area. This practice received occasional mention in other sites as well, where it was sometimes supplemented by the application of herbal and other medicines on the abdomen.

There was also mention of more primitive methods being used occasionally. In Maharashtra, 1 key informant spoke about a male abortionist who aborted pregnancies of over 4 to 5 months' gestation. It was reported that he would cut the embryo into pieces from below and because of the method he used, was known as the cutter (*kapya*). In Uttar Pradesh, too, one provider who was interviewed talked of occasionally using his bare hands lubricated with mustard oil in order to remove the embryo. However, the use of such methods was not common. As is evident from Table 10.4, such instances were more the exception than the rule, which is probably why people remember them so well.

Table 10.4: Use of invasive procedures as reported by informal providers

NGO partner	No. using	Sex	Methods used	Education or training	Place of learning abortion procedure	Place of practice
ARTH, Rajasthan	3/3	1F 2M	2 use D&C 1 uses catheter or EVA for pregnancies >3 months	1 nurse 1 DHMS[a] 1 BAMS[b]	Observation during govt service Apprenticeship with a senior physician	2 have clinics, one practices from home
BVS, Maharashtra	1/7	F	Medicated root	Illiterate	From family	At the clients' home only
CHSSS, Madhya Pradesh	8/20	2F 6M	D&C; MR; Scissors, Ovum forceps; Sharp metallic instruments	2 nurses 2 RMPs 1 BAMSs 2 vaidya-visharad 1 DBH	Apprenticeship with qualified doctors Repeated practice	
Karuna Trust, Karnataka	5/32	All 5F	1 trained dai uses sticks 2 use MRS 2 use D&C	1 illiterate 1 RMP 2 ANMs	1 from family 4 observation during govt service	1 clinic 4 from their own homes
Shramik Bharti; Uttar Pradesh	5/5	4F 1M	Catheter with glycerine Sharp instruments D&C	1 auxiliary nurse 1 dai 1 RMP 1 electro-homeopathy		Clinics (shops) Their own home

Note: None of the interviewed providers in the SORT or Swaasthya studies reported the use of invasive methods.
[a] DHMS: Diploma in Homeopathy Medicine and Surgery.
[b] BAMS: Bachelor of Ayurvedic Medicine and Surgery.

Invasive methods were mentioned more commonly in northern India. In both Rajasthan and Uttar Pradesh, all the interviewed providers used some form of invasive intervention in order to induce abortion. Two of the three providers in Rajasthan who acknowledged providing abortion services mentioned the use of D&C, while one provider indicated that he felt a sharp curette was not safe and so used the EVA technique that he had learned from a 'gynaecologist' friend. In Uttar Pradesh women and key informants reported that invasive procedures seemed to be the most common way in which informal abortion service providers induced abortion. All of the five interviewed providers used instillation of glycerine through a catheter to induce abortion. The same providers also mentioned that when women came to them in later stages of pregnancy, they used instruments like tweezers and artery forceps or a sharp curette. One provider mentioned that she owned an entire D&C kit.

Of the 20 interviewed providers in Madhya Pradesh, eight admitted to using instruments like scissors and other sharp metallic objects. Some performed abortion using a Menstrual Regulation (MR) syringe or a sharp curette. Key informants and community members said that unlike their counterparts in Haryana, Maharashtra and Karnataka, dais in Uttar Pradesh and Delhi used catheters and other instruments or 'machines'.

Paramedical providers learned invasive methods during their years of service in the formal sector, by observing doctors; others acquired this knowledge by doing a period of apprenticeship with experienced doctors. Skills were acquired over time and with repeated practice. As an informal provider (ARTH, Rajasthan) remarked: 'It has taken 15 years for my hands to become fully skilled. And now, even you [the researchers] have come inquiring about me!'

Accessing Clients

In general, most informal providers obtained clients through word of mouth. In most of our research sites, such providers were well known in the local community. However, in Maharashtra, two informal providers said that they used the service of 'touts' or middlemen (one of whom was actually a woman) in order to obtain and screen clients. This method of client procurement was not mentioned anywhere else.

Some providers used their formal jobs in order to refer clients to their informal practice. For example, the two nurses who were interviewed in Madhya Pradesh used the PHC where they worked to attract clients, whom they asked to come back to their homes for treatment. Clients were also referred to informal providers by other providers. For example, in Karnataka it was common for ANMs to refer clients to herbalists in the area.

Duration of Pregnancy

Most informal providers who prescribed oral concoctions, tablets or injections had self-imposed limits on the duration of pregnancy for which they offered treatment. In Haryana, they seemed not to go beyond two to three months of a missed period. Twelve weeks seemed to be the outer limit in Madhya Pradesh too, though many restricted their treatment to eight or nine weeks. This seems to reflect not only the widely-held perception that these drugs are less effective at higher pregnancy durations but also a concern for possible complications.

Informal providers who had had some exposure to, or training in, the formal health system showed willingness to induce abortion among women with higher pregnancy durations. One of the trained nurses in Madhya Pradesh conducted abortions up to 16 weeks. Several other providers who used invasive methods also occasionally performed abortions for higher gestations.

Place of Practice

Traditional herbalists generally practised from their residence, although for a higher fee many of them were also willing to make home visits when necessary. Such practitioners appeared to be in great demand among clients whose mobility was limited but who placed a premium on secrecy: 'Even big people come in jeeps and cars and take me to their place for giving abortion medicines, said an informal provider. (BVS, Maharashtra)

Other informal providers often set up shop (*dukan*) in the community. This 'dukan' phenomenon was particularly common in northern India, especially in Haryana, Delhi and Uttar Pradesh. Although informal providers in Rajasthan and Madhya Pradesh also often functioned out of 'clinics', these were not referred to as 'shops'.

While a few paramedical workers functioned from home, most seemed to use the infrastructure and facilities available at the PHCs where they were employed to conduct abortions after the PHCs' regular functioning hours.

Clients rarely stayed at a provider's clinic or home for more than the minimum required time and the actual abortion often took place in the client's own home. A family member usually reported back to the provider about the success of the method used or to ask for a repeat abortion in case of failure.

Cost of Abortion

While the actual cost of abortion varied from location to location (ranging, on an average, from Rs 50 to Rs 700), informal providers in most of our study areas usually charged less than formal private providers and the cost of availing services from them was often even lower than the rate prevalent in the public sector.

In all seven research sites we found that informal providers frequently extended credit facilities to poor clients. Payments could be made in instalments and often only after the treatment was demonstrably successful. In Karnataka, instead of cash, herbalist providers often accepted payment in kind (rice or wheat). These same providers also sometimes waived their charges for women from their own village, especially young unmarried girls or widows, because they felt it was their duty to protect their community's honour. The same providers, on the other hand, had exorbitant charges for women who did not belong to the community.

Lower costs and flexibility in the mode of payment were very likely the most important reasons why informal providers were preferred over formal ones, even when the latter were physically accessible. Nevertheless, even among informal providers, charges varied by pregnancy duration and the marital status of the client. Some providers charged per month of pregnancy duration. In all research sites it was mentioned that unmarried clients had to pay considerably more than married clients with the same pregnancy duration, often five times higher. Charges also varied by the type of method providers used and those using instruments and other types of interventions generally charged more than those who used oral preparations.

Treatment of Complications

No informal provider claimed to be successful in inducing abortion in every case. Though perceptions of success varied from provider to provider, in general most reported that they were successful at least six to eight times out of ten. The failure rate for oral medication (especially if the pregnancy duration was beyond six to seven weeks) was perceived to be higher than that for invasive procedures. When providers failed to induce abortion they often repeated the oral medication in higher doses, shifted to more invasive methods or referred the women to a formal hospital.

Informal providers also seemed to be aware of the complications that could arise from improperly performed abortions. Providers in the tribal area of Nashik spoke of skin burns that result from overzealous application of herbal pastes to the abdomen. Several providers in Madhya Pradesh spoke of perforation that can result from using sharp instruments, whereas those in Rajasthan mentioned life-threatening bleeding and other complications.

> One has to be careful with this [procedure]; if things go wrong death can result. The intestine might get injured, the kidney might get injured. Yes sir! One has to be careful. (Informal provider [ARTH, Rajasthan])

Many providers prevented complications by restricting their practice to early pregnancy when complications are likely to be fewer, or by avoiding intervening in cases they felt might be risky. Many did take some measures (however inadequate from a scientific point of view) to prevent infections. In all seven sites, providers who used instruments 'sterilised' them by either boiling them or washing them with boiled water or with Dettol. All the interviewed providers in Rajasthan prescribed antibiotics to be taken post-abortion.

While awareness of complications was high, few providers admitted to any complication having occurred in cases that they themselves had treated and for which they were therefore responsible. Only 1 female provider in Uttar Pradesh mentioned that in the past year she had 'spoiled' four to five cases.

Several providers said that they treated minor problems themselves, either with oral or intra-muscular antibiotics or with an injection of methergine to control bleeding. More often than not, though, they tended to refer clients to the formal health services in both the government and private sectors. Most informal providers cultivated linkages with ANMs and other health functionaries working in PHCs or nearby private hospitals. A few of the better-established providers even took women with complications to city clinics in their own vehicles.

FGDs revealed that women often reported back to the provider who had conducted the abortion for minor post-abortion complications ('normal' bleeding, mild infection); however when complications were perceived to be serious, family members generally took the pregnant woman directly to a formal provider in the city.

Inducing Menstruation or Inducing Abortion?

Most informal providers used 'hot medicines'—often in the form of tablets or injections—to bring on a delayed period. They did not confirm pregnancy prior to providing these medicines, as most felt that treating delayed periods was distinct from performing an abortion. This was partly due to the fact that women themselves often sought services for regulation of menstruation as opposed to abortion, partly because it allowed providers to remain outside the purview of the legal provisions of abortion service regulations, and also because many of them were males and for them to do even a physical examination, much less an internal one, of women was not culturally acceptable.

In more urbanised areas like Delhi, however, awareness of pregnancy confirmation by pregnancy tests seemed to be increasing. For many women a delayed period meant a visit to a provider or chemist in order to obtain a pregnancy test. Women in Haryana villages too seemed to be aware of the existence of such tests and several informal providers mentioned that they used them as well.

Knowledge of Legal Issues

Awareness about the legal aspects of abortion varied across the different research sites and among different types of informal providers. Though the providers were not directly questioned on this aspect, it was clear from interactions with them that other than traditional herbalists, most providers were aware of at least some aspects of the law, and a few were knowledgeable even of the most minute details. As one ISM abortion provider in Uttar Pradesh said, illegal abortion practice could result in imprisonment for seven years.

The publicity around the Prenatal Diagnostic Techniques (PNDT) Act has led many communities—not only women and men in general, but also formal and informal providers—to believe that all abortions are now illegal. This was especially noticeable in Delhi and Haryana where the PNDT Act has received the maximum publicity. In some settings informal providers, who felt they were practising comfortably and without fear of legal repercussions, said that they had now become conscious of the illegality of their practice.

SECURING PRACTICE WITHIN THE COMMUNITY

By and large, communities viewed the services of informal, village-level providers as essential and as meeting a felt need. In a sense, therefore, the community itself became their protector. Informal providers appeared to be well known within the community; secrecy and confidentiality were maintained only with respect to outsiders. In an FGD with SORT, Haryana, an ANM commented: 'Matters of the village must remain in the village.'

Informal providers used multiple strategies and methods to secure their practice and preserve their status within the community. Maintaining a congenial relationship with the community was one such strategy. Some relied on the goodwill built by the 'medical' practice of their family elders: 'My father was a famous vaidya [ayurvedic practitioner] in this village, said an informal provider (ARTH, Rajasthan). 'Because of his name people come to me for treatment.'

In rural settings, the flexibility that many providers showed in terms of the fee they charged and their willingness to accept it in instalments or waive it altogether in certain circumstances enhanced their standing in the community in which they lived and worked.

They also maintained a congenial relationship with the formal health system. For instance, in Karnataka we found that informal providers enjoyed a good relationship with the ANMs and sometimes also helped them in their routine work. In return, ANMs rarely interfered with the providers and at times even referred clients to them. In addition, many informal providers cultivated connections with private hospitals. This enabled them to refer clients who developed complications to these hospitals, with the assurance that their cases would be handled quickly and without the embarrassment of inconvenient questions. Some informal providers also used their role in the formal health system (as ANMs or trained Reproductive and Child Health [RCH] workers) as an effective cover for their role as abortion service providers.

Some providers adopted other ways to protect themselves from law enforcers. In Delhi, we found that some informal practitioners camouflaged their illegal status by displaying framed certificates and flashy signboards listing various degrees (usually displayed only during the hours that the clinic was open) as this was perceived to be an indicator of their being respectable and highly qualified. A woman recognised as a doctor in the community carried a signboard that described her as a 'gynaecologist'. However, during the course of the interview with her it became evident that she had only a B. Sc. degree.

Others protected themselves by keeping a low profile and offering abortion services only in their own homes or in the homes of their clients. They did not open a clinic or 'shop' that could be identified as their workplace, and all of them screened their clients carefully to ensure that they were not law enforcers in disguise.

It is only when things went wrong, such as the occurrence of a serious complication or death, that the equilibrium was upset. Although this proved to be too sensitive an issue to probe, the existence of a nexus between informal providers and the police was mentioned by several respondents. As a tout for an informal abortion provider (BVS, Maharashtra) said: I know all the police, no problem!

Women participating in the FGDs in Delhi said that informal/illegal providers bribed the police so that no action was taken even if their intervention resulted in a complication or death. In Rajasthan many providers were careful to cultivate and nurture political connections as well. They generally faced no trouble from the community: the process of proving that injury or death occurred at the hands of a provider is so complex that community members are more often than not wary of even attempting it.

> They do not give any receipt or anything, even if someone wants to file a case, they would need some proof. When there is no proof there is no legal case. (FGD with women [Swaasthya, Delhi])

> People think, 'We have lost our loved one. Now what can be done?' (FGD with women [Swaasthya, Delhi])

These informal providers did not restrict their medical practice to treating delayed periods or inducing abortion. Even if general medical practice was not their primary occupation, all 79 of the informal providers interviewed also treated other types of clients—men, women and children. This was a successful way of camouflaging the fact that they provided abortion services. Since providing abortion services was never their sole activity, the pretence of being general practitioners provided both themselves and their clients with the necessary cover.

Circumstances in which Services of Informal Providers are Preferred

Married Women

In order to understand the role informal providers play in dealing with unwanted pregnancies, it is necessary to understand from the perspective of women the sequence of steps that they take when menstruation is delayed. It appears that dealing with a delayed period is a first step, distinct from dealing with an unwanted pregnancy.

Women who participated in the FGDs mentioned the use of herbal home remedies as a first response to bringing on a delayed period. The use of kadha was mentioned in rural Haryana, peri-urban Uttar Pradesh as well as Delhi. While the actual composition of the kadha varied across different areas, it usually (as mentioned earlier) consisted of a mixture of what were assumed to be 'hot' foods and spices that could aid the resumption of menstruation (see Table 10.3 above). It was generally believed that these homemade herbal remedies were effective only when taken within the first 15 to 20 days after a missed period. However, belief in the efficacy of home remedies differed across areas: most participants in FGDs as well as key informants in Uttar Pradesh said that though such methods were effective in the past, they were no longer as effective as they used to be.

When herbal remedies did not work, the next option, at least for many rural women, was informal providers (including chemists) located nearby and within the community. Opinions varied on the efficacy of the informal providers' treatment of delayed periods. Women believed that such treatment only worked if the delay in the onset of menstruation was not too long. The acceptable period of delay was defined variously as ranging between 15 to 20 days and two-and-a-half months.

A formal provider was sought when these two options did not work or caused problems like excessive bleeding. It was only at this stage that the process was thought of as being 'an abortion'. As was evident from FGDs in Haryana, only an invasive surgical procedure is perceived as an abortion or '*safai*'. And for such procedures the preference was clearly for formal providers as the first choice.

However, the distinction between treating delayed periods and having an abortion was not so clearcut and community men and women mentioned that women who suspect they are pregnant and do not want to continue with the pregnancy also take the same kadhas as those who are simply trying to regulate their menstruation. Informal providers, too, are well aware that many clients who come to them for delayed menstruation may in fact be pregnant but choose to conceal that fact in order to protect themselves.

While there seems to be increasing awareness among women that it is safer to use the services of formal providers and that the treatment offered by them is more likely to succeed (especially during the initial few weeks of a missed period), married women across the sites spoke of using informal providers in many situations, either as a preference or out of necessity. The following are some of the circumstances because of which women often prefer informal providers:

- No matter what the illness, most tribal women shy away from using the formal health system. Reproductive health problems are generally treated with home remedies. It is only when such remedies fail or it becomes clear that it is impossible to treat them at home that more formal providers are approached. Seeking abortion from informal providers seems to be a natural extension of this. This is true of tribal areas in Maharashtra and Karnataka as well.
- In Delhi, women said that though people in the community would prefer to use hospitals, obtaining the family's permission to go outside their immediate community is often a problem. Therefore, informal providers, who are generally more easily accessible, are the first option.
- Women also spoke of being comfortable with trying oral medicines (herbal, ayurvedic or allopathic) as a first measure as they have an inherent fear of invasive procedures. For many of them, even vaginally instilled medicines are a better option than the insertion of instruments. Such medication is perceived to be less risky, especially in early pregnancy.
- Informal providers are also cheaper than their counterparts in the organised sector. The flexibility in terms of payment options that they provide also makes their services more convenient to use. Given the fact that women do not usually have to travel far to access these providers and, in most cases, can continue to stay at home means additional savings in opportunity and time costs. Thus, for women without independent financial means, informal providers are a viable alternative to formal services.

- What women found most attractive about informal providers was their pleasant and respectful way of treating clients—a feature that was markedly less evident among doctors and nurses working in urban hospitals.

This last point was expressed by women as follows:

> K [name concealed] is a good nurse, she does not scold, she does not get irritated, no matter how many women reach her. We do not feel afraid of talking to her. (A woman who had an abortion with an informal provider [Shramik Bharti, Uttar Pradesh])

> We don't go to private hospitals because it is very expensive and we do not go to government hospitals because they don't listen to us. We therefore go to informal providers. (FGD with women [CHSSS, Madhya Pradesh])

Women did not always have a say in choosing providers, even where a choice was available. It was often the husband who made this choice. We found that in several areas husbands often chose providers with whom they or their network of male friends were familiar and they were more likely to opt for low-cost village providers or to consult and buy medication from a chemist.

Informal providers (even those who performed abortions in cases of advanced pregnancies) were rarely used when abortion was sought based on sex selection. In such cases the preference was invariably for formal providers, no matter how faraway they were located or how expensive their services were. This was because formal providers were considered more likely to perform a successful abortion; women who wanted sex-selective abortions did not want to take any chances.

While there was no gender preference with respect to the type of provider in the case of orally administered medication, notions of shame generally led to the choice of female providers for invasive procedures, particularly in Delhi, Uttar Pradesh and Haryana.

Communities seemed well aware of the complications that could ensue from the use of informal providers. In Maharashtra, for example, community members reported the death of one client that had taken place while under the care of an informal provider and the fact that a police enquiry was ongoing. A similar incident was reported in Madhya Pradesh. Respondents in Uttar Pradesh frequently mentioned consequences like excessive bleeding and infection, and linked illnesses such as cancer of the uterus to injury caused by the instruments used by informal providers for the abortion. In the FGD in Maharashtra, women spoke of the 'womb decaying' as a result of improperly conducted abortions. Unfortunately and perhaps ironically, many women thought of these risks as inevitable and/or acceptable. This may have been due to the perceived lack of options available to them.

Unmarried Women

In most rural areas, community members mentioned that unmarried girls or widowed women went to informal providers mainly because they felt that such providers could be trusted to maintain confidentiality. For example, during the FGDs with community members in Karnataka, it was learnt that while most married women were increasingly using the services of formal providers, almost all abortions among unmarried and widowed women were conducted by informal providers.

Interestingly, the finding from urban Delhi was the opposite: respondents were confident that unmarried women in their area did not use the services of informal providers. They would prefer formal providers in spite of the expense involved and the distance to be travelled to reach formal facilities. Families and communities in the area were more concerned about making sure that the pregnancy was safely terminated. Thus, it appears that considerations for choosing a provider are quite different in urban areas compared to those in rural areas.

Another interesting feature that surfaced was that in certain circumstances the general preference for female providers was sometimes overridden. With the exception of rural Karnataka, male informal providers were also used for abortion and related services by unmarried women. Male providers in Uttar Pradesh indicated that unmarried and widowed women felt comfortable approaching them for these services because they ensured confidentiality.

> The maintenance of full confidentiality of the women who come here for abortions is our responsibility. That is why in spite of our being male members of the village community, more women come to us for abortions. (Informal provider [Shramik Bharti, Uttar Pradesh])

However, while confidentiality was guaranteed by informal providers, it was not uncommon for them, like their counterparts in the private sector, to exploit the situation. They usually increased their charges substantially when they provided services to unmarried and widowed women.

> Married women do not care. If they [informal providers] do not do the abortion, someone else will. Unmarried girls are compelled [to use them]. They are afraid of society and the doctors take advantage of this fact. (Key informant [Shramik Bharti, Uttar Pradesh])

Changing Roles

Across the research sites in both rural and urban settings, there seems to be a shift towards using formal providers when they are easily accessible, when confidentiality is not a major issue and when women can afford their services. In both Maharashtra and Karnataka, respondents talked of formal services being better in the long run, given the higher possibility of failure and complications with informal methods.

In addition, the younger generation of informal providers is not always in favour of continuing with the herbal tradition because they feel it is not economically viable. Also, in both Maharashtra and Karnataka several informal providers reported pressure from family members to discontinue their practice because many of them felt that the 'sin' of conducting abortions had led to their children or other close family members remaining childless.

The increase in the use of formal services, especially in the southern states and the consequent decline in their own clientele has prompted many informal providers in rural Karnataka to switch from being service providers to becoming 'referral' agents who serve as a link (often for a fee) between women and the formal health service system (Bharathi 2003). This role has been documented in other southern states like Tamil Nadu (Ramachandar and Pelto 2002), as also in less developed areas like Jharkhand (Barnes 2003). In some cases, the heightened consciousness of their illegal status and the perceived threat of being 'caught' (brought about in part by the PNDT Act, even though these providers are not involved in sex-selective abortions) has also led providers to either minimise their practice or to change their role.

CONCLUSION

Informal providers for abortions exist and practice in all seven geographical areas—tribal, rural or urban—where we conducted our research. Both providers and women seemed to make a distinction between the services provided for regulating menstruation (bringing on a delayed period) and those for actually inducing abortions. At times this distinction might be real and at times just serve as a convenient camouflage, allowing providers to remain out of the purview of the legal stipulations and helping women bypass the difficult decision-making and permission-seeking scenarios that they would otherwise encounter.

Informal provision of services is not uniform. A wide variety of methods were reported to be used by providers. Those that limited their practice to early gestations using oral, herbal or other traditionally handed-down medicines appeared to be functioning with relative safety and apparent efficacy. Instead of dismissing them out of hand, it is necessary for us to evaluate the possible abortifacient properties of many of these traditional preparations scientifically. Nevertheless, it cannot be assumed that all non-invasive methods are safe or without any side effects or complications. While it heartening to note that the use of invasive methods like inserting roots and sticks into the vagina is not very common, the use of 'modern' methods by those who are not trained to use them is potentially quite dangerous.

The fact that sometimes informal providers are used only because the formal providers are not easily accessible, are too costly or do not treat clients with respect or dignity speaks volumes for the failure of the formal health system. Personalised service, ready availability, congenial behaviour and convenience appeared to be important considerations in the choice of informal providers, despite the fact that the medical risks involved or the chances of failure were often perceived to be higher. Formal facilities need to learn from informal providers the necessity for maintaining confidentiality and for making women's needs the fulcrum around which their services revolve. It is also imperative to regulate formal services more strictly in order to prevent their misuse for profitable informal provision of services.

The potential implications of the preference for and the widespread use of oral allopathic medicines, due to the recent advent and legalisation of medical abortion drugs like mifepristone and misoprostol, are of immense relevance for public health policy and issues. While our research (which was done in 2002 soon after these drugs were legalised) may not have found much evidence of their use, the potential for providers replacing less effective drugs with these drugs is high.

As long as informal providers fulfil a felt need in the community, legal measures against those using potentially harmful practices are unlikely to make any real difference to the situation. The real challenge lies in how we can integrate informal providers into the more formal health systems without losing the advantage of their unique position of closeness to and respect within the community. Their transition from being informal providers to serving as an effective referral link between communities and safe services—as seen in Karnataka—seems a promising trend.

It would be worthwhile to also explore whether some categories of informal providers (those that have been trained as nurses or in ISM) can become legal mid-level providers of abortion services. This would not only provide them access to formal training opportunities but also make them legally accountable.

Notes

We are grateful to Vimala Ramachandran and Shveta Kalyanwala of HealthWatch, who contributed significantly to the management of our research and the preparation of this document, as we are to Ravi Duggal and his team at CEHAT. Our thanks to colleagues at the Ipas, India office, who provided logistic and technical support throughout the study and during the preparation of the report. Particular thanks to V. S. Chandrashekar, Gladson Paul and Mallika Bhattacharya. All the study partners answered our queries without hesitation or delays when we were preparing the synthesis of their reports. Without their willing participation, this document would not have been possible. However, any errors that may have crept in are solely our own.

1. The Abortion Assessment Project, India undertaken jointly by HealthWatch and CEHAT, has supported several studies in the country to create evidence-based knowledge on abortion issues. Abortion Facility-based studies were multi-centric and aimed to assess and analyse abortion services, including organisation, management, facilities, technology, registration, training, certification and utilisation in the public and private sector. For a summary of findings based on the studies, see Duggal and Barge (2004).

2. The principal investigators for the seven research studies were Sharad and Kirti Iyengar (ARTH, Udaipur), Shyam Ashtekar (BVS, Nashik), Alex George (CHSSS, Secunderabad), H. Sudarshan (Karuna Trust, Karnataka), Ganesh Pandey and Jayanta Upadhyay (Shramik Bharti, Kanpur), Sandhya Barge and Wajahat Khan (SORT, Vadodara) and Geeta Sodhi (Swaasthya, New Delhi).
3. For detailed reports of the various locations where the studies were conducted, the reader should consult the individual reports, whose titles are given in the References.
4. ARTH did not begin its data collection until February 2003 and CHSSS joined the partnership only in April 2003.

References

Study Reports from Individual Sites

ARTH

Iyengar, Sharad and Kirti Iyengar. 2003. 'Informal Providers of Abortion Services in Rajasthan: A Draft Report'. Udaipur: ARTH.

BVS

Ashtekar, Shyam, Shakuntala Mankad and Sarika Mankar. 2003. 'Study of Informal Abortion Providers in Nashik District'. Nashik: BVS.

CHSSS

George, Alex. 2003. 'Informal Providers of Abortion Care in Two Blocks of Madhya Pradesh and Social Perception of Them'. Secunderabad: CHSSS.

Karuna Trust

Sudarshan, K. and Vishnu H. 2003. 'Study of Informal Providers of Abortion Care in Rural Karnataka'. Bangalore: Karuna Trust.

SORT

Barge, Sandhya, Wajahat Ullah Khan, Yamini Venkatachalam, Jashoda Sharma and Shweta Shahane. 2003. 'Role of Informal Providers in Abortion: A Case Study of Two Villages of Jind District in Haryana'. Vadodra: SORT.

Shramik Bharti

Upadhyay, Jayanta and Ganesh Pandey. 2003. 'A Qualitative Study of Informal Providers of Abortion in Kanpur District, Uttar Pradesh'. Kanpur: Shramik Bharti.

Swaasthya

Swaasthya. 2004. 'A Study of Informal Providers of Abortion Services in a Resettlement Colony of Delhi'. New Delhi: Swaasthya.

Works Cited

Barnes, Lindsay. 2003. 'Abortion Options for Rural Women: Case Studies from the Villages of Bokaro District, Jharkahnd'. Abortion Assessment Project—India (AAP–I) Working Paper. Mumbai: CEHAT.

Bharathi, Veena. 2003. 'A Note', *Seminar* 532: 75–76.

CINI (Child in Need Institute). 2004. 'A Multicentric Study on Provider Related Issues in the State of Orissa'. Kolkata: Child in Need Institute.

Duggal, R. and S. Barge. 2004. *Abortion Services in India: Report of a Multicentric Enquiry*. Mumbai: Abortion Assessment Project—India, Centre for Enquiry into Health and Allied Themes (CEHAT) and HealthWatch Trust.

Ganatra, B. and S. Hirve. 2002. 'Induced Abortions among Adolescent Women in Rural Maharashtra, India', *Reproductive Health Matters* 10 (19): 76–85.

George, Alex. 2003. 'From Decoctions to Instruments', *Seminar* 532: 52–56.

———. 2004. 'An Enquiry into Provision of Abortion Services in Madhya Pradesh'. Bangalore: Manasa.

Iyengar, Sharad and Kirti Iyengar. 2004. 'Situation Analysis of Abortion Services in Rajasthan'. Udaipur: ARTH.

Johnston, Heidi, Rajani Ved, Neena Lyall and Kavita Agarwal. 2004. 'Where Do Rural Women Obtain Post Abortion Care? The Case of Uttar Pradesh, India', *International Family Planning Perspectives* 29 (4): 182–87.

Radkar, A. 2003. 'Family Matters', *Seminar* 532: 57–60.

Ramachandar, Lakshmi and Pertti Pelto. 2002. 'The Role of Village Health Nurses in Mediating Abortions in Rural Tamil Nadu, India', *Reproductive Health Matters* 10 (19): 64–75.

SORT (Society for Operations Research and Training). 2004. 'Situation Analysis of MTP Facilities in Haryana'. Vadodra: Centre for Research in Development and Change (A Division of SORT).

Varkey, P., P. P. Balakrishna, J. H. Prasad, S. Abraham and A. Joseph. 2000. 'The Reality of Unsafe Abortion in a Rural Community in South India', *Reproductive Health Matters* 8 (6): 83–91.

About the Editors

Leela Visaria holds a Ph.D. from Princeton University, and has been closely associated with the Gujarat Institute of Development Research, Ahmedabad, first as Professor (since 1987), and then as Director (from 2004 to 2006). Her research interests include historical demography, health, education, and demographic transition. She is presently Coordinator, HealthWatch.

Dr Visaria's articles have appeared in many scholarly journals. She is co-author of *Contraceptive Use and Fertility*, and co-editor of *Maternal Education and Child Survival*, and *Twenty-first Century India: Population, Economy, Human Development, and the Environment*.

Vimala Ramachandran of Educational Resource Unit, has extensive experience in qualitative research, policy and programme development and process documentation. She works on women's education and health, and on elementary education. She is Founder-Member and Trustee of HealthWatch, a network of NGOs and researchers working with women and health.

Ms Ramachandran's recent publications include *Bridging the Gap between Intention and Action: Girl's and Women's Education in South Asia; Hierarchies of Access: Gender and Social Equity in Primary Education;* and *Getting Children Back to School: Case Studies in Primary Education.*

Index